Basic and Clinical Science Course
Section 5

Neuro-Ophthalmology

1999-2000

(Last major revision 1997-1998)

LIFELONG
EDUCATION FOR THE
OPHTHALMOLOGIST

American Academy of Ophthalmology

The Basic and Clinical Science Course is one component of the Lifelong Education for the Ophthalmologist (LEO) framework, which assists members in planning their continuing medical education. LEO includes an array of clinical education products that members may select to form individualized, self-directed learning plans for updating their clinical knowledge. Active members or fellows who use LEO components may accumulate sufficient CME credits to earn the LEO Award. Contact the Academy's Clinical Education Division for further information on LEO.

This CME activity was planned and produced in accordance with the ACCME Essentials.

The Academy provides this material for educational purposes only. It is not intended to represent the only or best method or procedure in every case, nor to replace a physician's own judgment or give specific advice for case management. Including all indications, contraindications, side effects, and alternative agents for each drug or treatment is beyond the scope of this material. All information and recommendations should be verified, prior to use, with current information included in the manufacturers' package inserts or other independent sources, and considered in light of the patient's condition and history. Reference to certain drugs, instruments, and other products in this publication is made for illustrative purposes only and is not intended to constitute an endorsement of such. Some material may include information on applications that are not considered community standard, that reflect indications not included in approved FDA labeling, or that are approved for use only in restricted research settings. The FDA has stated that it is the responsibility of the physician to determine the FDA status of each drug or device he or she wishes to use, and to use them with appropriate patient consent in compliance with applicable law. The Academy specifically disclaims any and all liability for injury or other damages of any kind, from negligence or otherwise, for any and all claims that may arise from the use of any recommendations or other information contained herein.

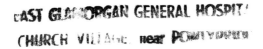

Basic and Clinical Science Course

Thomas A. Weingeist, PhD, MD, Iowa City, Iowa
Senior Secretary for Clinical Education

Thomas J. Liesegang, MD, Jacksonville, Florida
Secretary for Instruction

M. Gilbert Grand, MD, St. Louis, Missouri
BCSC Course Chair

Section 5

Faculty Responsible for This Edition

Thomas R. Hedges III, MD, *Chair,* Boston, Massachusetts

Deborah I. Friedman, MD, *Consultant,* Syracuse, New York

Jonathan C. Horton, MD, PhD, San Francisco, California

Steven A. Newman, MD, Charlottesville, Virginia

Gerald G. Striph, MD, Toledo, Ohio

Marilyn C. Kay, MD, Milwaukee, Wisconsin
Practicing Ophthalmologists Advisory Committee for Education

Recent Past Faculty

Roy W. Beck, MD	Nancy J. Newman, MD
Terry A. Cox, MD	Alfredo A. Sadun, MD
Steven E. Feldon, MD	Peter J. Savino, MD
Craig W. George, MD	Lyn A. Sedwick, MD
Mark J. Kupersmith, MD	Thomas L. Slamovits, MD
Kenneth H. Musson, MD	

In addition, the Academy gratefully acknowledges the contributions of numerous past faculty and advisory committee members who have played an important role in the development of previous editions of the Basic and Clinical Science Course.

American Academy of Ophthalmology Staff

Kathryn A. Hecht, EdD
Vice President, Clinical Education

Hal Straus
Director, Publications Department

Margaret Denny
Managing Editor

Fran Taylor
Medical Editor

Maxine Garrett
Administrative Coordinator

American Academy of Ophthalmology
655 Beach Street
Box 7424
San Francisco, CA 94120-7424

CONTENTS

GENERAL INTRODUCTION

The Basic and Clinical Science Course (BCSC) is designed to provide residents and practitioners with a comprehensive yet concise curriculum of the field of ophthalmology. The BCSC has developed from its original brief outline format, which relied heavily on outside readings, to a more convenient and educationally useful self-contained text. The Academy regularly updates and revises the course, with the goals of integrating the basic science and clinical practice of ophthalmology and of keeping current with new developments in the various subspecialties.

The BCSC incorporates the effort and expertise of more than 70 ophthalmologists, organized into 12 section faculties, working with Academy editorial staff. In addition, the course continues to benefit from many lasting contributions made by the faculties of previous editions. Members of the Academy's Practicing Ophthalmologists Advisory Committee for Education serve on each faculty and, as a group, review every volume before and after major revisions.

Organization of the Course

The 12 sections of the Basic and Clinical Science Course are numbered as follows to reflect a logical order of study, proceeding from fundamental subjects to anatomic subdivisions:

1. Update on General Medicine
2. Fundamentals and Principles of Ophthalmology
3. Optics, Refraction, and Contact Lenses
4. Ophthalmic Pathology and Intraocular Tumors
5. Neuro-Ophthalmology
6. Pediatric Ophthalmology and Strabismus
7. Orbit, Eyelids, and Lacrimal System
8. External Disease and Cornea
9. Intraocular Inflammation and Uveitis
10. Glaucoma
11. Lens and Cataract
12. Retina and Vitreous

In addition, a comprehensive Master Index allows the reader to easily locate subjects throughout the entire series.

References

Readers who wish to explore specific topics in greater detail may consult the journal references cited within each chapter and the Basic Texts listed at the back of the book. These references are intended to be selective rather than exhaustive, chosen by the BCSC faculty as being important, current, and readily available to residents and practitioners.

Related Academy educational materials are also listed in the appropriate sections. They include books, audiovisual materials, self-assessment programs, clinical modules, and interactive programs.

Study Questions and CME Credit

Each volume includes multiple-choice study questions designed to be used as a closed-book exercise. The answers are accompanied by explanations to enhance the learning experience. Completing the study questions allows readers both to test their understanding of the material and to demonstrate section completion for the purpose of CME credit, if desired.

The Academy is accredited by the Accreditation Council for Continuing Medical Education to sponsor continuing medical education for physicians. CME credit hours in Category 1 of the Physician's Recognition Award of the AMA may be earned for completing the study of any section of the BCSC. The Academy designates the number of credit hours for each section based upon the scope and complexity of the material covered (see the Credit Reporting Form in each individual section for the maximum number of hours that may be claimed).

Based upon return of the Credit Reporting Form at the back of each book, the Academy will maintain a record, for up to 3 years, of credits earned by Academy members. Upon request, the Academy will send a transcript of credits earned.

Conclusion

The Basic and Clinical Science Course has expanded greatly over the years, with the addition of much new text and numerous illustrations. Recent editions have sought to place a greater emphasis on clinical applicability, while maintaining a solid foundation in basic science. As with any educational program, it reflects the experience of its authors. As its faculties change and as medicine progresses, new viewpoints are always emerging on controversial subjects and techniques. Not all alternate approaches can be included in this series; as with any educational endeavor, the learner should seek additional sources, including such carefully balanced opinions as the Academy's Preferred Practice Patterns.

The BCSC faculty and staff are continuously striving to improve the educational usefulness of the course; you, the reader, can contribute to this ongoing process. If you have any suggestions or questions about the series, please do not hesitate to contact the faculty or the managing editor.

The authors, editors, and reviewers hope that your study of the BCSC will be of lasting value and that each section will serve as a practical resource for quality patient care.

OBJECTIVES FOR BCSC SECTION 5

Upon completion of BCSC Section 5, *Neuro-Ophthalmology,* the reader should be able to:

- Explain the importance of an accurate and detailed history to the differential diagnosis of neuro-ophthalmic disease
- Describe the critical importance of follow-up and its potential for modifying the diagnosis
- Outline the necessity of tailoring the neuro-ophthalmic examination
- Select the most appropriate tests in order to manage the neuro-ophthalmic problem in a cost-effective manner
- Explain possible systemic implications of ophthalmic disorders
- Appraise the anatomy of the visual pathway in order to localize lesions
- Define the anatomy of the vascular system and the importance of it to neuro-ophthalmic pathology
- Describe the association between pupil and eyelid position and ocular motor pathology
- Review pathophysiology and management of diplopia and central ocular motor disorders
- Assess eye movement disorders and the ocular motor system
- Review anatomy of other cranial nerves
- Identify the effects of systemic disorders on visual and ocular motor pathways

A Brief History of Neuro-Ophthalmology and Visual Field Testing

Tumors, strokes, and inflammations that produce hemianopias, cranial nerve palsies, and sudden blindness have, of course, always existed. But their relationships with each other remained mysterious until the relevant neuroanatomy and neurophysiology were understood.

Just 150 years ago, it was probably possible to teach everything there was to know about neuro-ophthalmology in 10 or 15 minutes, but in the 1990s neuro-ophthalmology has grown into a rich and complex field of study. The history of neuro-ophthalmology contains bits of the history of neurology, of ophthalmology, and of all the related basic medical sciences.

In the 1930s and 1940s a few American ophthalmologists were beginning to take an interest in the borderland between neurology and ophthalmology. They started to publish papers on clinical neuro-ophthalmology. In this early group were David G. Cogan of Boston; Frank B. Walsh of Baltimore; Donald J. Lyle of Cincinnati; C. Wilbur Rucker of Rochester, Minnesota; Alfred Kestenbaum of New York; and P. J. Leinfelder of Iowa City. It was during these years that the word *neuro-ophthalmology* began to appear in the titles of textbooks: Rea, 1938; Lyle, 1945; Kestenbaum, 1946; Walsh, 1947.

Frank B. Walsh (1895–1978), more than anyone else, was responsible for identifying neuro-ophthalmology as a plausible medical subspecialty. At The Johns Hopkins University, he brought together everything he had learned about neuro-ophthalmology, organized it, tempered it with his own experience, and published it as a fat, red-bound book called *Clinical Neuro-Ophthalmology* in 1947. The second edition of Walsh's book came out in 1957. Walsh's book and his personal example led a number of young doctors to the realization that the subject matter in neuro-ophthalmology could keep them busy for a lifetime.

What follows is a chronological overview of a small part of the history of neuro-ophthalmology. It is the story of how the discovery of the decussation at the chiasm contributed to awareness of visual field loss and led to the clinical testing of visual fields.

One of the questions that troubled ancient philosophers was "Why, when we are equipped with two good eyes, do we not see two of everything?" Gradually, thinkers came to agree that images from the two eyes must come together somewhere in the brain and become fused into one.

450 BC   Hippocrates described a patient with a hemianopia.

150 BC   Ptolemy is credited with estimating the outer limits of the visual field.

AD 130   It was known by the Greeks that the two optic nerves come together inside the head. This juncture was called the χιασμα (chiasma) by the anatomist and physician Rufus of Ephesus. The Greek word *chiasma* means the mark of the letter X *(chi)*, so the crossing of the optic nerves was named after the letter of the Greek alphabet that it physically resembles.

AD 165   A generation or two after Rufus of Ephesus, Galen of Pergamon saw the chiasm as a potential hydraulic connection between the two eyes and as the dividing point in the visual pathway that serves to distribute the vital fluid from the ventricles to both eyes.

200–1200   Arab medical knowledge, based chiefly on Galen's writings, was the best medical knowledge available during the European Middle Ages. Arab physicians clarified many of Galen's ideas: the hollowness of the optic nerves, their merging in the chiasm "so that their two cavities become one," the "origin" of the optic nerves from the cerebral ventricles, and the existence of a "pneuma constantly circulating from the ventricles to the eye."

1500   Leonardo da Vinci, curious about the eyes and the brain, based his drawings on Galen rather than on dissection.

1555   Andreas Vesalius, the Belgian anatomist, marked the turning point in neuroanatomy. His drawings were based on personal dissections of the brain, and those who followed him (Eustachio, Varolius, Laurentius, Vieussens) were careful to dissect for themselves.

1604, 1610   Johannes Kepler published his reasons for believing the retina to be the essential percipient element in the eye.

1630   René Descartes (1596–1650), French philosopher and mathematician, still accepted most of Galen's anatomy, but he devised a mechanistic physiology. He had the visual spirits ("impulses") passing from the retina along the optic nerve, not decussating at the chiasm, and arriving at a retinotopic array in the lateral ventricle, where they were transferred to the centrally located pineal gland ("the seat of the soul"). Here in the pineal gland, according to Descartes, each image met its fellow from the other eye, so that the two images became combined into a single visual experience. From the pineal gland these fused images were deposited in the brain for future recall as visual memory.

1660   Thomas Willis, a busy Oxford physician, undertook a major study of the anatomy of the brain. In his book *Cerebri Anatome* (1664), Willis described the circle of vessels at the base of the brain that now bears his name.

   In the 17th century, it was not known whether the optic nerves intermingled and exchanged fibers at the chiasm or whether they were just briefly bound together at the base before proceeding, each nerve to its own side of the brain.

1667   Willis spoke of visual field defects in patients with ocular disease.

1668   Edmé Mariotte reported that there was a nonseeing area in the visual field of every normal eye and demonstrated that it was caused by the entrance of the optic nerve into the eye at that location.

1682   Isaac Newton (1642–1727), the celebrated mathematician, physicist, and philosopher of Cambridge and London, deduced that there must be a hemidecussation at the chiasm; it was the best way to get the images from the two eyes together in the brain.

1682   William Briggs (1650–1704), a fellow of Cambridge University and a physician at St. Thomas Hospital in London, described the retinal fibers as converging within the eye upon the "optic papilla" and then traveling along the optic nerve and passing through the chiasma without any decussation of the fibers.

Briggs was 8 years younger than Newton and must have known him from his days at Cambridge. After Briggs said at the Royal Society that there was no mixing of optic nerve fibers at the chiasm, Newton wrote a letter to Briggs dated September 12, 1682, suggesting that Briggs was wrong: ". . . how is this coincidence [of the pictures from the two eyes] made? Perhaps by the mixing of the marrow of the nerves in their juncture [that is, at the chiasm] before they enter the brain, the fibers on the right side of each eye going to the right side of the head and those on the left side to the left."

1704   Twenty-two years later, Newton published this hemidecussation hypothesis in his book *Opticks* as one of a series of "queries" and thus became the first to indicate clearly in print that a partial decussation of the optic nerves in the chiasm could be the basis of single binocular vision.

1710   Hermann Boerhaave spoke of scotomata and tried to get patients to fix on a small spot and then describe where the dark areas were.

1719   Giovanni Battista Morgagni (1682–1771), Professor of Anatomy in Bologna and Padua, has been called "the Prince of Anatomists" and "the Founder of Pathological Anatomy." He described a case of impaired vision in both eyes caused by a unilateral lesion in the brain. This seems to have been the earliest correct interpretation of a homonymous hemianopia.

1723   Abraham Vater and J. Christian Heinecke published a thesis in which they described at some length the case of a young man who suffered sudden onset of a homonymous hemianopia. Upon finding that with either eye, or with both together, he could see only half of what he was looking at, "his spirit was not a little perturbed." His vision returned to normal in about an hour. (From a distance of 270 years, his symptoms suggest migraine.) The authors then argued that this kind of symptom could only occur if there is a hemidecussation of the optic nerves at the chiasm. Not surprisingly, they had not noticed Newton's brief mention of this thought buried at the back of a difficult English-language optics book.

1738   Chevalier John Taylor (1703–1772), English Ophthalmiatric Knight-Errant, Travelling Cataract Coucher, and Charlatan-Oculist Extraordinaire, published the first diagram illustrating the concept of a hemidecussation at the chiasm. Posterity may have a low opinion of Taylor's character and professional accomplishments, but his views on the anatomical basis of single binocular vision were remarkably modern. Taylor appears to have accepted Newton's chiasmal hemidecussation (1704), Morgagni's autopsied case (1719), and Vater and Heinecke's clinical case (1723), but he gave no credit to any of them. Some internal evidence—the discussion of chameleons' eyes—suggests that Taylor had read Newton. In any case, Taylor made the further suggestion that fibers originating at corresponding points in the two retinas meet at a single point in the brain to produce a single subjective visual experience.

1759   William Porterfield spoke of the wide horizontal visual field of birds and rabbits.

1801   Thomas Young measured the limits of the visual field at 90° temporally, 60° medially, 50° up, and 70° down.

1817   Joseph Beer of Vienna spoke of central and paracentral scotomata, concentric contractions, and half-field loss.

1824   William Hyde Wollaston (1766–1828), a chemist and metallurgist famous for his work with the platinum metals, conceived the idea of a hemidecussation at the chiasm, strictly on the basis of his own transient loss of vision to one side and apparently without knowledge of Newton's ideas or the clinical cases of the 18th century. He wrote,

> It is now more than 20 years since I was first affected with the peculiar state of vision to which I allude, in consequence of violent exercise I had taken for 2 or 3 hours before. I suddenly found that I could see but half of the face of a man whom I met: and it was the same with respect to every object I looked at. In attempting to read the name JOHNSON over a door, I saw only SON; the commencement of the name being wholly obliterated to my view. In this instance the loss of sight was toward my left. This blindness was not so complete as to amount to absolute blackness, but was a shaded darkness without definite outline. The complaint was of short duration, and in about a quarter of an hour might be said to be wholly gone, having receded with a gradual motion from the center of vision obliquely upwards toward the left.
>
> It is now about 15 months since a similar affection occurred again to myself, without my being able to assign any cause to it whatever, or to connect it with any previous or subsequent indisposition. The blindness was first observed, as before, in looking at the face of a person I met, whose left eye was to my sight obliterated. My blindness was in this instance the reverse of the former, being to my right (instead of the left) of the spot to which my eyes were directed; so that I have no reason to suppose it in any manner connected with the former affection.
>
> In reflecting upon this subject, a certain arrangement of the optic nerves has suggested itself to me, which appears to afford a very probable interpretation of a set of facts, which are not consistent with the generally received hypothesis of the decussation of the optic nerves.

He then argued persuasively that a homonymous field loss would be impossible without such a hemidecussation. In retrospect, these episodes were almost certainly migrainous scotomata without headache. In fact, Wollaston himself went on (in the same paper) to describe five other cases of a similar nature, several of which were associated with migraine.

> Wollaston WH. On semi-decussation of the optic nerves. *Phil Tr Roy Soc London.* 1824;114:222.

Three years later, late in 1827, Wollaston's left arm became numb, and in July 1828 his left pupil became fixed. He described these symptoms to a medical friend as if they were those of another person, and on hearing that they suggested a terminal brain tumor, he went home and started to dictate papers for publication on all of his completed work. Most of these papers were published posthumously. In his final weeks, he remained alert and his vision and hearing were good, but he was unable to speak. He died later that year, and his autopsy report described an intraventricular hemorrhage. The recurrent homonymous hemianopic scotomata that set him thinking about chiasmal hemidecussation were probably not related in any way to his final illness.

Wollaston's publication aroused widespread interest in the chiasmal crossing of the optic nerves. Johannes Müller showed in 1826 that the lateral fibers of the chiasm do *not* cross, and the 19th century microscopists were soon to demonstrate that Wollaston, Chevalier Taylor, Vater and Heinecke, and Isaac Newton were right in suggesting a complete hemidecussation of optic nerve fibers at the chiasm.

1825   Purkinje pointed out that not only did visual acuity deteriorate in the peripheral visual field, but so did the quality of color perception as well. Purkinje contrived an apparatus for estimating the limits of the visual field, but it was never put to clinical use.

1842   Himly, of Göttingen, spoke of "amaurosis periphica" as opposed to "amaurosis centralis."

1847   Desmarres, of Paris, described loss of the upper field in retinal detachment.

Clearly, some practicing ophthalmologists of this period knew about visual field defects, but clinical use of perimetry was not widespread until von Graefe.

1856   Albrecht von Graefe, 28, published a paper called "Examination of the Field of Vision in Amblyopic Disease" (*von Graefe's Archiv.* 1856;2/2:258–298). He used a blackboard as a tangent screen and worked at a distance of 18 inches with a piece of chalk held in a wire as a test object. He gave examples of central scotoma; ring scotomata; concentric narrowing of the field; enlargement of the blind spot; and homonymous, bitemporal, and binasal hemianopia. He suggested that homonymous hemianopias are caused by unilateral cerebral disease and heteronymous hemianopias by growths at the base of the brain. von Graefe's pioneering paper started the trend that finally put visual field testing equipment into the ophthalmologist's office.

1857   Hermann Aubert and Richard Förster of Breslau began a group of papers under the title "Contributions to the Knowledge of Indirect Vision," using a tangent screen like von Graefe's. The test was done in a darkened room, and, to keep fixation from wandering, the screen and the test object were only briefly illuminated by the arc from a Reis bottle. The patient watched the screen through a short tube lined with black felt so that the tested eye was not exposed to the flash. Aubert and Förster soon decided that it was important to keep the target at a constant distance from the eye in different parts of the visual field; they made a simple arc perimeter and continued their studies.

1869   Förster and Aubert developed an arc perimeter for the practicing ophthalmologist. It was very popular and became known as the Förster perimeter.

1871   De Wecker improved von Graefe's tangent screen by equipping it with a chin rest and a stand and marking it with concentric circles, starting at 10°.
   Until Brudenell Carter's instrument became available in 1873, all perimeters and campimeters had the blind spot at the zero point and fixation at 15° to the right in the left eye and 15° to the left in the right eye. This convention was started by von Graefe in an effort to match the field to the fundus picture. In 1856 von Graefe was still trying to get practicing ophthalmologists to use Helmholtz's ophthalmoscope routinely, and his paper on visual field testing stressed that fundus lesions had matching visual field defects. Putting the blind spot at zero helped to make this clinical point, because it got rid of the horizontal ambiguities and left only the vertical inversion.

Fifteen years later, there was no longer any doubt that major retinal lesions produced matching field defects. Carter's innovation, locating the fixation point at zero, proved to be popular. This new way of plotting the field required the doctor to imagine both vertical *and* horizontal flips—from the point of view of the patient—in order to locate a retinal lesion in the visual field. However, it seemed to make better physiologic sense to measure the distances from the fovea, and it was easier to set the right blind spot to the right of fixation and the left blind spot to the left. This new convention won the day and became the universally accepted way to plot visual fields.

1872   Scherk developed a bowl perimeter to eliminate the distracting background always present in an arc perimeter. He solved the technical problem of how to illuminate the surface evenly by splitting the bowl at the zero meridian (i.e., through the blind spot) and connecting the two halves with a double hinge. This allowed him to let light onto the section being used.

1874   The first book devoted entirely to visual field testing was written by Wilhelm Schön (*Die Lehre vom Gesichtsfelde und seinen Anomalien*, Berlin, 1874). Schön used an arc perimeter and did not work too closely with the central 10°. He discussed the characteristic kinds of field loss found in glaucoma, retinitis pigmentosa, detachment of the retina, embolism of the central artery of the retina, retrobulbar neuritis, intoxication amblyopia, and chiasmal disease.

1875   The next book on the subject, by Richard Pauli, came out in Münich and was entitled *Beiträge zur Lehre vom Gesichtfeld* (Contribution to the Science of Visual Fields).

1875   Julius Hirschberg used a screen marked with rings out to 45°. He studied his patients' visual fields very carefully with this device and coined the term *campimetry* for the tangent screen technique to distinguish it from *perimetry*.

1881   Uhthoff mounted a small campimeter screen onto the Förster arc perimeter.

During the 1880s, it became generally accepted that the arc perimeter, although designed for peripheral field mapping, was also satisfactory for central field defects. From this assumption came the idea that no central defects of any clinical importance existed, and that the perimeter was the only proper way to plot visual fields.

1893   Groenouw coined the term *isopter* for a line on a perimetric chart joining points of equal sensitivity.

1889   Jannik Peterson Bjerrum (1851–1920), professor of ophthalmology in Copenhagen, reintroduced and popularized campimetry. Bjerrum found that mapping the subtleties of the central 30° was far more useful than the routine outlining of the perimeter of the visual field, as then commonly done. He scorned the available perimetric instruments, mounting a tangent screen on the back of his office door. Bjerrum's screen grew to 2 meters across, of black velvet with concentric rings and radial lines of inconspicuous black, and was used at 1 and 2 meters. Bjerrum used a series of small test objects of increasing subtlety. These careful techniques restored some of von Graefe's emphasis on the central visual field, and Bjerrum and Rønne were able to demonstrate the characteristics of the earliest field loss in glaucoma with which their names are still associated. The simplicity and sensitivity of the tangent screen were very appealing, and dust covers were put over many arc perimeters.

1900   Hermann Wilbrand's authoritative article on perimetry in the four-volume work of Norris and Oliver made a plea for paying attention to retinal physiology, also emphasizing the importance of thorough quantitative perimetry.

1909–1927   Henning Rønne, working in Bjerrum's clinic, stressed the importance of using a graduated series of test objects.

In the United States Alexander Duane, Harry Friedenwald, Clifford B. Walker, and Luther C. Peter popularized the work of Bjerrum and Rønne. Duane and Friedenwald put their stamp of approval on the new techniques, and Peter wrote a popular book on the subject, *The Principles and Practice of Perimetry* (Lea & Febiger, 1916). Walker made many important contributions to the science of perimetry.

In Scotland important figures included A. H. H. Sinclair and Harry Moss Traquair. Traquair of Edinburgh used an arc perimeter and a 2-meter tangent screen. His many astute insights into visual field interpretation made his book *An Introduction to Clinical Perimetry* (1927) very popular.

The perimeter of Feree and Rand (1924) not only supplied its own controlled illumination but had a small campimeter attached to the arc. This little tangent screen could be used for careful central field testing but could also be slipped along the arc so that freehand scotoma mapping could be done anywhere in the periphery.

Ralph I. Lloyd developed the stereocampimeter, a device that made it possible to fix with one eye and plot the suppression scotoma in the other, amblyopic, eye.

1945   Hans Goldmann of Bern devised a hemispheric bowl, self-illuminated, projection perimeter in which fixation, retinal adaptation, and stimulus size and intensity could be precisely controlled. The field could be readily recorded by means of an ingenious pantograph. This dependable instrument, made by Haag-Streit of Bern, became the standard kinetic perimeter.

1956   David O. Harrington's book *Visual Fields* emphasized careful tangent screen work and clinical interpretation. The book came out in several new editions over the next 30 years.

1959   Harms and Elfriede Aulhorn developed a perimeter specifically designed to do static threshold perimetry, commonly called the Tübinger Perimeter and made by Oculus. Cross sections of the "island of vision" were made by finding the threshold sensitivity at various locations along a single meridian. The advantages of static threshold perimetry had been pointed out in 1933 by Louise L. Sloan.

1971   Mansour Armaly and Stephen Drance developed screening tactics for glaucoma detection using suprathreshold static testing with Goldmann's perimeter.

As the technology gradually became available, computer-controlled automated static threshold perimetry was developed. Credit goes especially to Franz Fankhauser, John Lynn, Anders Heijl, E. C. T. Krakau, Stephen Drance, and Lars Frisén. Instruments made by Octopus and Humphrey are now in use in the offices of almost every ophthalmologist and optometrist in North America.

The trouble with perimetry, automated or not, is that it is, of course, a psychophysical test—always dependent on the mood, fears, and alertness of the subject. To quote Harvey Cushing: "Good perimetry depends not so much upon the perimeter, as on the man behind the perimeter."

H. Stanley Thompson, MD

CHAPTER I

The Neuro-Ophthalmic Examination

History

A carefully elicited history can often lead to the diagnosis of a neuro-ophthalmic disorder even prior to the examination. The main purpose of the history is to help generate a differential diagnosis that can efficiently guide the examination and testing of the patient. Common neuro-ophthalmic chief complaints include visual loss, transient visual phenomena, diplopia, ptosis, unequal pupils, headache, or periocular pain. Occasionally patients without specific ophthalmologic complaints are referred to be screened for the effects of a systemic or neurologic disease.

The ophthalmologist needs to develop a history-taking procedure that provides enough structure to review the possibilities completely yet enough flexibility to respond to the individual without exhausting the patient or incurring unnecessary expenses.

Allow the patient to relate the story with as little prompting as possible, limiting examiner bias. Clarify the history, as needed, after the patient has finished. Repeating and rephrasing the patient's words helps ensure that the clinician's understanding is accurate. Questioning about the chief complaint and present history must establish whether the onset was acute or gradual and whether the course or symptoms have remained stable, deteriorated, or spontaneously improved since the onset. Are there other associated systemic, ocular, or neurologic complaints? Has any treatment or other factor altered the course?

A history pointing toward specific diagnoses will suggest related questions discussed below. The examiner should obtain pertinent history from the classic past medical, family, social, and system review areas. Many examiners prefer to delay reviewing prior evaluations and test results until they have developed an independent opinion.

Visual Disturbances

Establish whether the visual disturbance is unilateral or bilateral. If visual loss is monocular, the problem is very likely anterior to the chiasm. Bilateral visual loss may be caused by bilateral ocular or optic nerve disease or a disorder at or posterior to the chiasm. Patients often erroneously equate homonymous visual loss with a monocular problem on the side of the temporal field defect. It is important to ask whether the patient actually closed each eye to determine if the problem was with one eye or the homonymous hemifield of both eyes. This information is so crucial to the differential diagnosis and further history-taking that it may be worthwhile to stop and ask the patient to cover each eye to assess the disturbance before continuing.

Inquire whether the loss of vision was gradual or sudden. Acute onset of visual loss over minutes to days is typical of an ischemic or inflammatory process. Compressive or toxic lesions tend to be gradual and progressive, except when acute expansion or rupture of an aneurysm or pituitary apoplexy occurs. Slowly progressive visual loss may be discovered suddenly and misinterpreted as having an abrupt onset. The patient might have covered the normal seeing eye and discovered the visual loss in the affected eye without warning. Or a patient may become suddenly aware of long-standing visual loss only when the second eye becomes involved.

The duration of visual loss can also suggest certain diagnoses. For example, transient visual obscurations lasting seconds might suggest papilledema, whereas monocular visual loss lasting several minutes might suggest embolic disease in the retinal circulation. Progressive visual loss over several days that lasts weeks suggests optic neuritis.

Monocular pain with eye movement and visual loss is a common presentation of optic neuritis; however, pain and motility problems with visual loss are also typical of inflammatory lesions in the orbit and cavernous sinus. Further investigation is required to determine the cause. Pain unrelated to eye movement or obvious intraocular disease may indicate an intracranial lesion. Question patients with eye pain about neurologic and systemic symptoms associated with headache as well as about other ocular symptoms related to external disease and uveitis.

Diplopia

Double vision is a frequent manifestation of neuro-ophthalmic disease. The patient may see a distinct second image or only a shadow or ghost image. Diplopia is sometimes described as blurred vision or difficulty seeing to one side. At times, the second image is so far off to the periphery that a patient with significant ocular misalignment is unaware of the diplopia.

A key question in the diplopia patient's history is whether the double vision is monocular or binocular. Binocular diplopia is present only with both eyes open; it disappears when *either* eye is covered. This distinction is so crucial to the differential diagnosis that the examiner may need to pause during the history and ask the patient to cover each eye while fixating on a target to determine the answer.

Monocular diplopia, which persists with one eye covered, almost always indicates an ophthalmologic, rather than a neurologic, problem. Common causes include refractive error, keratoconus, cataract, and iridectomy. Monocular diplopia is frequently described as a ghost image; more than one image may be seen, and the phenomenon may change with ambient lighting. Occasionally, monocular diplopia can coexist with binocular diplopia (e.g., a diabetic patient with cataract and a sixth nerve palsy). In such cases, the examiner may need to conduct the history and physical examination along multiple lines. Very rarely, monocular diplopia that is identical in each eye can be caused by disease affecting the occipital-parietal visual cortex (see chapter III).

Binocular diplopia results from misalignment of the eyes. Possible causes include the following:

- Neurologic disease (e.g., cranial nerve palsy)
- Disease of the neuromuscular junction (e.g., myasthenia gravis)
- Muscular disorder (e.g., Graves disease)
- Displacement of the globe (e.g., intraconal tumor)

Ask the patient if the images are separated horizontally, vertically, or obliquely. Is the separation of the images worse in certain gaze positions, at distance or at near, or with head tilting? Such questions help distinguish which muscles or nerves are involved. Determine if the severity or presence of diplopia varies with the time of day or is associated with fatigue or ptosis.

Neurologic Disturbances

The presence or absence of neurologic signs and symptoms not involving vision can also provide clues to the location of underlying disease. For example, amaurosis fugax associated with episodes of contralateral extremity weakness suggests ischemic disease in the territory of the ipsilateral internal carotid artery. In contrast, multiple cranial nerve deficits with homonymous field loss might suggest disease in the territory of the posterior circulation. The clinician's goal is to correlate the patient's symptoms with syndromes having a common neurologic localization or a common etiology.

Functional Visual Loss

Neuro-ophthalmologists frequently examine patients whose subjective complaints seem to contradict the objective findings. In addition to visual loss, diplopia, or pain, complaints may include atypical visual phenomena. In contradictory cases, the examiner must consider the possibility that the problem is functional, or not attributable to an organic cause.

Patients who feign visual difficulty for secondary gain (often financial) may be malingering. Often patients who are unaware that the visual difficulty is nonorganic may have an underlying psychiatric disorder. The ophthalmologist's role is to establish that the complaints are nonorganic and to determine the level of visual function; the precise diagnosis and management may be left to the primary care physician or psychiatrist.

The history often provides a clue to the functional nature of the visual loss. The onset of symptoms is not typical of known organic disease and is often related to an event such as trauma or to a procedure that the patient claims to be the cause. The chief complaint may be incompatible with the findings. For example, the patient may give responses suggestive of decreased vision in the right eye yet complain spontaneously of "not seeing anything to the right" with both eyes open.

During history taking, observe whether the patient makes visually elicited movements or fixates on objects in the room. Malingerers may bump into objects or fall softly but rarely hurt themselves. Other functional patients tend to avoid objects in their path altogether. The examiner needs to be alert to a discrepancy between the visual function suggested by the history and that observed during the history, the examination, and candid moments (such as while the patient is in the waiting area during pupillary dilation). Specific tests are discussed in detail later in this chapter; see pp 32–36.

Examination and Testing

Visual Acuity

Visual acuity is the most common measure of central visual function. The best-corrected visual acuity should be determined with careful refraction. A pinhole visual acuity may be useful in situations where refraction is difficult, such as keratoconus. However, the functional accuracy of pinhole acuities can be misleading. A pinhole acuity significantly better than the acuity obtained by other methods is suggestive of an undiagnosed refractive or ocular media problem such as oil-drop cataract.

For patients with reduced vision, move the chart as close as necessary for the patient to see. Letters or numbers are recorded with the numerator representing the distance from the eye and the denominator indicating the line that is read. Rather than obtaining "finger-counting" vision, obtain a reproducible numeric acuity. The examiner using a 20/200 letter on a card that the patient is able to read at 2 feet can record the acuity as 2/200. Observe if the patient requires eccentric fixation (possible macular disease), tends to read only one side of the eye chart (possible visual field defect), or reads single optotypes much better than whole lines (possible amblyopia).

Color Vision

Clinical evaluation of color perception can include testing with specialized color materials or with large colored objects. Detailed testing of color vision can confirm known and detect unrecognized congenital color discrimination defects as well as rare progressive cone dystrophies. Acquired disturbances of the macula, optic nerve, and chiasm may cause less specific loss of color appreciation.

The majority of color vision deficits are nonspecific, and only on occasion will acquired color vision defects predominantly disturb a single color axis. For example, acquired macular disease may diminish blue/yellow discrimination in its early stages, because blue cones are concentrated in the perifoveal ring. Yet red/green defects have historically, if not accurately, been associated with optic nerve disease. The relative importance of the fovea, which has few blue cones, and the predominance of red/green cones feeding the optic nerve make the easily measured red/green confusion more apparent in many optic nerve diseases.

Testing of color vision is complementary to assessment of visual acuity. It is useful in the demonstration and assessment of reduced visual function, especially if visual acuity is relatively normal in the presence of optic nerve disease. Persistent dyschromatopsia is common even after recovery of visual acuity in optic neuropathies.

Perform color vision testing with each eye separately in order to detect unilateral disease. The *Farnsworth-Munsell 100-hue test* gives a comprehensive characterization of a color vision defect and can help distinguish acquired from congenital abnormalities. However, the patient must order 84 colored disks and the test must be scored; the time-consuming nature limits this test's clinical use. The *Farnsworth Panel D-15*, a shorter version using 15 plates, is more practical but less sensitive.

Pseudoisochromatic color plate testing (e.g., *Ishihara* or *Hardy-Rand-Rittler*) was designed to screen for congenital red/green color deficiencies. *Lanthony tritan* plates may be used to detect blue/yellow defects. These tests are frequently used for a gross estimate of acquired color loss and central visual dysfunction. They have never been validated for that use and are often given in suboptimal lighting situations. However, they are quick, commonly available, and can be clinically useful.

Color desaturation can be tested using a brightly colored object (commonly a red mydriatic bottle cap) to compare the function of the two eyes. Ask the patient to compare the saturation, or "redness," of the object as perceived by each eye. It is important to verify that the patient is describing the richness of the color (e.g., deep red or washed out) rather than the brightness (see below). Subjective desaturation of colors in one eye often indicates an acquired dyschromatopsia, a sign of optic nerve dysfunction. See also BCSC Section 12, *Retina and Vitreous,* chapter III.

Hart WM Jr. Acquired dyschromatopsias. *Surv Ophthalmol.* 1987;32:10–31.

Brightness Comparison

Brightness comparison is also a subjective test. After shining a bright light into first one and then the other eye, ask the patient, "In which eye is the light brighter: right or left?" Ascribe a value of 100 cents to the "brighter eye" and then ask the patient to assign a value in cents to the dimmer eye (e.g., 50 cents if the light seems half as bright). The subjective difference between the two eyes can be quantified on the chart as RE100/LE50.

Brightness perception can also be quantified by putting a sequence of darker neutral-density filters before the better-seeing eye until the patient states that the brightness is the same between the eyes. This method is useful for two reasons: the patient may not accurately use the 100-point scale, and the patient is masked toward the neutral-density value of the lens and may be less biased.

Brightness comparison testing has many limitations, including the nonstandard brightness of the light, the varying background illumination, the subjective nature of assigning a "brightness" value for gradations along the 100-point scale, and the variability of the patient's emotional state during subsequent visits for comparison. Nevertheless, it does correlate with the more objective relative afferent pupillary defect (RAPD), helps patients describe their deficit to the examiner, provides another measure of central visual function, and can be used in patients in whom the RAPD is difficult to measure.

Browning DJ, Buckley EG. Reliability of brightness comparison testing in predicting afferent pupillary defects. *Arch Ophthalmol.* 1988;106:341–343.

Sadun AA, Lessell S. Brightness-sense and optic nerve disease. *Arch Ophthalmol.* 1985;103:39–43.

Photostress Recovery Test

The photostress recovery test helps to differentiate between optic nerve disease and visual loss caused by a macular process. Determine the patient's best-corrected visual acuity and note the line on the eye chart. Ask the patient to look for about 10 seconds directly into a strong light (e.g., direct ophthalmoscope) held 2–3 cm in front of the eye to be tested. Record the number of seconds required for the patient to recover and be able to read the same or next larger line on the eye chart. With optic nerve disease the recovery time is frequently normal (less than 60 seconds). But with a maculopathy recovery time may be considerably prolonged (90–180 seconds). Each eye is tested separately. The test is invalid for eyes with acuity of less than 20/80.

Glaser JS, Savino PJ, Sumers KD, et al. The photostress recovery test in the clinical assessment of visual function. *Am J Ophthalmol.* 1977;83:255–260.

Spatial Contrast Sensitivity

The *contrast threshold,* the lowest amount of contrast needed to see a grating, can be determined for a range of gratings of various sizes to give a *contrast sensitivity function* (CSF). The examiner varies the contrast between similarly sized targets and the background on a wall chart or TV monitor. Because acuity measurement is only one point on the CSF curve, a CSF provides another viewpoint on central visual function.

Patients with vague visual complaints, such as cloudy or misty vision, often have elevated contrast thresholds even though they have 20/20 Snellen acuity. Such complaints are heard from patients with a variety of clinical problems including cataracts, glaucoma, macular lesions, optic neuropathies, and cerebral diseases. CSF determinations can reveal and quantify subtle degrees of central visual loss and can be useful in the serial follow-up of patients with optic neuropathies. As in many threshold tests, the results do not always show a clear-cut delineation between normal and abnormal patients.

> Moseley MJ, Hill AR. Contrast sensitivity testing in clinical practice. *Br J Ophthalmol.* 1994;78:795–797.

Visually Evoked Cortical Potentials

The visually evoked cortical potential (VECP) is an electrical signal recorded from the scalp overlying the occipital cortex following visual stimulation of the retina. The VECP (also VEP or VER for visually evoked response) is buried in the ongoing electroencephalogram (EEG), which is a summation of cortical activity. If a series of identical time-locked photic or contrast pattern stimuli are presented, and the electrical signal measured from occipital area electrodes is amplified and averaged with a linear averager, the underlying EEG "noise" can be subtracted, leaving only the visually related electrical activity. The VECP is chiefly a measure of macular visual function, because the foveal area is represented by a much larger area in the superficial and posterior occipital cortex, close to the recording electrodes, while the smaller area representing the more peripheral retina lies deep within the calcarine fissure.

The VECP may be generated by different stimuli. A stroboscopic light is the stimulus for the *flash VECP.* A checkerboard pattern or bar grating can be reversed, or the pattern can be flashed on and off to produce the *pattern VECP.* Different stimuli produce different wave forms. When the stimulus is presented at a low reversal rate, a discrete response called the *transient VECP* can be demonstrated with discrete reproducible wave shapes (Fig I-1).

The wave most often studied in the clinic is the positive deflection that occurs approximately at 100 msec after the stimulus, called the P100 wave. The *amplitude* of this response is defined as the height of the potential as measured from peak to trough. The *latency* of the P100 wave is the time from the onset of the stimulus to the peak of the response. In toxic and compressive optic neuropathies reduction in the amplitude of this wave seems to be more pronounced than is lengthening of latency. In demyelinating disease the changes are reversed: the latency is relatively more prolonged than the amplitude is reduced.

The VECP should be standardized for a given set of stimulus conditions in age-matched controls for each laboratory. The VECP amplitude may be decreased if refractive errors are uncorrected or if the patient does not concentrate on the pattern, limiting the utility of electrophysiologic testing in the diagnosis of functional disease.

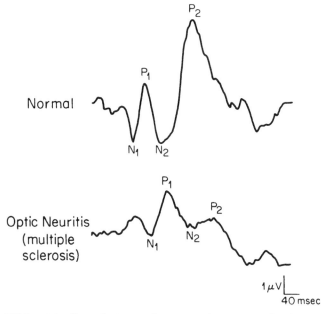

FIG I-1—Visually evoked cortical responses from a normal individual (top) and a patient with optic neuropathy from multiple sclerosis (bottom) who shows not only a reduced amplitude but a marked delay in the appearance of the peaks.

Electrical techniques may test the integrity of the visual pathways in nonverbal patients such as infants. A normal VECP, especially when combined with a normal electroretinogram (ERG), is good evidence of intact visual pathways. Specialized VECP testing can estimate visual acuity in preverbal infants.

Some clinicians use VECP to detect or verify an optic neuropathy, particularly optic neuritis as a second subclinical lesion in multiple sclerosis. However, as other modalities, such as neuroimaging and automated perimetry, have improved, the need for electrophysiologic testing in neuro-ophthalmology has decreased (see chapter II).

Baker RS, Schmeisser ET, Epstein AD. Visual system electrodiagnosis in neurologic disease of childhood. *Pediatr Neurol.* 1995;12:99–110.

Fishman GA, Sokol S. *Electrophysiologic Testing in Disorders of the Retina, Optic Nerve, and Visual Pathway.* Ophthalmology Monograph 2. San Francisco: American Academy of Ophthlmology; 1990.

Gottlob I, Fendick MG, Guo S, et al. Visual acuity measurements by swept spatial frequency visual-evoked-cortical potentials (VECPs): clinical application in children with various visual disorders. *J Pediatr Ophthalmol Strabismus.* 1990;27:40–47.

Pattern Electroretinogram

The pattern electroretinogram (PERG) is the electrical potential measured from the retina in response to a reversing check or grating pattern. The PERG disappears as the ganglion cell layer in the retina degenerates in patients with an optic neuropathy and in experimental animals following section of the optic nerve. The flash ERG remains intact in the eye that is blind from an optic neuropathy. Unfortunately, the variability of the PERG has limited its clinical utility. PERG has been useful experimentally in assessing prognosis of acute optic neuropathies. Newer focal ERG techniques allow discrete areas of the macula, including the fovea, to be tested selectively. These techniques can be useful in differentiating optic nerve from macular disease.

Fishman GA, Sokol S. *Electrophysiologic Testing in Disorders of the Retina, Optic Nerve, and Visual Pathway.* Ophthalmology Monograph 2. San Francisco: American Academy of Ophthlmology; 1990.

Kaufman DI, Lorance RW, Woods M, et al. The pattern electroretinogram: a long-term study in acute optic neuropathy. *Neurology.* 1988;38:1767–1774.

Matthews GP, Sandberg MA, Berson EL. Foveal cone electroretinograms in patients with central visual loss of unexplained etiology. *Arch Ophthalmol.* 1992;110:1568–1570.

Visual Field Testing

Testing of the central and peripheral visual field is performed for the following three reasons:

□ To detect an abnormality in vision

□ To localize the defect along the afferent visual pathway

□ To quantitate the defect and measure change over time

Perimetry is thus useful in limiting the differential diagnosis and following the progression of disease. It evaluates another aspect of visual function and is complementary to assessments of Snellen acuity, color perception, and other aspects of vision.

Screening of the visual field by some method is essential in all patients with vision complaints. The clinician must select from various techniques depending on the purpose of the test and the attention span, health, and age of the patient. Each test has advantages and disadvantages discussed below.

The key questions in neurologic localization of visual field deficits are the following:

□ Is the problem in one eye, one visual field, or both?

□ If monocular, is the problem related primarily to the optic nerve?

Patients frequently report that they have lost vision in one eye when, in reality, they have lost vision in a homonymous field. Visual field testing will clarify this confusion. Visual field defects that respect the vertical midline, or meridian, are a result of disease at or posterior to the chiasm. Defects that stop abruptly at the horizontal meridian are generally caused by optic nerve rather than retinal disease. If bilateral, such altitudinal defects may be a result of occipital lobe disease. The answers that visual field testing can provide will considerably alter the differential diagnosis and guide further testing. Localization of field defects is covered in greater detail in chapter III.

TABLE I-1

PERIMETRIC TERMS

TERM	CHARACTERISTICS
Characteristics of the visual field defect	
Absolute	No stimulus perceived in the affected area
Relative	Bigger and brighter stimuli may be perceived in the affected field, but smaller, dimmer targets are not seen. The size and shape of the field defect, therefore, change inversely with changes in size and/or intensity of the presented stimulus. Defects may be described as shallow when only the smallest or dimmest targets fail to be identified or deep if bright objects are not detected in the central portion of the defect.
Terms describing visual field defects	
Scotoma	Area of depressed visual function surrounded by normal visual function (e.g., the blind spot)
Central	Involves fixation only
Cecocentral	Extends from fixation temporally to the blind spot
Paracentral	Involves a region next to, but not including, fixation
Pericentral	Involves a region symmetrically surrounding, but not involving, fixation
Arcuate	Corresponds to and represents nerve fiber bundle loss
Altitudinal	Involves two quadrants in either the superior or inferior field
Quadrantanopia	One quadrant of visual field involved
Hemianopia	One half of visual field involved, either nasal or temporal
Description of bilateral visual field defects with respect to spatial localization and extent	
Homonymous	Same side of visual space affected in each eye
Bitemporal	Opposite temporal sides of visual field space affected in each eye
Complete	Entire field affected
Incomplete	A portion of the field spared
Congruity	Tendency for homonymous field defect to be symmetrical (i.e., to have a similar size, location, and shape in each eye's field)

Common terms used to describe visual field defects appear in Table I-1. It is helpful to divide visual fields in each eye into four quadrants: superior temporal, superior nasal, inferior temporal, and inferior nasal. The vertical and horizontal meridians go through the central fixation point.

Samples of visual field results and their clinical correlates can be found throughout this volume. A detailed discussion of the interpretation of visual fields and the evolving field of automated perimetry is beyond the scope of this text, but it is an important topic in neuro-ophthalmology. The reader is strongly advised to review the Academy's monograph on visual fields or another textbook on the subject. BCSC Section 10, *Glaucoma,* also discusses visual fields in detail in chapter IV.

> Walsh TJ, ed. *Visual Fields: Examination and Interpretation.* Ophthalmology Monograph 3. 2nd ed. San Francisco: American Academy of Ophthalmology; 1996.

The following tests are all part of the repertoire commonly referred to as visual field testing.

Confrontation testing A variety of confrontation techniques can be useful. However, they all lack sensitivity and should be followed, when possible, with a more sensitive field test. Confrontation tests are very useful for training patients prior to more sophisticated testing and may enhance the productivity of other testing. A simple way to begin is to have the patient cover one eye with the palm of one hand (not the fingers as the patient might peek through the spaces) and look at the examiner's nose from a few feet away. Some examiners close their own eye opposite from the patient's covered eye and have the patient fixate instead on the examiner's remaining open eye; the field that the examiner can still see acts as a gross check of the patient's possible visual field. Ask if the patient, while fixating, can still see the examiner's eyes, ears, hair, chin, mouth, etc. This method can easily identify large scotomata and is useful in rapidly finding altitudinal hemifield loss.

The patient is then shown a moving hand in each quadrant of the field and asked if the moving hand is visible. With nonverbal patients, the examiner can note which quadrants elicit patient eye movements to fixate on the examiner's hand. The resulting field is described according to the quadrant in which the patient is able to detect hand movement (e.g., hand movement only inferonasally). The examiner can determine if the patient scans rather than fixates before moving on to other techniques.

Hand comparison, a form of subjective clarity comparison, can be performed with two hands, one placed in the nasal and one in the temporal hemifield. Similarly, comparison can be made between the hands located superiorly and inferiorly. The examiner presents both hands to the patient at the same time while one of the patient's eyes is covered. The patient is asked to identify the hand that appears "less clear." In this manner, a relative field defect can be detected.

Color comparison testing can be performed in a similar fashion while the patient occludes one eye. The examiner holds identical red objects in each hand (e.g., red-topped mydriatic bottles) and asks the patient if the red objects appear the same in each hand. Within a relative scotoma one object may appear washed out or as a color other than red. Normally, colors in the center are more intense than those in the periphery. Thus, a relative central scotoma may be detected by holding one red object in front of the examiner's nose and the other eccentrically. Patients with a central defect may see the eccentric object as more red. Illumination of the hands or colored objects must remain equal across the visual field when performing comparison testing.

Finger-count testing is similar to hand-motion testing except that the patient is asked to identify the number of fingers presented in each quadrant by the examiner. Use 1, 2, or 5 fingers; 3 or 4 fingers are not identified as reliably. Children can play a game of mimicking the examiner. If responses seem reliable at this point, the patient is then asked to add up the fingers of two hands presented in opposing quadrants (double simultaneous stimulation). The latter test may indicate a subtle visual field defect, extinction caused by disease in the parietal lobe near the optic radiations, or dyscalculia.

Kodsi SR, Younge BR. The four-meter confrontation visual field test. *Trans Am Ophthalmol Soc.* 1992;90:373–380.

Trobe JD, Acosta PC, Krischer JP, et al. Confrontation visual field techniques in the detection of anterior visual pathway lesions. *Ann Neurol.* 1981;10:28–34.

Amsler grid   Amsler grid testing is useful as a rapid screening suprathreshold test of the central 20° of the visual field (about 10° from fixation). The Amsler grid plate is held at 14 inches. The patient, optically corrected for near vision, covers one eye and looks at a fixation point in the center of a grid. The examiner asks the patient to describe any areas of metamorphopsia and uses the information to help distinguish optic nerve from macular disease. Ask the patient to describe any scotomata. It is important to watch the patient for scanning rather than fixating on the central point and to avoid suggesting a field defect during patient instruction. Cross-polarizing filters used to lower luminance may increase sensitivity, but sensitivity with Amsler grid testing is low and correlation with areas of pathology is variable. In spite of this, its simplicity makes it useful to some clinicians. Defects identified with the Amsler grid can be confirmed with other techniques.

Schuchard RA. Validity and interpretation of Amsler grid reports. *Arch Ophthalmol.* 1993;111:776–780.

Wall M, Sadun AA. Threshold Amsler grid testing. Cross-polarizing lenses enhance yield. *Arch Ophthalmol.* 1986;104:520–523.

Tangent screen   The tangent screen is an inexpensive method of evaluating the central visual field. It is most useful in guiding differential diagnosis by rapidly delineating the shape and location of defects. The tangent screen can identify scotomata too small to be measured by other perimetric devices. It can be used with patients who are poor candidates for more rigorous testing, such as those with short attention spans. It is easily used with patients in wheelchairs. Once a defect is identified with a tangent screen, other visual field techniques may be more appropriate for quantification and serial follow-up.

The patient gazes with one eye at a black screen 1–2 meters away in good lighting and fixes on a central spot. The examiner uses a thin black wand with various targets on the tip. Typically, these targets can be rotated to present either a white/colored surface of a specified size that can potentially be seen by the patient or a black surface not seen by the patient as it blends into the screen. The patient signals when the target is seen as it is moved about. A good examiner can rapidly identify scotomata smaller than the physiologic blind spot.

Fixation is difficult to enforce or measure, and the examiner must take care not to distract the patient from fixation. The examiner's arm and moving wand can tip off the patient. In areas without a tangent screen, an examiner can perform a variant of this test with a handheld laser pointer on the ceiling or wall.

Manual bowl perimetry   The Goldmann perimeter is useful for evaluating both the central and peripheral fields. Optical near correction is used for the central field testing. The perimeter can be used with a moving target (*kinetic perimetry*) or a stationary target (*static perimetry*).

In kinetic perimetry a target is chosen with fixed size and luminance. While the patient fixates centrally, the target is moved inward from the nonseeing periphery, and the patient signals when it is seen. The entire periphery is probed in discrete locations defining an *isopter,* the outer limit of visibility of a particular target. The examiner tests points within the isopter statically, by transiently displaying the target and verifying that it can be seen as expected. Inability to see the target indicates a scotoma or island of relatively poorer vision within the isopter. The kinetic target is then moved outward from the scotoma until it can again be identified, and the boundaries are plotted.

Varying the size and luminance of the target creates differing isopters. This method helps differentiate *relative* defects, in which larger, brighter targets are seen, from *absolute* defects, in which no target can be perceived. By serially following the smallest size and dimmest luminance of targets identified within a scotoma or the relative size of peripheral isopters, progression or regression of visual loss can be monitored over time.

In the hands of an experienced perimetrist, manual field machines can be used for rapid, sensitive, reproducible evaluations of the visual field for diagnosis or disease follow-up. Goldmann perimetry also has the advantage of allowing the perimetrist to observe the patient's fixation and fatigue level and to adjust the test accordingly. However, a perimetrist's skill and bias can have a large effect on test accuracy.

Anderson DR. *Testing the Field of Vision.* St Louis: Mosby; 1982.

Automated bowl perimetry Automated perimetry has become the standard method of evaluating the visual field. Reasons for this include the following:

- Difficulty in finding trained perimetrists
- Improved standardization that allows better serial and interinstitutional comparisons of fields
- Improved sensitivity
- Statistical evaluation of the data in an individual field and comparisons of serial fields
- More efficient management of patient data
- Electronic data storage and transmission
- Low cost of operation, although the machine itself is costly

Automated perimeters usually perform static perimetry, although kinetic models are available. Most devices display a series of targets in multiple, predetermined locations to identify the *threshold of vision.* Threshold is commonly defined as the dimmest target identified 50% of the time at a given location. This reading is compared to age-related norms and to the same patient's perception over time. To increase test reliability, the automated perimeter varies the location and luminance of the targets, so they seem randomly presented to the patient.

The machine tests only a limited number of discrete points, and a gray-scale depiction of the field can be derived by interpolating between the measured regions. The machine also displays the actual level of luminance identified and a comparison with normal values. It can perform a point-by-point comparison with previous fields and statistically evaluate whether change has occurred. Patient test reliability is assessed by identifying the following:

- False positive response rate: how frequently the patient signals when no light is displayed

- False negative response rate: how often the patient fails to signal when a target much brighter than the known threshold for that spot is displayed

- Loss of fixation: how often the patient signals when a target is displayed within the physiologic blind spot

It is important to review these and other reliability measures when interpreting a visual field.

Automated perimeters can be programmed to provide rapid screening examinations, to perform more detailed threshold evaluations, or to concentrate efforts within selected areas of the field. Screening studies are of limited utility in diagnosis and serial follow-up; threshold perimetry is the standard used in neuro-ophthalmology. Software is available to help guide interpretation (at least with glaucoma patients). Compared to manual perimeters, however, these machines are less forgiving of patients with shorter attention spans or slow reaction times, and they can therefore be less useful in some neuro-ophthalmic settings.

Anderson DR. *Automated Static Perimetry.* St Louis: Mosby–Year Book; 1992.

Newman SA. Automated perimetry in neuro-ophthalmology. In: *Focal Points: Clinical Modules for Ophthalmologists.* San Francisco: American Academy of Ophthalmology; 1995;13:6.

Techniques of Pupil Examination

In dim light ask the patient to fixate on a distant accommodative target. With a handheld *bright* light (e.g., halogen direct or indirect ophthalmoscope), diffusely illuminate the pupils from below. Note the size (mm), shape (round, peaked, etc.), and position (central, eccentric) of each pupil. If *anisocoria,* a difference in pupillary size, is noted, examine the pupils in brighter light. Ascertain if the degree of anisocoria is accentuated in light, indicating parasympathetic paresis, or in darkness, indicating sympathetic paresis. At the slit lamp, determine if synechiae, sphincter rupture, abnormal segmental movements, or iris atrophy are present.

Evaluate the reactivity of each pupil to direct light. Descriptions can be verbal (e.g., sluggish, brisk) or numerical (e.g., 2 out of 4). Check the *rate* of dilation as well; dilation lag can be a sign of sympathetic nerve dysfunction. In addition to light reactivity, assess the reaction to a near accommodative target.

The swinging-light test can detect a *relative afferent pupillary defect* (RAPD). RAPD, commonly known as a *Marcus Gunn pupil,* is objective evidence of asymmetric optic nerve conduction. In a dimly lit room, have the patient fixate on a distant accommodative target. Shine a bright light into one pupil from below. Briskly and rhythmically swing the light from one eye to the other. In normal eyes both optic nerves transmit the same afferent information regarding the light intensity. As both pupils are already constricted (direct and consensual response) from the light entering the first eye, there is either no pupil movement or a similar degree of constriction as the light is moved to the second eye. After initial illumination of either eye, some pupillary movement may occur (physiologic pupillary unrest).

In the case of unequal optic nerve conduction, however, the pupils will paradoxically dilate each time the light is swung to the affected side, which is transmitting less light information to the Edinger-Westphal nucleus than the previously established consensual baseline. Conversely, the pupils will constrict when the light is moved to the unaffected eye as a result of the transmission of more light information. Minimal cases may display only slower constriction or faster dilation on one side when the light is swung. See Figures IV-3, IV-4, and IV-5 on pp 101–103. Chapter IV discusses the pupils in detail.

The degree of an RAPD may be roughly quantitated with various scales such as "marked" or 2+, or it may be more precisely measured with neutral-density filters. Various filters placed in front of the normal eye reduce the amount of light it can perceive, until it is equal to the unfiltered light level of the affected eye. As the density of the filters is increased, the RAPD will gradually diminish until it is observed in the other eye.

The presence of an RAPD is an extremely reliable and sensitive indicator of asymmetric optic nerve function. The lack of an expected RAPD should cause reevaluation of a working diagnosis of optic neuropathy. An RAPD is not seen with symmetric optic nerve disease or with dysfunction posterior to the lateral geniculate bodies. Any disease that markedly reduces the conduction of light information to the Edinger-Westphal nucleus can result in a Marcus Gunn pupil. An RAPD can occur with extensive, asymmetric macular disease or large retinal detachments involving the papillomacular bundle. Optic tract lesions result in mild RAPDs contralaterally (i.e., in the eye with the temporal field loss), as a majority of nerve fibers have already crossed in the chiasm. With extremely rare exceptions, a Marcus Gunn pupil is *not* found with media opacities such as cataract or vitreous hemorrhage.

Monocular blindness unaccompanied by damage to the pupil does not cause anisocoria. Although a pupil in a blind eye fails to react to direct light, it will constrict consensually when the normal contralateral eye is stimulated. Therefore, the pupil on the amaurotic side will not be larger than on the normal side. However, the swinging flashlight test can still demonstrate an RAPD in the blind eye.

The finding of an RAPD in a patient with known or suspected amblyopia should be approached with caution. A minimal RAPD seen in this setting may represent subtle optic nerve hypoplasia or retinal ganglion cell damage that is underlying the amblyopia. Other neuro-ophthalmic evaluations, such as ophthalmoscopy and perimetry, are appropriate to confirm that the RAPD is a result of amblyopia and not another, potentially treatable, condition. Follow-up evaluation should be performed to assess any increase in the RAPD or development of other signs and symptoms.

Bell RA, Waggoner PM, Boyd WM, et al. Clinical grading of relative afferent pupillary defects. *Arch Ophthalmol.* 1993;111:938–942.

Thompson HS, Montague P, Cox TA, et al. The relationship between visual acuity, pupillary defect, and visual field loss. *Am J Ophthalmol.* 1982;93:681–688.

Ocular Motility

Begin the examination of a patient with ocular motility dysfunction such as binocular diplopia by watching the patient during the history. Does the patient adopt a head tilt or face turn? Does the patient close one eye? Are such findings present in old photographs? A patient may be unaware of, or may deny, a long-standing head tilt.

Is head bobbing present? Do sudden head movements accompany shifts in fixation? Test each eye's ability to fixate on a target and record the fixation as central and maintained, unsteady, or wandering.

Eye Movements

Eye movements are covered extensively in BCSC Section 6, *Pediatric Ophthalmology and Strabismus.* See also chapter V for a detailed discussion of the anatomy and physiology of the ocular motor system and ocular motility.

Test *ductions* (monocular eye movements) by having the patient look with the uncovered eye in various directions on command (*saccades*) and by having the patient follow an object being moved by the examiner (*smooth pursuit*). Testing ductions before measuring misalignment with prisms will frequently reveal the involved muscle or muscles. Grade dysfunction from 1+ to 4+ underaction, by percentage of normal, or in degrees using a kinetic perimeter.

Versions are binocular eye movements. The two eyes move in the same direction with conjugate versions (e.g., to the right in dextroversion) or in opposite directions with disconjugate versions (e.g., both eyes moving toward the nose with convergence). When testing versions, look for relative overaction, unusual shooting movements, or eyelid fissure changes in certain gaze positions.

Test convergence, especially in the presence of pupillary abnormalities that may signify a periaqueductal syndrome or with complaints of headache or reading difficulty. Convergence should be specifically assessed when internuclear ophthalmoplegia is suspected.

When a patient cannot voluntarily move his or her eyes into a desired position, the examiner should attempt to move the eyes using the oculocephalic reflex (doll's head phenomenon) or caloric testing. Oculocephalic testing uses the vestibular system to drive the eyes in a particular direction. If the eyes move into the paretic field of gaze with these tests, the lesion is probably supranuclear in nature (i.e., the neurologic wiring from the cranial nerve nucleus to the muscle is probably intact). Thus, a patient with progressive supranuclear palsy may be unable to look up or down with saccades or pursuit but may have full versions with the head rotation accompanying flexion and extension of the neck. Failure of an oculocephalic maneuver to drive the eyes into a selected position does not necessarily indicate an infranuclear paresis, however. Restrictive disease must be excluded with forced duction testing, which is discussed on pp 28–30.

To perform an oculocephalic test on a conscious person, have the patient fixate on an object while rotating the head horizontally and vertically. If the patient continues to fixate, the eyes will move in the direction opposite to the head movement. This maneuver usually suffices for vestibular stimulation in the ophthalmologist's office, precluding the need for caloric testing. A full discussion of caloric nystagmus is beyond the scope of this book.

> Berger JR. Clinical approach to stupor and coma. In: Bradley WG, Daroff RB, Fenichel GM, et al, eds. *Neurology in Clinical Practice.* Boston: Butterworth-Heinemann; 1996:51–53.

Bell's phenomenon is the upward turning of the eyes with the closure of the eyelids. It is assessed by having the patient close the eyelids tightly. While forcing separation of the eyelids, note if the eyes are upturned. Eyes that rotate up would suggest a supranuclear lesion rather than other causes of upgaze paresis, as would normal vertical doll's head responses. Bell's phenomenon is an important finding in patients with seventh (facial) nerve palsies, as it suggests that their corneas will be partially protected when eyelid closure is inadequate.

Testing of optokinetic nystagmus (OKN) can be helpful in evaluating saccades and localizing cerebral lesions. An OKN drum of alternating stripes or a tape of alternating 2-inch colored squares provides the stimulus. Pass the targets right, left, up, and down to elicit optokinetic nystagmus. The patient's eyes will pursue the moving target, then rapidly saccade back, to fixate on the next moving target in sequence. OKN testing is useful in the following clinical settings:

☐ Evaluation of internuclear ophthalmoplegia by exaggerating slowed adduction using an OKN target moving toward the side of the medial longitudinal fasciculus lesion

☐ Congenital nystagmus showing an OKN response in the opposite of the expected direction

☐ Evaluation of dorsal midbrain syndrome using downward-moving OKN targets to bring on convergence-retraction nystagmus

☐ Testing of functional visual loss by eliciting normal responses despite the subjective loss of vision

Diplopia

Binocular diplopia can be characterized accurately with prism cover or Maddox rod testing in the nine standard gaze positions and with head tilt. This testing helps identify whether the strabismus is comitant and quantitates the degree of deviation in different directions of gaze. This information helps the examiner formulate the differential diagnosis of strabismus and can also create a baseline for judging change over time.

Alternate prism cover testing is performed by having the patient fixate on an accommodative target. A cover is alternated from one eye to the other, and refixation eye movements are noted as the cover is moved. Vertical and horizontal prisms are placed in front of one or both eyes until refixation movements stop when the cover is alternated. This test can be repeated in each of the nine diagnostic gaze positions as well as with head tilt.

A Maddox rod can be used in a similar fashion. Place a red Maddox rod in front of one eye with the cylinders in the same direction as the deviation to be measured (e.g., cylinders horizontal to measure horizontal deviation). Have the patient fixate on a white light with the opposite eye. If horizontal binocular diplopia is present, the patient will see a white light separate from a vertical red line. Place loose prisms or a prism bar in front of the fixating eye until the white light is superimposed on the red line created by the Maddox rod. Once the horizontal deviation is measured, it can be corrected by a prism placed in the trial frame. Rotate the Maddox rod 90° and measure vertical deviations in the same fashion.

Vector, or oblique, prism measurements can determine the net deviation in any gaze position faster than separate vertical and horizontal prism readings. Vector measurements are useful for both diagnosis and treatment with prism glasses or Fresnel adhesive prisms. Put the patient's corrective lenses in the back of a trial frame. Place a red Maddox rod lens with axis marker in the rotating portion of the trial frame over the eye with poorer visual acuity. The patient fixates on a distant or near white target and sees a white light separated from a red line. The patient or the examiner rotates the Maddox rod until the red line passes through the white light. Rotate the Maddox rod 90° and the axis marker will show the prism correction axis. Using loose prisms or a prism bar, place a prism over the Maddox rod aligned with the axis marker. Ask the patient if placing this prism moved the light closer to the red line; if the light is farther away, rotate the loose prism or bar 180°. Change prism power until the white light is superimposed on the red line. This result is the power, base orientation, and axis for correcting the deviation.

Measuring a field of binocular single vision is a fast, but less precise, method of serially following the progress of a patient with diplopia. Seat the patient with both eyes open at a kinetic bowl perimeter and set the chin rest in the midposition horizontally. Display a large (e.g., III-4e) target in a region of single vision. Move the target out in all directions and mark the field as soon as the patient notes diplopia. The normal shape of the field of binocular single vision is an inverted triangle. With a deficit such as a sixth nerve palsy, one horizontal half of the field will be truncated as diplopia occurs in gaze to the affected side (Fig I-2). In patients with normal retinal correspondence, other alternatives for serial measurement include the Hess-Lees screen and Lancaster red-green tests.

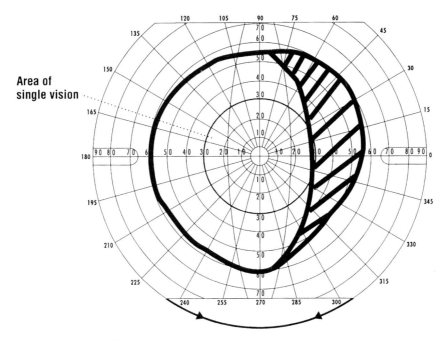

FIG I-2—A field of binocular single vision in a patient with a right sixth nerve palsy. Note the area of diplopia in right gaze (right side of field) and single vision in left gaze. The shaded region signifies diplopia. This qualitative plot can be scored for subsequent comparison.

Paralytic strabismus   Red-glass testing may provide sufficient information for diagnosis in less time than detailed prism measurements. Place the red glass over the
patient's right eye and turn on the white light. Ask the patient to point to the two
lights and determine from the response if the diplopia is horizontal, vertical, or
oblique. Have the patient look at the red image and show, using both hands, the
distance between the two images. Repeat the process by moving the red filter in front
of the left eye or asking the patient to fixate on the white image instead of the red
one. The deviation is larger when the patient fixates with the paretic eye. With time,
this sign disappears.

Suspected paresis of one muscle can be confirmed by analysis of the position
of the two images seen with a red filter over one eye. For example, in a horizontal
deviation, the patient is either esotropic or exotropic. With a red glass over the
patient's right eye, ask if the red light is on the right side of the white light. A yes
answer means the patient is esotropic (uncrossed diplopia) and a no answer
indicates exotropia. In paralytic esotropes, either the right or the left lateral rectus
muscle is weak; and in paralytic exotropes, one of the medial rectus muscles is
weak. Move the fixation target to the right and left side. The lights will be farthest
apart in the field of action of the paretic muscle. There may be single binocular
vision in gaze away from the paretic field.

Cyclovertical deviations can be localized using a three-step test to determine
maximal deviation in horizontal, vertical, and oblique gaze and with right and left
head tilt (Fig I-3). Although useful in confirming a fourth nerve palsy, this test is inac-
curate when a single muscle paresis is not the correct diagnosis, as in the case of
restrictive myopathies or multiple nerve involvement.

Patients suspected of cyclovertical deviations should undergo double Maddox
rod testing for torsional deviation. Place red and white Maddox rod lenses in a trial
frame and ask the patient to adjust them until the lines are parallel. The torsional
deviation can be read off the lens axis marker on the trial frame. If the patient has
difficulty in distinguishing both the white and red lines, insert a 4.0 D base-down
prism over one eye to separate the lines for easier viewing.

Nonparalytic strabismus   The tests described above can fail to identify isolated
muscle dysfunction causing diplopia for a number of reasons. First, cranial nerve
III (oculomotor), whose subnuclei control several muscles, may be partially or
completely involved. Second, multiple ocular motor nerves may be variably affected. Third, compensatory changes in affected and antagonist muscles may occur
over time, resulting in a misleading pattern of eye movements. Fourth, diplopia may
result from generalized disease of the muscles or neuromuscular junction. Finally,
diplopia may be restrictive (e.g., the infiltrative myopathy in Graves disease) rather
than paralytic.

The *forced duction test* is essential to differentiate a neurogenic ocular motility
imbalance from a restrictive disorder such as muscle entrapment or thyroid ophthalmopathy. One of the various techniques for performing this test involves placing a
cotton-tipped applicator at the limbus of an anesthetized eye and pushing the eye
into the field of limited duction. Alternatively, the examiner can soak a cotton-tipped
applicator in topical anesthetic and hold it near the limbus for approximately 1
minute. Using fine-toothed forceps, the examiner grasps the conjunctiva and Tenon's
capsule near the limbus, where they form a tight adhesion, and moves the eye in the
direction of paretic gaze. Some clinicians prefer to grasp the muscle insertion rather

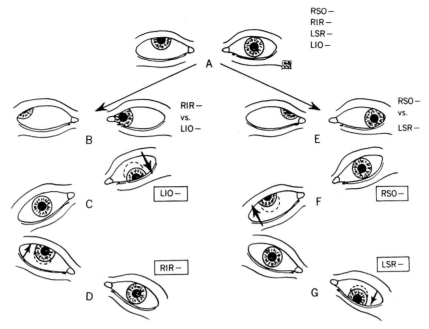

RSO –
RIR –
LSR –
LIO –

A

RIR –
vs.
LIO –

B

LIO –

C

RIR –

D

E

RSO –
vs.
LSR –

RSO –

F

LSR –

G

FIG I-3—Demonstration of the three-step test. *A,* Patient has a right hypertropia. One of the following four muscles is paretic: right superior oblique (RSO), right inferior rectus (RIR), left superior rectus (LSR), or left inferior oblique (LIO). *B,* The hypertropia increases in right gaze, implicating either the RIR or LIO. *C,* If the LIO is the paretic muscle, the vertical deviation will increase on head tilt right. *D,* If the RIR is the paretic muscle, the hypertropia increases on head tilt left, when the right eye must extort. *E,* If the hyperdeviation increases in left gaze, then either the RSO or the LSR must be paretic. *F,* Paretic RSO with hyperdeviation increasing on right head tilt. *G,* Paretic LSR with hyperdeviation increasing on left head tilt. Note that after the second step either two intorters or two extorters are isolate. If this is not the case, examiner returns to step one and reevaluates. (Reproduced with permission from von Noorden GK. *Atlas of Strabismus.* 4th ed. St Louis: Mosby–Year Book; 1983:149.)

than the limbus (Fig I-4). This procedure requires a strong topical anesthetic, such as 10% cocaine or 4% Xylocaine, whereas the other techniques can be performed with proparacaine hydrochloride.

If the ocular rotation is easily performed by the examiner, the defect is likely neurogenic; if resistance is met, the problem is probably restrictive or mechanical. However, anatomic changes may occur with long-standing neurogenic paresis, leading to ipsilateral antagonist contracture and thus resulting in a positive forced duction test.

An active *force generation test* is used clinically to make a qualitative judgment of muscle force. Anesthetize the eye as described in the forced duction test. Grasp the limbus and ask the patient to look in the direction of paretic gaze. The examiner can sense the amount of force generated by the tested muscle and determine whether normal forces are being generated against a mechanical restriction. In cases

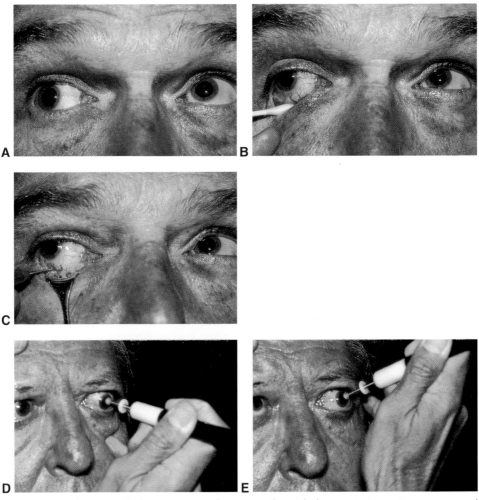

FIG I-4—*A*, This patient had an incomitant deviation with a right hypotropia increasing on attempted upgaze. *B*, 4% Xylocaine was applied to the eye in drop form and then with a cotton tip held over the muscle for 1–2 minutes. *C*, The eye is then grasped. Grasping may be at the limbus, although it is better done at the insertion of the presumed restricted muscle. The patient is instructed to look in the direction of maximal deviation, and an attempt is made to manually rotate the globe in that direction, taking care not to press the eye into the orbit. *D-E*, Alternatively, pneumotonometry or handheld applanation tensions may be taken in primary position and with the patient looking into eccentric gaze. Elevation of more than 4 mm Hg suggests restriction of the opposite muscle. Although less accurate, a Goldmann applanator can be used in a similar fashion at a slit lamp.

of neurogenic paresis, the test allows a qualitative estimate of the degree of paresis. Testing the same muscle in the opposite eye offers the examiner a comparison.

Feibel RM, Roper-Hall G. Evaluation of the field of binocular single vision in incomitant strabismus. *Am J Ophthalmol.* 1974;78:800–805.

Kushner BJ. Errors in the three-step test in the diagnosis of vertical strabismus. *Ophthalmology.* 1989;96:127–132.

Moradiellos DP, Parrish DE. A clinical technique for correcting diplopia with prism. *J Amer Optom Assoc.* 1986;57:740–743.

Spector RH. Vertical diplopia. *Surv Ophthalmol.* 1993;38:31–62.

Sullivan TJ, Kraft SP, Burack C, et al. A functional scoring method for the field of binocular single vision. *Ophthalmology.* 1992;99:575–581.

Ocular Sensation

Cranial nerve V, the trigeminal nerve, carries sensory information from the eye and face. A cotton wisp, typically a cotton applicator tip twisted to a fine point, can be used to test corneal as well as facial sensation. Corneal sensation must be checked prior to instillation of topical anesthetics used for applanation tonometry or forced duction testing. It should be tested in patients with the following:

☐ Paresthesias involving the face

☐ Unexplained keratitis

☐ Dysfunction of any of the cranial nerves

☐ Other signs of parasellar, cavernous sinus, or orbital disease

The cornea should not be touched if pharmacologic agents are to be applied topically as part of a work-up for anisocoria.

All three branches of cranial nerve V should be tested and motor function assessed. The patient's jaw should open and close in the midline, and the pterygoid muscle should move the jaw to the opposite side. The masseter muscles should be palpated during facial jaw closure. Fifth nerve damage may occasionally result in hearing defects (tensor tympani dysfunction).

Eyelid Function and Facial Movement

Observation of the eyelids can be helpful in identifying the nature and cause of an ocular motor problem. Examination of the eyelids begins with observation of their general shape and appearance (an S shape may indicate neurofibromatosis), blink rate (low in Parkinson disease and high in blepharospasm), and abnormal movements (synkinesis with other facial muscles). Measure the opening of the palpebral fissure in primary position (adult normal is 9–12 mm with the upper eyelid covering 1 mm of the limbus and the lower eyelid just touching it). Verify that unilateral ptosis is not an artifact of vertical strabismus. The eyelids should be everted to rule out a local cause of ptosis such as a retained contact lens or giant papillary conjunctivitis. If the ptosis is asymmetric, and especially if the higher eyelid appears retracted, lift the ptotic eyelid manually and see if the higher eyelid drops to a new position.

The examiner evaluates the functional ability of the levator by measuring the total excursion of the eyelid margin, from downgaze to upgaze, while firmly pressing on the patient's eyebrow to prevent frontalis action. Normal upper eyelid excursion is 12–16 mm. Watch the eyelid during target pursuit from up- to downgaze. Normally this motion is smoothly accomplished, but the eyelid may hang up or move downward with jerky movements in thyroid disease or as a result of aberrant third nerve regeneration (lid lag).

In cases of suspected fatigable ptosis caused by myasthenia gravis, look for progressive ptosis by having the patient fixate on the examiner's hand elevated to provoke extreme upgaze; the patient should be able to hold this position without sinking of the eyelid for about 1 minute (the time for the examiner to start to feel fatigue!). Test for an eyelid twitch sign by having the patient fixate in downgaze for a few seconds, then rapidly refixate straight ahead. Look for overshoot upward of the eyelid and fluttering while it settles into position.

Evaluation of facial motor function includes assessment of orbicularis oculi and other facial muscle strength. Reinnervation phenomena such as synkinesis with eyelid closure and facial tics may be signs of a previous seventh nerve injury.

Assessment of the Orbit

Patients suspected of having orbital disease or arteriovenous shunting in the region of the cavernous sinus should be examined for the following:

□ Degree of proptosis

□ Orientation of the globe

□ Presence of a bruit

□ Arteriolization of the conjunctival and scleral veins

□ Signs of congestion or infiltration of orbital tissue

□ Effects of head position and Valsalva maneuver on the proptosis

An abnormally elevated pulse pressure can be identified by noting the pulsation of the mires during applanation tonometry or measured with a pneumotonometer tracing. The amount of resistance to manual retropulsion of the globe can be compared to the patient's contralateral orbit or to the examiner's own. Proptosis can be measured for serial comparison with an exophthalmometer. It may be helpful to compare the patient's current appearance with old photographs.

Verifying Functional Visual Loss

Some patients complain of monocularly decreased vision when examination reveals no relative afferent pupillary defect, normal retina and optic nerve appearance, equal or near equal retinoscopic findings, and the absence of a heterotropia. Consider functional visual loss in these cases. To justify this diagnosis the examiner must demonstrate that the patient has better vision than the subjective responses indicate. This usually requires tricking the patient.

Patients suspected of functional visual loss are often difficult to examine because of defensive and uncooperative behavior. Typically, they have already had multiple examinations. The examiner must be patient, persistent, and facile with the tests being used, so that the patient remains unaware of the examiner's goal: demonstrating better sight than claimed. This type of examination may require a certain amount of showmanship! One or more of the tests described below might be used depending on the clinical circumstances. For example, if a patient complains of monocular loss of vision, the examiner might use a test based on confusion of the two eyes so the patient is not sure which eye is being tested. Of course, if these tests fail to demonstrate better vision, the clinician should reconsider the diagnosis of functional disease. In addition to decreased vision, other neuro-ophthalmic complaints such as diplopia, lost peripheral vision, or periocular pain may be functional as well. It is important to remember that patients with a functional component to their presentation may have an underlying physical disease.

"Bottom-up" Acuity

The examination begins with acuity determination at the smallest line of the Snellen chart (i.e., 20/10). If the patient cannot see these letters, the examiner announces the use of a "larger line" and then uses the 20/15 line and several different 20/20 lines. The examiner continually expresses disbelief that such "large" letters cannot be identified. If the patient still denies being able to read the letters, he or she is asked to determine the number of characters present and whether they are round, square, etc. Once the count is established, the examiner might suggest that the characters are letters and that the first one is easier to identify than the others. By the time the "very large letters" (i.e., 20/50) are reached, the patient often can be cajoled into reading optotypes much smaller than those read on initial acuity testing. The examiner might have the patient wear trial frames with four lenses equaling the correct prescription and suggest that these are special magnifying lenses that might permit improved vision.

Deception of the Eye Tested

Using a phoropter or trial frame, announce that the "good" eye is to be tested, although neither eye is occluded. As the patient slowly reads down the Snellen chart, progressively fog the "good" eye without the patient's knowledge. The "bad" eye is then occluded, and the vision is tested in the "good" eye with the previously used fogging lens in place. If the patient cannot read better than 20/200 with the fogged unaffected eye but had done so with both eyes unoccluded, it becomes obvious that the smaller optotypes were read with the "bad" eye. This finding indicates that the visual loss is functional.

One method of fogging is to gradually introduce plus-power sphere, using a phoropter, in front of the "good" eye. Another method is to place high-power (2.00–6.00 D) cylinders of opposite sign at the same axis (net power: zero) in the trial frame. As the patient reads binocularly, the axis of one of the cylinders is gradually changed, thus fogging the "good" eye.

Red-green glasses used with the duochrome filter of the projection chart allow monocular acuity testing with both eyes open. The letters in the red zone are seen with the eye behind the red lens, those in the green zone with the eye behind the green lens. Since the green filter is more efficient, it is placed before the better eye.

A special testing set, Binocular Integrated Multicolored Vision Assessment Test (BIMVAT), is available for this purpose. It consists of red and blue filters to be fitted over the patient's near correction in trial frames and a test booklet of variously sized letters made up of orange, brown, and blue components. The orange components are seen through the blue filter but not the red filter. Some of the test letters are constructed so that they could be read as two different letters (e.g., either *P* or *R*) depending on whether all of the components are seen. The blue filter is placed over the "blind" eye. Any letter with all orange components then read correctly was read with the "blind" eye through the blue filter. Based on the decreasing size of the letters, a visual acuity may be determined.

Although the BIMVAT is similar to the distance duochrome test in theory, it makes it more difficult for the patient to deceive the examiner because the test letters are mixed by eye and the letters visualized change depending on whether they are seen with one or both eyes. In contrast, the letters in the duochrome test are seen by one eye only and segregated by side of the eye chart.

Stereoscopic vision requires binocularity. A nomogram has been created that correlates stereoacuity with the necessary visual acuity of each eye. Vectographs viewed with polarizing lenses allow each eye to be tested separately with neither eye occluded. Also useful is the Titmus stereoacuity test with stereoscopic circles, which requires good near acuity in each eye to identify the smallest circles. Presbyopic patients being tested must have near correction.

The examiner can also quantitate the visual acuity in the "bad" eye by using the prism dissociation test. Place a small vertical prism in front of one eye and ask the patient to compare the clarity of the two lines seen; watch carefully that the patient does not close one eye. It may be helpful to place the prism in front of the "good" eye while suggesting that the upper and lower vision of the "good" eye is being tested. The minimum target size when both lines can be read indicates the true acuity of the "bad" eye.

"Complete Blindness"

Testing a patient complaining of monocular blindness is somewhat different from and, in most instances, easier than testing a patient claiming partial loss of vision. The examiner must show only that some vision persists in a "blind" eye to document a functional component to the visual loss. In addition to the tests described above, the following are helpful.

Optokinetic testing Targets can be used to test each eye for vision separately. The production of optokinetic nystagmus in a "blind" eye is evidence that the eye has useful sight.

Place a large mirror before the "blind" eye while its fellow eye is occluded. Rocking the mirror horizontally and then vertically will cause the patient's entire visible environment to tilt. If vision is present, the eye will move. Introduce a prism before the "blind" eye while the patient is reading binocularly. If removal of the prism causes a refixational movement of the eyes, binocularity has been demonstrated.

Color-blind testing Ask if the patient was born color-blind. If the answer is no, offhandedly occlude the "good" eye and ask the patient to read a color plate book. Surprisingly, this trick can work if carried off well!

Nonvisual tests The following additional tests do not establish vision, but they can help the clinician confirm a suspicion of functional disease. Have the patient sign his or her name. Truly blind patients do so with little difficulty. Test proprioception by having the patient use an index finger to touch the nose or other index finger. The patient with functional disease may mistake this for a visual task and be unable to perform it.

Electrophysiologic testing The diagnosis of functional visual loss can be established clinically in most patients who claim their loss is severe. However, electrophysiologic studies (electroretinogram and VECP) may be used to confirm that the retinal-cortical pathway is generally intact in patients suspected of feigning severe loss. These tests, although occasionally helpful, can have both false positive and false negative results in this setting. Failure to document good visual function after several attempts should cause reevaluation of the diagnosis.

Visual field testing Visual field testing is helpful, since nonphysiologic perimetric responses are often present. A spiral, or tunnel, visual field on perimetry is a classic example (Fig I-5). A tangent screen isopter that fails to expand when tested at increasing distances (e.g., smaller at 2 meters than at 1 meter) along with inconsistencies throughout the visual field are also typical. Both manual kinetic and automated static perimeters can be easily "fooled" by a patient feigning vision loss. A high index of suspicion is needed when a field defect does not correspond to other clinical findings. Monocular hemianopia may be revealed as functional when the defect persists during a binocular field test.

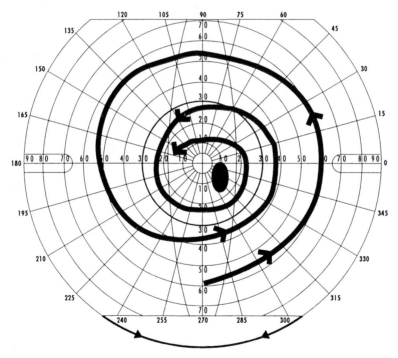

FIG I-5—A spiral field from a patient with functional visual field loss. As the test continues, the isopter continues to shrink. Sometimes this result can be reduced by testing with the target moving outward instead of inward.

Donzis PB, Rappazzo JA, Burde RM, et al. Effect of binocular variations of Snellen's visual acuity on Titmus stereoacuity. *Arch Ophthalmol.* 1983;101:930–932.

Gittinger JW Jr. Functional hemianopsia: A historical perspective. *Surv Ophthalmol.* 1988;32:427–432.

Keane JR. Neuro-ophthalmic signs and symptoms of hysteria. *Neurology.* 1982;32: 757–762.

Kramer KK, La Piana FC, Appleton B. Ocular malingering and hysteria: diagnosis and management. *Surv Ophthalmol.* 1979;24:89–96.

Slavin ML. Functional visual loss. In: *Focal Points: Clinical Modules for Ophthalmologists.* San Francisco: American Academy of Ophthalmology; 1991;9:2.

Slavin ML. The prism dissociation test in detecting unilateral functional visual loss. *J Clin Neuroophthalmol.* 1990;10:127–130.

Thompson HS. Functional visual loss. *Am J Ophthalmol.* 1985;100:209–213.

Thompson JC, Kosmorsky GS, Ellis BD. Fields of dreamers and dreamed-up fields: functional and fake perimetry. *Ophthalmology.* 1996;103:117–125.

Conclusion

A complete neuro-ophthalmic history and examination can be time-consuming, but it need not be. The history frequently provides the strongest guide to the diagnosis. Decide which components of the physical examination techniques described are appropriate for each patient and plan ahead during the examination, as the order of the tests might be important (e.g., pharmacologic testing of anisocoric pupils should be performed before applanation tonometry). It may not be possible to do all tests desired during one visit; the clinician must select the most applicable subset of available tests based on the differential diagnosis and other constraints such as time. Table I-2 provides a useful checklist. *It is unlikely that all of these tests would be necessary in any one examination.*

TABLE I-2

NEURO-OPHTHALMIC HISTORY AND EXAMINATION

History

Chief Complaint
Present Illness
Past Medical and Ophthalmologic History
Family History
Social History
Systems Review

Physical Examination

Observation of the patient for clues during the history
Visual function testing
      Visual acuity
      Color vision
      Contrast sensitivity
      Brightness comparison
      Color (red) desaturation
      Stereoacuity
      Photostress test
      Perimetry
            Confrontation fields
            Amsler grid
            Tangent screen
            Static or kinetic manual fields
            Automated threshold fields
Eyelid position and function
Pupil evaluation
      Appearance
      Reactivity to a light source
      Reactivity to a near target
      Relative afferent pupillary defect
Alignment and motility
      Ductions and versions
      Saccades and pursuit
      Convergence
      Prism measurements
      Maddox rod testing
      Forced duction testing
Nystagmus and fixation evaluation
Facial, trigeminal, and other nerve testing
Slit-lamp evaluation
Tonometry
Fundus examination
Imaging, laboratory tests, and other special exams

CHAPTER II

Neuroimaging in Neuro-Ophthalmology

Neuro-Ophthalmic Indications

Imaging studies complement the patient history and physical examination. Neuro-ophthalmic indications for ordering neuroradiologic tests include the diagnosis and follow-up of

- Unexplained or progressive proptosis
- Acquired visual loss of uncertain etiology
- Cranial neuropathies
- Papilledema
- Supranuclear eye movement disorders
- Acquired nystagmus
- Intracranial vascular anomalies, mass lesions, demyelinating lesions, or other abnormalities thought to be related to systemic disease with intracranial involvement such as sarcoidosis

In order to promote cost-efficient resource use, the ophthalmologist should select the most appropriate test based on the differential diagnosis, rather than ordering a general scan of the orbit or head. Discussing the case with the radiologist is helpful in selecting imaging techniques that will answer specific clinical questions best. Viewing films with the radiologist, particularly when the radiologist's interpretation differs from the clinical expectations, can help the clinician identify many subtle findings or "normal variants" that correlate with clinical findings. It is crucial to verify that a "negative" scan has adequately imaged the region of expected pathology. Frequently, scans ordered for optic nerve disease fully image the brain but have only one or two relevant views at the optic nerve level and may not be formatted for maximum sensitivity of disease detection in that region (e.g., using contrast material or suppressing the signal of orbital fat).

Computed Tomography

Computed tomography (CT) was the first radiographic imaging technique able to create views of the soft tissues of the brain in cross section (Fig II-1). The patient is moved through a circular structure with an x-ray emitter located across from a detector. In any position the x-ray beam is attenuated by the density of the intervening target tissue. The emitter is rotated 180°, and the computer reconstructs an image by calculating the density of the target from the collected set of attenuation values. A gray-scale image is created by assigning a shade to these various values.

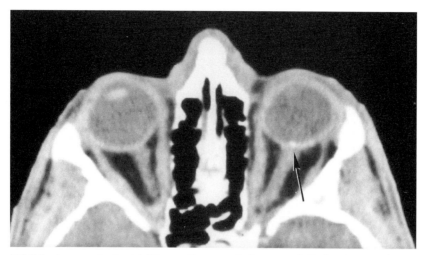

FIG II-1—A noncontrast axial CT scan. The arrow indicates a calcified optic nerve drusen. Note the excellent visibility of bone, muscles, and optic nerve. The patient's head is slightly tilted, allowing visibility of the lens in one eye but not the other. A small portion of the brain is visible; note the relatively poor soft-tissue contrast between gray matter, white matter, muscle, optic nerve, and sclera.

Different windows, created by the total range of attenuation values shown in the entire image and the range of values shown in each shade of gray, may be produced to emphasize selected soft tissue or bone. CT scanning with intravenous contrast enhancement improves visualization of most tumors, large blood vessels, and inflammatory processes. CT safely delivers between 3 and 10 rads (cGy) to the target tissue without risk to the adult lens, which is damaged with exposure at the 200 cGy level.

Magnetic Resonance Imaging

Magnetic resonance imaging (MRI) is the neuroimaging study of choice for demonstration of intracranial soft-tissue anatomy and pathology. MRI does not use ionizing radiation to render an image. Rather, the target tissue is subjected to a strong magnetic pulse, and the energy emitted from the recovering tissue is converted to an image. Images are produced by assigning a gray-scale value to the various levels of magnetic field thus measured. Views can be obtained directly in any plane (e.g., axial, coronal, sagittal, etc.), allowing excellent localization and three-dimensional reconstruction of lesions. Further, the technique of scanning can be modified to highlight different tissues in the same area or to accentuate various pathologic states. A radiologist's consultation is invaluable in maximizing the efficiency of the scan for a particular clinical use.

The contrast between central nervous system white and gray matter is considerably greater on MRI than CT. Air, cortical bone, and rapidly flowing fluids such as blood in an artery, arterial aneurysm, or an arteriovenous shunt give no signal or appear black on an MRI, unless special pulse sequences are used. Structures containing flowing blood appear bright on a CT scan performed with contrast enhancement.

MRI Terminology

The MRI process applies a large static magnetic field to the area to be imaged, causing many of the tissue's protons to align parallel and with the field. The protons may be tipped perpendicular to this static field by selective excitation from a radio frequency (RF) pulse. As the protons return to their original state (relaxation), the energy they emit can be detected. Relaxation occurs longitudinally, against the magnetic field, and in the transverse plane. The protons spin like tops and gradually settle down as they lose energy.

The time required for 63% of the protons to realign with the main magnetic field is termed *T1,* the *spin-lattice time.* The *spin-spin relaxation time* of a tissue, *T2,* is the time required for 63% of the protons to relax with the plane perpendicular to the main magnetic field.

Different tissues have inherently different T1 and T2 properties. Gray matter of the brain has a T1 of 920 msec and T2 of 101 msec; white matter has a T1 of 790 msec and T2 of 92 msec. To create the image, a series of RF bursts is sent through the tissue; the time between bursts is known as the *repetition time (TR),* and the pattern of bursts is termed a *pulse sequence.* The *echo time, TE,* is the interval from the first RF pulse to the measurement of the signal. Various TR and TE combinations emphasize contrast differences between tissues of varying T1 and T2 characteristics and result in images that highlight certain tissues or pathologic states.

T1-weighted images (T1WI) have relatively short TR (≤1000 msec) and TE (≤20 msec) values and show excellent anatomic detail but may fail to distinguish pathologic states (Fig II-2). White matter has a relatively high signal intensity (bright on T1WI), whereas water, cerebrospinal fluid, and vitreous have a relatively low signal intensity (dark on T1WI). Conversely, longer TR (≥2000 msec) and TE (≥40 msec) values emphasize the T2 differences of the various tissues (Fig II-3). A T2-weighted image (T2WI) shows cerebrospinal fluid, water, and vitreous with a high (bright) signal relative to the brain's white matter.

Because signal intensity is related to the tissue's water content or magnetically alterable proton density, a long TR and short TE are used to create proton-density-weighted images. These images have low contrast, but they highlight edema and other pathologic states. Numerous pulse sequences have been developed to optimize the imaging of certain regions such as the orbit with its high fat content.

Magnetic contrast media such as gadolinium-DTPA are also available to enhance MRIs. Gadolinium is paramagnetic because of its unpaired electrons. Any tissue or structure containing gadolinium will appear much brighter than normal on a T1-weighted image. The blood-brain barrier prevents accumulation of gadolinium in the normal brain or optic nerves. However, areas of inflammation, tumor, or breakdown of the blood-brain barrier allow gadolinium to persist within these tissues, and its presence will heighten the signal on a T1WI.

Orbital fat has high signal (bright image) on a T1WI and contrasts with the darker optic nerve, sheath, and extraocular muscles. Enhancement of any intra-orbital structure with gadolinium may be counteracted by the brightness of the adjacent orbital fat. Fat-suppressed T1-weighted pulse sequences selectively darken the signal of all fat yet preserve the T1 signal of the other orbital structures. Fat-suppressed gadolinium-enhanced T1-weighted images show good contrast between

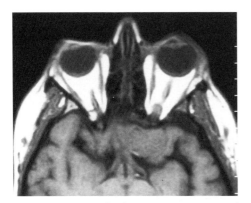

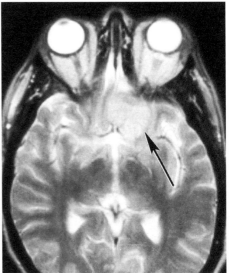

FIG II-2—A T1-weighted MRI. A meningioma of the left optic nerve and cavernous sinus is poorly visible. Note that the vitreous and cerebrospinal fluid are hypointense and the orbital fat is hyperintense on T1-weighted images. Image shows some contrast between white and gray matter, but bone is not well seen.

FIG II-3—A T2-weighted MRI of the patient shown in Figure II-2. Note that the vitreous and cerebrospinal fluid are now hyperintense. The meningioma (arrow) is much more visible with T2 weighting. The relative brightness of orbital fat lowers contrast within the orbit.

enhanced structures that are brightened by the gadolinium effect and fat that is darkened through suppression from the pulse sequence employed (Fig II-4).

Kent DL, Haynor DR, Longstreth WT Jr, et al. The clinical efficacy of magnetic resonance imaging in neuroimaging. *Ann Intern Med.* 1994;120:856–871.

Wirtschafter JD, Berman EL, McDonald CS. *Magnetic Resonance Imaging and Computed Tomography: Clinical Neuro-Orbital Anatomy.* Ophthalmology Monograph 6. San Francisco: American Academy of Ophthalmology; 1992.

MRI vs CT Scanning

MRI has largely supplanted CT in the examination of the intracranial contents. In comparison to MRI, however, CT does have relative advantages as well as disadvantages. Images can be obtained with CT in less time, making it a useful modality in non-sedated children. Newer CT scanners can obtain an image in less than 1 sec per view with spatial resolution of better than 1 mm^3. CT is superior in detecting calcification, imaging bone, and detecting acute intracranial hemorrhage. Computed tomography has wider availability than MRI and generally costs less. CT scanning usually does not miss significant lesions in the orbit or central nervous system, although it may not image them as well as MRI.

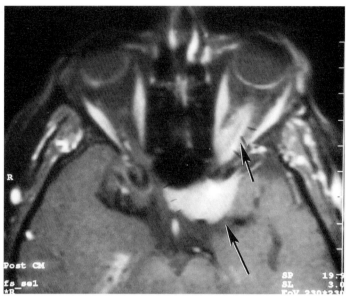

FIG II-4—A fat-suppressed gadolinium-enhanced T1-weighted image of the patient shown in Figures II-2 and II-3. The long arrow points to the meningioma, which is easily seen in comparison with the standard T1 image of Figure II-2. The short arrow points to the meningioma encasing the optic nerve. The fat suppression renders the orbital fat hypointense, permitting better visualization of the optic nerve and extraocular muscles than with the standard T1 image.

The main disadvantages of CT are relatively poor soft-tissue contrast, particularly in the brain; artifacts from cortical bone and metallic objects such as dental fillings; and the lack of direct sagittal scanning capability. Additional disadvantages include difficulties in positioning patients to perform a coronal scan; potential side effects of intravenous contrast administration, which is more problematic than with MRI contrast material; and the accumulated radiation dose for many studies.

Some clinicians primarily employ CT in the acute setting or as a screening study (e.g., prior to an emergent lumbar puncture) and subsequently obtain an MRI as a follow-up study. Other clinicians find that a preliminary CT is less cost effective than simply obtaining the more expensive, yet more definitive, MRI alone. The decision depends on the relative price and availability of facilities. At times CT and MRI can be complementary.

Because of its multiplanar capability and increased soft-tissue contrast, MRI is superior to CT in the evaluation of most intracranial conditions not involving bone. MRI is also preferred for demonstration of vascular malformations and aneurysms except when the presence of intraparenchymal or subarachnoid hemorrhage or calcification is important in the differential diagnosis. MRI currently requires a scanning time of several minutes per sequence, long enough to lead to motion artifact and problems with very ill patients. Newer programs have reduced the scanning time significantly. Claustrophobic patients can have difficulty being surrounded by the MRI machinery and may benefit from sedation. Some scanners with an open gantry are more accommodating to claustrophobic patients. Intramuscular sedatives or even general anesthesia with life support can be employed with an MRI-compatible ventilator. The presence of a cardiac pacemaker is still an absolute contraindication for MRI. Other relative contraindications include the presence of intracranial aneurysm clips and other potentially movable metallic intraocular or intracranial foreign bodies, although many institutions will scan patients with clips known to be nonmagnetic or materials felt to be very securely in position. Even if metallic foreign bodies such as braces on teeth do not pose a risk of movement during MRI scanning, they may induce extensive artifact in the adjacent tissues.

Orbit

CT scanning generally produces imaging of the orbit that is adequate for most purposes and is faster and less expensive than magnetic resonance techniques. Cortical bone and orbital fat provide excellent contrast for CT images. Axial slices 1.5 mm–3.0 mm in thickness detect the majority of orbital lesions. Directly obtained coronal scans, rather than reformatted axial scans, are helpful in imaging the superior and inferior orbital walls, the paranasal sinuses, and the extraocular muscles and in showing their relationship to the posterior optic nerve. However, these scans may be difficult to obtain in elderly patients or those with cervical disease because of the position required.

Four common indications for orbital/facial CT are the following:

□ To determine the extent of trauma

□ To diagnose thyroid ophthalmopathy or myositis

□ To search for calcification or metallic foreign bodies

□ To evaluate paranasal sinusitis

Both direct axial and coronal views should be obtained. Calcifications, as in optic nerve drusen or nerve sheath meningiomas, may be seen without contrast material (see Figure II-1, p 39).

Contrast material is useful when a mass lesion is suspected, but it is not needed in all settings. The contrast-enhanced CT scan shows an increased signal intensity in a nonspecific pattern of involved orbital tissues with inflammatory, infiltrative, and neoplastic disorders. An enlarged superior orbital vein can usually be seen in cases of orbital arteriovenous shunting.

The anatomic appearance of the extraocular muscles usually allows thyroid ophthalmopathy and orbital inflammatory syndromes to be distinguished with CT scanning. Classically, thyroid ophthalmopathy (Graves disease) is associated with enlargement of the muscle belly but sparing of the tendinous insertion. While the muscle tendons remain normal in appearance, the orbital fat commonly shows an increase in volume and "graying." On the other hand, myositis causes muscle enlargement that generally includes involvement of the tendon.

With the use of surface coils, MRI can render soft-tissue contrast and spatial resolution superior to that of CT scanning within the orbit. Although surface coils improve orbital magnetic resonance imaging, they do not allow simultaneous viewing of the brain because of the limited depth of penetration. Orbital surface coils are useful in imaging the anterior orbit but, unfortunately, do not penetrate sufficiently to visualize the apex well. Surface-coil technology, although beyond the pure research stage, is not yet widespread. In spite of MRI's better soft-tissue contrast, the less expensive CT usually provides soft-tissue imaging within the orbit sufficient for clinical use as well as superior bone imaging.

Parasellar and Cavernous Sinus Regions

MRI is the study of choice for the cavernous sinus region, sella, and suprasellar cistern. This technique can often accomplish the following:

□ Demonstrate individual cranial nerves within the cavernous sinus

□ Show the cavernous sinus venous plexus and areas of thrombosis

□ Distinguish the carotid artery with flowing blood or intravascular thrombosis

□ Image both intracranial optic nerves, the chiasm, and the optic tracts in a single axial plane

□ Distinguish an aneurysm with a "flow void" from a solid lesion (see discussion of MR angiography, p 47)

Gadolinium enhancement is useful in evaluation of neoplasms in the sella and suprasellar region. Multiplanar views allow excellent assessment of compressive visual pathway lesions near the sella.

The regions of the sella and cavernous sinus can also be assessed with contrast-enhanced, thin-section coronal and axial CT. However, bony artifact, decreased soft-tissue contrast, and difficulty in imaging the sagittal plane make CT a less attractive choice than MRI. CT is often used as a complement to assess bony destruction or calcification, which may be found in craniopharyngiomas, for example.

Intracranial Tumors

Although most intracranial neoplasms can be visualized with a contrast-enhanced CT scan, MRI's superior soft-tissue contrast, resolution, and lack of bony artifact usually make it the test of choice. However, CT may be useful in the evaluation of adjacent bones or in the detection of calcification. Each lesion is evaluated for the following:

□ Whether it is intra-axial or arises from the dura mater

□ The presence of calcification or hemorrhage within the tumor

□ The extent of the mass effect

□ The presence of cerebral edema

□ The number and location of lesions

□ Whether it appears to be infiltrative

For example, a meningioma often arises from the adjacent dura mater, enhances uniformly, causes hyperostosis in the adjacent bone, and may or may not be accompanied by cerebral edema. Gadolinium administration is essential to differentiate the signals of intraparenchymal tumors such as gliomas, meningiomas, and metastatic lesions from the often similar signals of the brain. Contrast enhancement may cause a bright signal in the meninges in carcinomatosis and inflammatory diseases such as meningitis or sarcoidosis.

The posterior fossa and skull base are ideal regions for MRI, which produces no artifacts from adjacent bone, unlike CT. MRI is thus the preferred study for evaluating lesions such as acoustic neuroma. Most infarcts (depending on age), hemorrhages, demyelinating plaques, and neoplasms of the brain stem are easily visualized on high-resolution MRI.

Vascular Lesions

Fresh blood is well visualized by computed tomography. CT is an excellent screening study for subarachnoid hemorrhage. On the other hand, nonhemorrhagic cerebral infarcts often are not detectable by CT scan within 24–48 hours of onset. Once the lesion appears, it has a low attenuation signal (appearing darker than the adjacent brain) and little, if any, mass effect. After approximately 3–7 days, an infarct can enhance with contrast. If an infarct becomes hemorrhagic, it will appear hyperdense initially, isodense within days, and hypodense gradually over 2–6 weeks. Though small lacunar infarcts can appear in the deep gray and white matter, most infarcts involve the cortical tissue. An acute intracerebral hematoma appears hyperdense in a CT image and may have an area of low attenuation from the edema in the adjacent brain. A breakdown in the blood-brain barrier adjacent to the hemorrhage may enhance with contrast. Infarcts and small hemorrhages of the brain stem are often difficult to demonstrate because of their small size and also because of artifacts induced by adjacent petrous bone.

Arteriovenous malformations (AVM) of the brain that have not hemorrhaged may still be visible on a noncontrast CT scan with a high attenuation signal as a result of the intravascular blood. The serpiginous shape of this signal, which enhances with contrast material, is typical of this vascular lesion. Mass effect may be present, especially following an intracerebral hemorrhage. Similarly, arterial aneurysms can cause an intracerebral hemorrhage as well as the more commonly seen subarachnoid hemorrhage. A subarachnoid hemorrhage following aneurysm rupture may be seen in the cisterns and in the interhemispheric fissures during the first 24 hours. The aneurysm itself is rarely visualized unless it is larger than 2.5 cm (a so-called giant aneurysm).

The age of a cerebral infarct or hemorrhage affects the appearance of the lesion on MRI. As time passes, the iron-containing components of blood react chemically, altering their magnetic properties. In the first few hours, an acute bleed is largely isointense with surrounding cerebral tissue and thus invisible on MRI. Therefore, CT is the imaging technique of choice for an acute intracerebral hemorrhage. With time, the T1 and T2 characteristics of the iron-containing structures evolve in a predictable pattern, enabling the clinician to date the duration of the lesion. The presence of deoxyhemoglobin renders acute intracerebral bleeds and hemorrhagic infarctions centrally hypointense on T2-weighted images. As the hemorrhage ages, more deoxyhemoglobin changes into methemoglobin, subsequently increasing the signal intensity on both T1 and T2 images. As breakdown continues to hemosiderin, the T2 images again become hypointense. Chronic hematomas can have a hyperintense, fluid-filled center on T2-weighted images.

Hayman LA, Taber KH, Ford JJ, et al. Mechanisms of MR signal alteration by acute intracerebral blood: old concepts and new theories. *Am J Neuroradiol.* 1991;12: 899–907.

MR imaging characteristics are quite different in the setting of flowing blood, because hemoglobin acted upon by the magnetic pulse is carried away before the signal generated can be measured. The result is a hypointense *flow void* in patent blood vessels with rapidly moving blood. The increased blood flow in brain AVMs causes flow voids in many of the affected vessels, including the arterialized venous drainage. Because of the different rates of blood flow, these lesions often have a heterogeneous appearance. MRI provides better anatomical detail of the location of an AVM than does CT. Areas of flow void can be difficult to distinguish from areas of calcification, as both are hypointense. Attempts to use MRI to determine whether an AVM has bled in the distant past have been disappointing because the imaging characteristics found in chronic intracerebral hemorrhages are similar.

MRI can be diagnostic of other intracranial vascular lesions such as venous malformations in Sturge-Weber syndrome, dural venous sinus or cortical vein thrombosis, telangiectasia, and venous anomalies. MRI can also determine whether a dural AVM shows significant arterialized drainage into the ophthalmic or cortical venous circulations. Although MRI is excellent for imaging vascular lesions, it can completely miss some large items such as dural fistulas. Traditional cerebral angiography remains the standard for direct visualization and evaluation of intracranial vascular lesions. The special case of arterial aneurysms is discussed under Magnetic Resonance Angiography, p 47.

Multiple Sclerosis

CT, particularly using a high-volume ("double dose") delayed technique, can adequately demonstrate demyelinating plaques seen in multiple sclerosis (MS). However, MRI is more sensitive, in both symptomatic and asymptomatic patients. MS plaques have prolonged T2 (hyperintense) relaxation time and are best demonstrated on a T2-weighted image (T2WI). The plaques appear mainly in white matter anywhere within the central nervous system and have a tendency to occur in the periventricular region. Plaques found in the region of the corpus callosum are highly suggestive of multiple sclerosis. MS plaques with high signal on T2WI and areas of contrast enhancement with gadolinium on T1WI may be seen in the optic nerves of patients with optic neuritis. Contrast enhancement is not necessary but will highlight acutely inflamed lesions and may help in dating them. When screening for multiple sclerosis, it is important to include imaging of the brain rather than selectively studying the optic nerves.

Transient white-matter lesions are common in, but not diagnostic of, multiple sclerosis. Similar-appearing lesions can occur with collagen vascular diseases that affect the brain, such as systemic lupus erythematosus. Use of these lesions to diagnose MS is controversial. Many clinicians feel that their presence, in the setting of acute optic neuritis or another single mononeuropathy, is highly suggestive of multiple sclerosis. Others require active lesions in a distinctly separate time frame or the presence of clinical signs and symptoms before diagnosing MS. The lack of enhancing lesions does not exclude the diagnosis of multiple sclerosis.

Francis GS, Evans AC, Arnold DL. Neuroimaging in multiple sclerosis. *Neurol Clin.* 1995;13:147–171.

Giang DW, Grow VM, Mooney C, et al. Clinical diagnosis of multiple sclerosis. The impact of magnetic resonance imaging and ancillary testing. Rochester-Toronto Magnetic Resonance Study Group. *Arch Neurol.* 1994;51:61–66.

Goodkin DE, Rudick RA, Ross JS. The use of brain magnetic resonance imaging in multiple sclerosis. *Arch Neurol.* 1994;51:505–516.

Magnetic Resonance Angiography

Phase-contrast magnetic resonance angiography (MRA) has grown out of techniques that can distinguish the phase shift related to the velocity of flowing blood from stationary tissue that lacks this shift. A newer MRA technique, *time of flight,* rapidly saturates the tissue with a repetition time shorter than local tissue T1 and directly images magnetized flowing blood. This method is currently used more often for intracranial and carotid MRA. Vascular narrowing caused by atherosclerosis or dissections and the abnormal globular signal from aneurysms are readily seen. Many cerebral aneurysms and most brain AVMs can be visualized with the time of flight technique (Fig II-5). The lesions can be seen in dynamic three-dimensional images and can be reconstructed for viewing from any angle. Further, both carotids and the venous system are imaged simultaneously.

The most common use of MRA in neuro-ophthalmology is to evaluate the possibility of an aneurysm causing a third nerve palsy or another parasellar syndrome. Although dependent on the skills of the technician and radiologist, MRA has good resolution and is capable of detecting aneurysms in the range of 3–4 mm (much smaller than aneurysms that typically cause third nerve palsies). In this setting MRA, in combination with standard spin-echo views of the brain, may detect about 95% of aneurysms.

Intra-arterial angiography, discussed below, has superior spatial resolution and sensitivity in aneurysm detection at the present time. Although standard angiography itself carries a higher morbidity risk than MRA, the life-threatening nature of a missed aneurysm makes invasive angiography the "gold standard" for ruling out aneurysm. However, MRA is becoming an increasingly acceptable substitute for conventional carotid arteriography. Many neurosurgeons still require a conventional angiogram in planning treatment, but this rule is beginning to change as experience with MRA grows.

Magnetic imaging, with its lower direct risks, may play an important role when the actual risk of aneurysm is lower, as in certain cases of pupil-sparing third nerve palsies. It has the advantage over conventional arteriography of screening for other intracranial processes that may be the cause of symptoms and signs. Occasionally, the two techniques are complementary; each has been reported to find aneurysms that the other missed.

Hamed LM, Silbiger J, Silbiger M, et al. Magnetic resonance angiography of vascular lesions causing neuro-ophthalmic deficits. *Surv Ophthalmol.* 1993;37:425–434.

Arteriography

Intracerebral angiography involves catheterizing the large arteries of the head and neck using a brachial or femoral approach, directly injecting contrast material, and taking standard radiographic images from various angles. Arteriography offers the highest sensitivity and specificity in detecting aneurysms, detects most AVMs, and can identify the vascular patterns of tumors (Fig II-6). In addition to diagnosis, the interventional radiologist can use angiographic techniques to treat lesions such as arteriovenous fistulas.

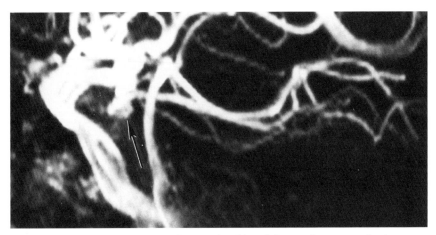

FIG II-5—A magnetic resonance angiogram showing a left posterior communicating artery aneurysm (arrow) at the junction with the internal carotid. Compare with Figure II-6.

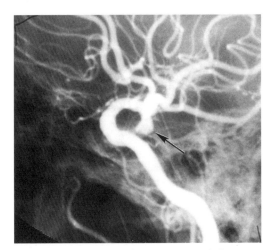

FIG II-6—A conventional arteriogram of the same patient shown in Figure II-5. The arrow indicates the posterior communicating artery aneurysm.

Standard angiography may have a small false-negative rate as a result of vaso-spasm, observer error, inadequate views, or partial thrombosis causing sluggish blood flow. Further, intra-arterial angiography is not without risk: mortality and permanent neurologic deficits may occur in 0.5%–1.5% of patients. However, given the risk of aneurysmal rupture (out-of-hospital mortality of about 50%), neuro-imaging is a necessity in cases of suspected aneurysm. CT scanning (or perhaps, MRI) followed by direct angiography is probably still the test sequence of choice in patients with high-risk characteristics. Increasingly, and particularly in patients without high-risk characteristics for aneurysm, MRI with MR angiography is becom-ing an acceptable alternative.

Functional MRI

In addition to providing anatomical images of the brain, magnetic techniques can image hemodynamic changes resulting from cerebral activity, including visual processing and other physiologic phenomena as well as pathologic states. Unlike other noninvasive imaging techniques of cerebral activity, such as positron emission tomography (PET) and single-photon emission computed tomography (SPECT), functional MRI (fMR) is relatively fast and does not require isotopes. Thus, it can produce rapidly repeated image sequences. An fMR image is created when the signal of an area of resting brain is compared to the signal following stimulation (e.g., a cognitive task or sensory input). The latter signal reflects changes in blood flow and microvascular oxygenation. It is detected and processed with specialized hardware and software additions to an MR scanner. At this point, fMR has limited availability and is strictly a research tool.

Moseley ME, Glover GH. Functional MR imaging: capabilities and limitations. *Neuroimaging Clin N Am.* 1995;5:161–191.

Color Flow Doppler Imaging

Color flow Doppler imaging maps color-coded Doppler information on the velocity of blood flow within vessels onto standard two-dimensional gray ultrasound images of nearby anatomic structures (Fig II-7). It is useful in identifying significant carotid artery stenosis and as an adjunct in evaluating retinal arterial occlusions, temporal arteritis, carotid artery dissection, and drug- or disease-induced changes in orbital blood flow. By demonstrating flow reversal in orbital vessels, color flow Doppler imaging identifies low-flow dural or carotid cavernous fistulas with high sensitivity and specificity and may even detect fistulas missed by angiography. The resolution is sufficient to diagnostically identify blood flow changes in patients with visual loss from ischemic optic neuropathy and retinal arterial occlusions. However, the equipment is expensive, and most information is obtainable by other techniques.

Aburn NS, Sergott RC. Orbital colour Doppler imaging. *Eye.* 1993;7:639–647.

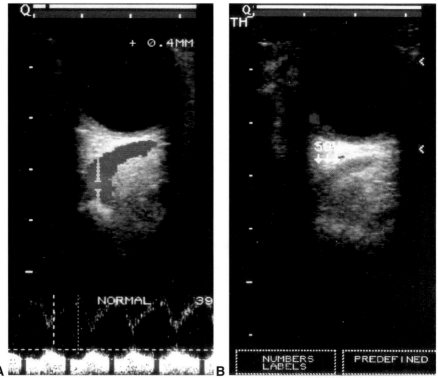

FIG II-7—Color flow Doppler images of the orbit in a patient before and after treatment of a dural shunt. *A,* The superior ophthalmic vein is enlarged and contains anterograde blood flow with an arteriolized (pulsatile) signal by spectral analysis. *B,* After treatment the thrombosed superior ophthalmic vein is visible by B-scan ultrasonography but contains no blood flow signal.

Orbital B-Scan Ultrasonography

B-scan ultrasonography of the eye is largely used to identify intraocular structures when the view of the fundus is obstructed or to diagnose subretinal lesions. With an experienced echographer, it is useful in distinguishing fluid within the optic nerve sheath from infiltrative lesions posterior to the globe. It can also be used to evaluate the extraocular muscles for enlargement.

CHAPTER III

The Sensory Visual System

The *retina* projects to a variety of visual nuclei in the thalamus, hypothalamus, and brain stem. Its major target is the *lateral geniculate body*, which relays visual information to the *primary visual cortex*. This pathway provides the neural substrate for visual perception.

Anatomy

Retina

The transduction of light to an electrical signal begins with the percipient elements of the retina: the rods and cones. The output of these photoreceptors activates a complex neuronal circuit within the retina. A detailed discussion of retinal anatomy and physiology is beyond the scope of this review. (See BCSC Section 12, *Retina and Vitreous.*) The following description focuses on the role the retina plays in the flow of visual information.

Considerable processing of visual information occurs at the level of the retina. More than 20 different types of neurons have been identified in the retina, grouped into five major classes:

□ Retinal ganglion cells

□ Amacrine cells

□ Bipolar cells

□ Horizontal cells

□ Photoreceptors

These cells are organized into distinct layers. Light passes through the full thickness of the retina to reach the photoreceptor outer segments, where absorption takes place. Information flows toward the inner retina, ultimately reaching the retinal ganglion cells. Each retinal ganglion cell contributes a single axon to the retinal nerve fiber layer. Along their intraretinal course, the axons remain unmyelinated, preserving the transparency of the retina. After passing through the lamina cribrosa, they become vested in myelin as they exit the globe to constitute the optic nerve.

Ganglion cells subserving central vision send their axons directly from the foveal area to the temporal aspect of the optic disc, forming the papillomacular bundle. Fibers from peripheral nasal ganglion cells enter the nasal portion of the optic disc directly. Fibers from the peripheral temporal retina enter the superior and inferior poles of the optic disc. Temporal retinal nerve fibers arising near the horizontal meridian run directly toward the disc until approximately 4 mm temporal to the fovea, where they diverge around the papillomacular bundle to become part of the superior and inferior arcuate nerve fiber bundles (Fig III-1).

Diseases of the retina, optic disc, optic nerve, and other portions of the anterior visual pathways can be expected to produce *anterograde* (downstream) or *retrograde*

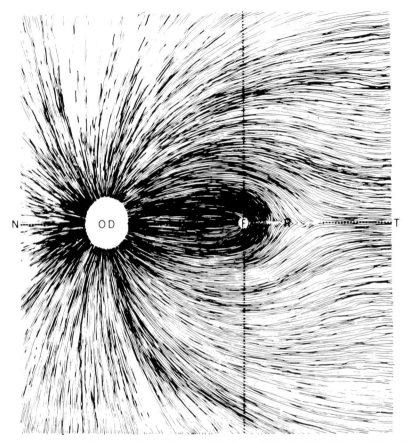

FIG III-1—Artist's drawing of normal nerve fiber layer. OD-optic disc; F-fovea; N-nasal retina; T-temporal retina; R-temporal raphe. (From Hogan MF, Alvarado JA, Weddell JE. *Histology of the Human Eye, an Atlas and Textbook.* Philadelphia: Saunders; 1971.)

(upstream) changes in the nerve fiber layer of the retina. These changes evolve weeks or months after the lesion occurs. They can be seen with the direct ophthalmoscope if the light is bright enough and the fundus has sufficient background pigmentation. The nerve fiber layer is more easily seen if the pupil is dilated and red-free (green) illumination is used.

Early focal defects of the nerve fiber layer produce fine slits or grooves most visible in the arcuate region. As atrophy progresses, the fine slits broaden to reveal a wider swath of dark-appearing retina devoid of normal linear nerve fiber layer striations. When atrophy is complete, visible nerve fiber layer is absent, and the region takes on a granular, dull appearance with complete loss of striations. Retinal vessels no longer covered by nerve fiber layer appear in sharp relief. In patients with disc edema, the normal striations in the peripapillary region become muddied and irregular, presumably because of axonal swelling.

Hoyt WF, Schlicke B, Eckelhoff RJ. Fundoscopic appearance of a nerve-fibre-bundle defect. *Br J Ophthalmol.* 1972;56:577–583.

Lundström M, Frisén L. Atrophy of optic nerve fibres in compression of the chiasm: Degree and distribution of ophthalmoscopic changes. *Acta Ophthalmol.* 1976;54: 623–640.

Ogden TE. Nerve fiber layer of the primate retina: morphometric analysis. *Invest Ophthalmol Vis Sci.* 1984;25:19–29.

Pollock SC, Miller NR. The retinal nerve fiber layer. *Int Ophthalmol Clin.* 1986;26: 201–221.

Rodieck R. *The Primate Retina.* New York: AR Liss; 1988:203–278.

Optic Disc

The optic disc is located in the nasal retina, 3–4 mm from the fovea. It averages 1.88 mm in vertical diameter and 1.76 mm in horizontal diameter. Because no photoreceptors overlie the optic disc, it gives rise to an absolute scotoma in the visual field called the blind spot. The blind spot is centered 15° from fixation and slightly below the horizontal meridian in the temporal visual field. It subtends 7° by 5°.

The retina and optic disc head derive their blood supply from different sources. The retina is fed by the central retinal artery, whereas the optic disc head ultimately receives its supply from the short posterior ciliary arteries. The blood supply to the optic nerve head is provided by an anastomotic ring of small arterioles, the *circle of Zinn-Haller,* that wreathes the intraocular end of the optic nerve (Fig III-2). The short posterior ciliary arteries provide the blood that flows through the circle of Zinn-Haller. Some collateral blood supply may also be received through the choroid. The precise anatomy of the blood supply to the optic nerve has been a subject of controversy. The considerable anatomical variation from subject to subject probably accounts for some of the confusion surrounding this topic.

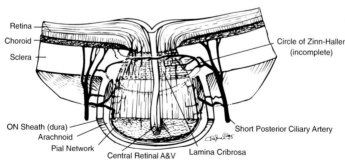

FIG III-2—Blood supply to anterior optic nerve. (Illustration by Craig A. Luce.)

Hayreh SS. Anatomy and physiology of the optic nerve head. *Trans Am Acad Ophthalmol Otolaryngol.* 1974;78:240–254.

Hayreh SS. Fluids in the anterior part of the optic nerve in health and disease. *Surv Ophthalmol.* 1978;23:1–25.

Hayreh SS. The role of optic nerve sheath fenestration in management of anterior ischemic optic neuropathy [letter]. *Arch Ophthalmol.* 1990;108:1063–1065.

Lieberman MF, Shahi A, Green WR. Embolic ischemic optic neuropathy. *Am J Ophthalmol.* 1978;86:206–210.

Quigley HA, Brown AE, Morrison JD, et al. The size and shape of the optic disc in normal human eyes. *Arch Ophthalmol.* 1990;108:51–57.

Optic Nerve

The optic nerve contains approximately 1 million nerve fibers and may be divided anatomically into four major portions:

□ Intraocular (1 mm)

□ Intraorbital (about 25 mm)

□ Intracanalicular (about 9 mm)

□ Intracranial (about 16 mm)

The orbital portion of the optic nerve extends from the globe to the optic canal. It is 3–4 mm in diameter, double the diameter of the intraocular portion as a result of the acquisition of myelin posterior to the lamina cribrosa. The orbital optic nerve normally follows an indirect, sinusoidal course to the optic canal. Its extra length allows the globe to rotate without stretching the nerve. When severe proptosis develops beyond 10 mm, the nerve becomes taut and the globe is tethered. Further proptosis often causes the back of the globe to tent at the attachment of the nerve.

Histologically, the optic nerve consists of bundles of myelinated axons interspersed with connective tissue septa containing blood vessels. The nerve is surrounded by three layers of meninges:

□ Dura mater, the outer layer that merges with the sclera

□ Arachnoid

□ Pia mater, which is fused to the outer surface of the nerve proper

Near the orbital apex, the optic nerve runs through a ring of connective tissue, the *annulus of Zinn*, which is composed of the tendinous origins of the rectus muscles. At the apex of the orbit the optic nerve enters the *optic canal*. The optic canal measures 5–10 mm long and 5–7 mm wide. The bony wall is thinnest medially where it separates the nerve from the ethmoid and sphenoid sinuses. Within the canal the optic nerve runs posteriorly and medially, forming an angle of approximately 35° with the midsagittal plane. In addition to the optic nerve, the canal contains the ophthalmic artery, some filaments of the sympathetic carotid plexus, and extensions of the intracranial meninges that form the sheath of the optic nerve.

In the canal the dura of the optic nerve and the periosteum of the bone are fused. In the orbit the optic nerve is relatively free to move, but in the optic canal it becomes anchored firmly. As a result, a small mass lesion in the optic canal can produce a compressive optic neuropathy, even before it becomes easily visible upon neuroimaging. The space between the pia and the arachnoid of the optic nerve communicates with the intracranial subarachnoid space and contains cerebrospinal fluid. Papilledema occurs when raised intracranial pressure is transmitted along this continuous cuff of fluid surrounding the optic nerve.

As the optic nerve exits the posterior opening of the optic canal, it passes through an unyielding falciform fold of dura, then continues posteriorly and medially, ascending at an angle of 45° to join the optic chiasm. The intracranial portion of each optic nerve ranges from 12 mm to 18 mm in length. Above the optic nerve lie the inferior surface of the frontal lobe of the brain (gyrus rectus), the olfactory tract, and the anterior cerebral and anterior communicating arteries. The lateral aspect of the optic nerve is often immediately adjacent to the internal carotid artery as it emerges from the cavernous sinus. Inferiorly and medially, the posterior ethmoid and sphenoid sinuses are adjacent to the nerve.

Hayreh SS. The ophthalmic artery III. Branches. *Br J Ophthalmol.* 1962;46:212–247.

Miller NR, ed. Anatomy and physiology of the optic nerve. In: *Walsh and Hoyt's Clinical Neuro-Ophthalmology.* 4th ed. Baltimore: Williams & Wilkins; 1995.

Optic Chiasm

Fibers from the two optic nerves merge to form the optic chiasm. Fibers from each nasal retina cross in the optic chiasm, whereas fibers from each temporal retina do not cross (Fig III-3). This *hemidecussation* in the chiasm means that each optic tract contains fibers from the contralateral nasal retina and the ipsilateral temporal retina, together representing the contralateral hemifield of vision. Slightly more than half the fibers (55%) in the optic nerve decussate because the nasal retina contains more ganglion cells than the temporal retina. Much of this difference is a result of the monocular crescent, corresponding to the extreme nasal retina, which has no counterpart in the temporal retina of the other eye.

The dorsal/posterior edge of the optic chiasm forms the floor of the third ventricle (Fig III-4). Carotid arteries bound it at either side. The chiasm measures about 8 mm in its anteroposterior direction, 13 mm wide, and 4 mm vertically. It is situated about 10 mm above the pituitary gland. The relatively large space between the chiasm and the pituitary, the inferior chiasmatic cistern, often allows suprasellar extension of a small pituitary tumor without evolution of a visual field defect. Only if a tumor grows large enough to obliterate this space and to impinge directly upon the optic chiasm will a visual field defect occur. The optic chiasm lies directly above the dorsum sella in most patients; however, it may be located more posteriorly or anteriorly. This variability in position helps to explain the range of visual field defects seen in patients with tumors in this area.

Miller NR, ed. Anatomy and physiology of the optic chiasm. In: *Walsh and Hoyt's Clinical Neuro-Ophthalmology.* 4th ed. Baltimore: Williams & Wilkins; 1995.

Optic Tracts

The optic tracts begin at the posterior aspect of the optic chiasm, diverge laterally, and continue posteriorly around the cerebral peduncles to terminate primarily in the *lateral geniculate bodies* (Fig III-5). Some fibers leave the primary optic pathway before reaching the lateral geniculate body, to innervate other subcortical visual areas. A special class of ganglion cells supplies the suprachiasmatic nucleus of the hypothalamus. This structure is located dorsal to the optic chiasm, on either side of the third ventricle. It is thought to provide visual input to neuroendocrine systems controlling diurnal rhythms.

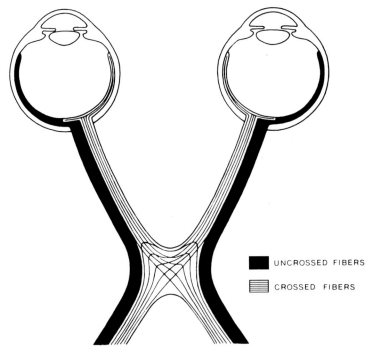

UNCROSSED FIBERS

CROSSED FIBERS

FIG III-3—Hemidecussation of fibers in the optic chiasm. (Hogan MJ, Alvarado JA, Weddell JE. *Histology of the Human Eye, an Atlas and Textbook.* Philadelphia: Saunders; 1971:394.)

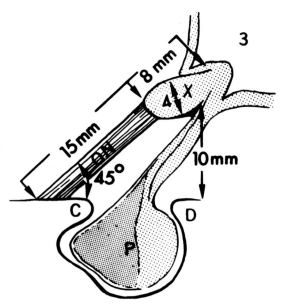

FIG III-4—Relationship of optic chiasm to third ventricle and pituitary fossa. 3-third ventricle; P-pituitary gland; C-anterior clinoid; D-posterior clinoid; ON-optic nerve; X-optic chiasm.

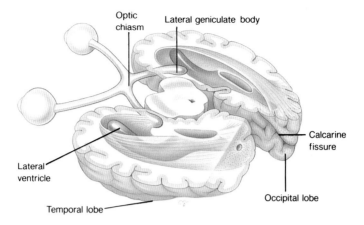

Optic chiasm

Lateral geniculate body

Calcarine fissure

Lateral ventricle

Occipital lobe

Temporal lobe

FIG III-5—Overview of the anterior and posterior visual system anatomy. (Illustration by Christine Gralapp.)

A major projection leaves the optic tract just before the lateral geniculate body to form the brachium of the *superior colliculus*. Also known as the optic tectum, the superior colliculus is involved in control of foveation reflexes. Injury to this structure disrupts eye movements and alignment, but it does not produce a visual field defect. Optic tract fibers terminate in the superficial gray layers of the superior colliculus. Others reach the midbrain through the brachium of the superior colliculus and terminate in the pretectal nuclear complex. The pretectal pathway controls light-mediated pupillary constriction. Projections from the pretectal nuclei go to the ipsilateral and contralateral Edinger-Westphal subnuclei of the oculomotor nucleus (see p 97). Finally, the optic tract conveys major retinal input to a visual nucleus in the thalamus of unknown function called the *pulvinar*.

Hendrickson A, Wilson ME, Toyne MJ. The distribution of optic nerve fibers in Macaca mulatta. *Brain Res.* 1970;23:425–427.

Sadun AA. Neuroanatomy of the human visual system. Part I. Retinal projections to the LGN and pretectum as demonstrated with a new stain. *Neuro-Ophthalmology.* 1986; 6:353–361.

Lateral Geniculate Body

The lateral geniculate body (LGB), or nucleus, is the part of the thalamus that is the site of termination for most of the afferent fibers of the primary visual pathway (Fig III-6). Neurons in the LGB receive retinal input and, in turn, relay it to the primary visual cortex in the occipital lobe. It is not known how the LGB modifies the retinal input to the visual cortex.

The cells of the LGB are organized in 6 major layers (Fig III-7). The *magnocellular neurons,* the largest ones, are found in layers 1 and 2; the *parvocellular,* or smallest, neurons appear in layers 3, 4, 5, and 6. Magnocellular neurons (*M-cells*) are thought to subserve motion detection, stereopsis, and low–spatial frequency

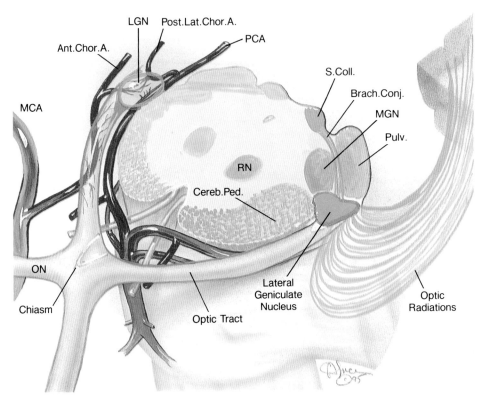

FIG III-6—The relationship of the lateral geniculate body (nucleus) to nearby structures and its blood supply. Abbreviations: Brach.Conj. = brachium conjunctivum; Cereb. Ped. = cerebral peduncles; MCA = middle cerebral artery; MGN = medial geniculate nucleus; PCA = posterior cerebral artery; Pulv. = pulvinar; RN = red nucleus; S.Coll. = superior colliculus. (Illustration by Craig A. Luce.)

contrast sensitivity. They project to layer 4C alpha of the primary visual cortex. Parvocellular neurons (*P-cells*) in the LGB probably serve fine spatial resolution and color vision. They project separately to layer 4C beta of the primary visual cortex.

Ganglion cell projections from the ipsilateral retina terminate in layers 2, 3, and 5 of the LGB; cells from the contralateral retina synapse in layers 1, 4, and 6. The cell projections rotate a quarter turn so that nerve fibers from the superior retina lie medially in the lateral geniculate body, while nerve fibers from inferior retina lie laterally. Rotation occurs again after the fibers leave the LGB so that superior and inferior retinal fibers again lie superior and inferior in the optic radiations and cerebral cortex. There is precise retinotopic order in the LGB.

Merigan WH, Katz LM, Maunsell JHR. The effect of parvocellular lateral geniculate lesions on the acuity and contrast sensitivity of Macaque monkeys. *J Neurosci.* 1987;11:994–1001.

Schiller PH, Logothetis NK, Charles ER. Functions of the colour-opponent and broadband channels of the visual system. *Nature.* 1990;343:68–70.

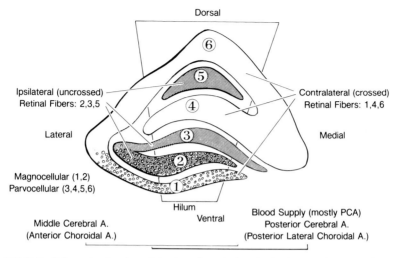

Dorsal

⑥

⑤

Ipsilateral (uncrossed)
Retinal Fibers: 2,3,5

④

Contralateral (crossed)
Retinal Fibers: 1,4,6

Lateral

③

Medial

②

Magnocellular (1,2)
Parvocellular (3,4,5,6)

①

Hilum

Ventral

Blood Supply (mostly PCA)
Posterior Cerebral A.
(Posterior Lateral Choroidal A.)

Middle Cerebral A.
(Anterior Choroidal A.)

FIG III-7—Schematic drawing of the lateral geniculate body showing layers of fibers from ipsilateral and contralateral retinal ganglion cells. (Illustration by Craig A. Luce, MS, CMI.)

Schiller PH, Malpeli JG. Functional specificity of lateral geniculate nucleus laminae of the rhesus monkey. *J Neurophysiol.* 1978;41:788–797.

Optic Radiations

The axons of geniculate neurons projecting to the primary visual cortex become the optic radiations. The optic radiations contain three main groups of fibers:

□ The superior portion containing fibers serving the inferior visual field

□ The inferior portion containing fibers serving the superior visual field

□ The central portion containing the macular fibers

Superior fibers leaving the LGB proceed posteriorly directly to the occipital cortex, running in the white matter underneath the parietal cortex. Inferior fibers, however, loop around the ventricular system into the temporal lobe, forming what is known as Meyer's loop. The most anterior fibers are found approximately 5 cm from the tip of the temporal lobe, but the distance may be variable. Removal of the anterior temporal lobe for the treatment of seizures or tumors often produces a homonymous visual field defect in the superior quadrant. The greater the amount of temporal lobe removed, the greater the risk of a visual field defect.

Anderson DR, Trobe JD, Hood TW, et al. Optic tract injury after anterior temporal lobectomy. *Ophthalmology.* 1989;96:1065–1070.

Occipital Cortex

The primary visual cortex, also called the *striate cortex, V1,* or *Brodmann's area 17,* receives the bulk of the projection from the LGB. It is situated along the calcarine fissure dividing the medial face of the occipital lobe (Fig III-8). The primary visual cortex contains a topographic map of the contralateral hemifield of vision. The representation of the central portion of the visual field is greatly magnified, whereas the representation of the peripheral visual field is relatively compressed. This exaggerated representation of central vision correlates with the higher acuity and greater density of photoreceptors and ganglion cells in the macula compared with the peripheral retina. The macular representation is located in the posterior half of the occipital lobe, extending slightly onto the lateral aspect of the cerebral hemisphere. The peripheral visual field is represented more anteriorly along the calcarine sulcus.

Despite the fact that humans have binocular vision, the visual fields of the two eyes do not overlap completely. There is a *temporal crescent* in each visual field, extending from an eccentricity of 55°–100°, which is seen by only the nasal retina of the ipsilateral eye. The primary visual cortex corresponding to this region is located in the most anterior portion of the calcarine cortex. This region of cortex is the only site in the visual pathway where a postchiasmal lesion can produce a monocular visual field defect. Conversely, the temporal crescent may be the only region spared after occipital cortex damage. The resultant hemianopia may give the appearance of being incongruous.

Surrounding the striate cortex is an extrastriate visual area known as *V2;* beyond V2 are visual areas V3, V4, V5, etc. Taken together, regions V2, V3, V4, and V5 occupy the region of cortex formerly known as Brodmann's areas 18 and 19 (Fig III-9). Several dozen extrastriate visual association areas have been identified in macaque monkeys. Their connections, arrangement, and function are currently the subject of intensive investigation. It is likely that different facets of visual function such as color, motion, stereopsis, and face recognition are segregated to some extent in different cortical extrastriate areas.

Horton JC, Hoyt WF. The representation of the visual field in human striate cortex. A revision of the classic Holmes map. *Arch Ophthalmol.* 1991;109:816–824.

Hubel DH. *Eye, Brain, and Vision.* New York: Scientific American Library; 1987.

Hubel DH, Wiesel TN. Brain mechanisms of vision. *Sci Am.* 1979;241:150–162.

Zeki S. *A Vision of the Brain.* Boston: Blackwell Scientific Publications; 1993.

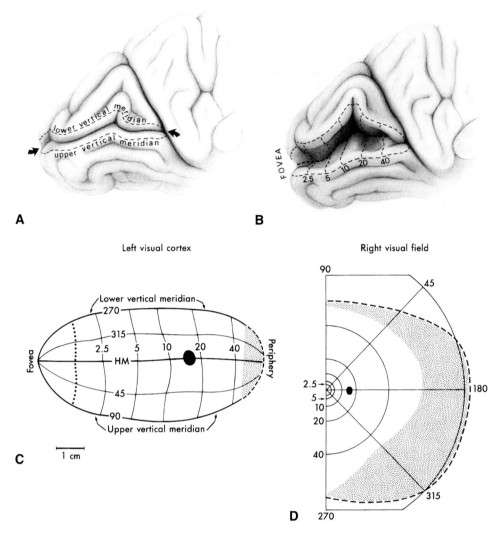

A

B

Left visual cortex

Right visual field

C 1 cm

D 270

FIG III-8—*A,* Left occipital cortex showing location of striate cortex within the calcarine fissure (running between arrows). The boundary (dashed line) between striate cortex (V1) and extrastriate cortex (V2) contains the representation of the vertical meridian. *B,* View of striate cortex after lips of the calcarine fissure are opened. The dashed lines indicate the coordinates of the visual field map. The representation of the horizontal meridian runs approximately along the base of the calcarine fissure. The vertical dashed lines mark the isoeccentricity contours from 2.5° to 40°. Striate cortex wraps around the occipital pole to extend about 1 cm onto the lateral convexity of the hemisphere, where the fovea is represented. *C,* Schematic, flattened map of the left striate cortex shown in *B* representing the right hemifield. The row of dots shows where striate cortex folds around the occipital tip. The black oval marks the region of striate cortex corresponding to the contralateral eye's blind spot. HM = horizontal meridian. *D,* Right visual hemifield, plotted with a Goldmann perimeter. The stippled area corresponds to the monocular temporal crescent, which is mapped in the most anterior ~ 8% of striate cortex. (Reprinted by permission of Horton JC, Hoyt WF. The representation of the visual field in human striate cortex. *Arch Ophthalmol.* 1991;109:822. Copyright © 1991, American Medical Association.)

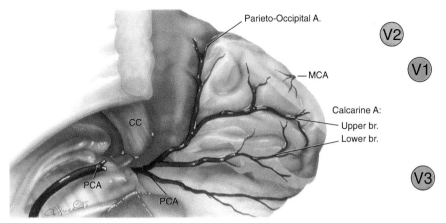

FIG III-9—The occipital cortex and its blood supply. Areas V1, V2, and V3 keyed by color. Abbreviations: CC = corpus callosum; MCA = middle cerebral artery; PCA = posterior cerebral artery. (Illustration by Craig A. Luce.)

Blood Supply of the Visual Pathways

Most areas of the visual system have more than one major vessel supplying them (Figs III-9, III-10, III-11). Table III-1 describes the blood supply for each region of the visual pathway.

TABLE III-1

BLOOD VESSELS SUPPLYING VISUAL PATHWAY

REGION OF PATHWAY	BLOOD SUPPLY
Optic nerve	
Orbital portion	Ophthalmic artery with meningeal anastomoses
Intracanalicular portion	Pial branches from the ophthalmic artery, possibly internal carotid
Intracranial portion	Small vessels from internal carotid, anterior cerebral, and anterior communicating arteries
Optic chiasm	Primarily by branches from internal carotid artery; occasionally by branches from anterior cerebral arteries and anterior communicating artery
	Posterior communicating and posterior cerebral arteries also likely
Optic tract	Anterior choroidal artery
	Branches from posterior communicating artery
Lateral geniculate body	Anterior and posterior choroidal arteries
Optic radiations and occipital cortex	Middle and posterior cerebral arteries

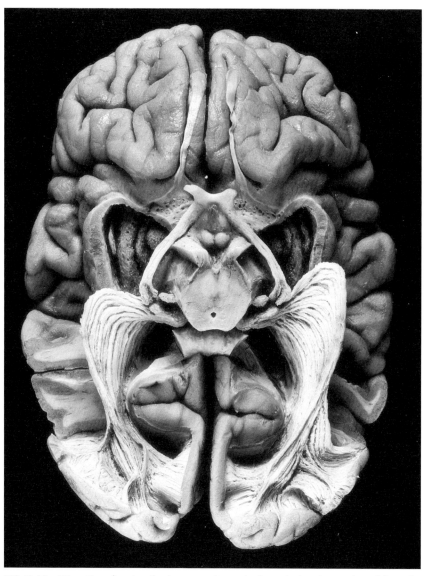

FIG III-10—Dissection showing the human retinogeniculocortical pathway viewed from the ventral aspect of the brain. The eyes and optic nerves have been removed just anterior to the optic chiasm. (Reprinted by permission from Gluhbegovic N, Williams TH. *The Human Brain*. Hagerstown, MD: Harper & Row; 1980.)

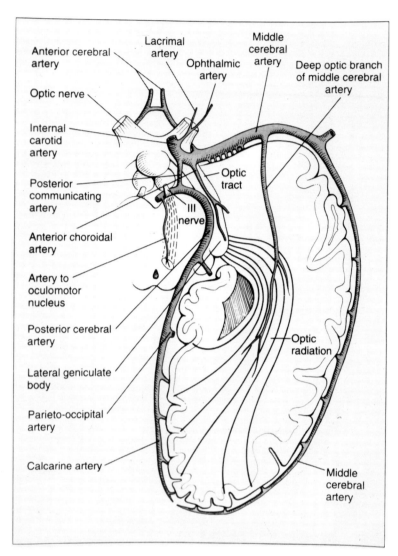

FIG III-11—The blood supply of the anterior and posterior visual systems. Note that each region of the visual system is supplied by multiple arteries. (Reprinted by permission from Podos SM, Yanoff M, eds. *Textbook of Ophthalmology.* Volume 6, *Neuro-ophthalmology.* St Louis: Mosby–Year Book; 1994.)

Visual Field Defects

Optic Disc/Optic Nerve

The arrangement of nerve fibers in the optic disc corresponds to their pattern of arrival from the retina. The upper retinal fibers are located in the upper portion of the optic disc, the lower fibers are below, and the nasal and temporal fibers enter on their respective sides. The fibers of the papillomacular bundle enter on the temporal side of the optic disc, displacing the fibers from the temporal retina into the superior and inferior poles of the disc. Figure III-1 on p 52 illustrates the arrangement of fibers entering the optic disc.

Moving from the optic disc toward the optic chiasm, retinotopic order becomes less precise in the optic nerve. Fibers from the temporal retina assume a more lateral position, while fibers from the nasal retina shift to a more medial position. About half the fibers in the optic nerve are derived from ganglion cells in the macula. These macular fibers are scattered throughout the retrobulbar optic nerve.

Visual field defects of the retina or optic nerve take several forms. Figure III-12 shows visual fields corresponding to each of the defects described below.

Cecocentral scotoma (Fig III-12A)   This field defect is classically found in patients with toxic optic neuropathies but can also be seen with any condition that produces a central scotoma. This defect may also be produced by an optic pit with serous retinal detachment.

Central scotoma (Fig III-12B)   When unilateral, this field defect is characteristically found in patients with optic neuritis, compressive lesions of the optic nerve, or any lesion that reduces central acuity (e.g., macular edema, disciform scar). When bilateral, this defect suggests a differential diagnosis of nutritional deficiencies, toxic optic neuropathies, or hereditary disorders.

Arcuate scotoma (Fig III-12C)   Fibers from the temporal retina arch over and under the papillomacular bundle to enter the superior and inferior poles of the optic disc respectively. Hence, lesions of the optic disc that damage these arcuate fiber bundles often produce arcuate scotomata that end abruptly along the horizontal midline. The most common diseases to cause this pattern of visual field loss are glaucoma, optic neuritis, anterior ischemic optic neuropathy (AION), branch retinal artery or vein occlusion, and optic disc drusen.

Altitudinal visual field defect (Fig III-12D)   An altitudinal field defect results from damage to the upper or lower pole of the optic disc. It can develop in optic neuritis, AION, or hemiretinal arterial or venous occlusive disease.

> Traustason OI, Feldon SE, Leemaster JE, et al. Anterior ischemic optic neuropathy: classification of field defects by Octopus automated static perimetry. *Graefes Arch Clin Exp Ophthalmol.* 1988;226:206–212.

All of these visual field defects can be produced by a lesion in either the optic nerve or the retina. Investigation of any patient with a visual field defect must include a careful examination of both the retina and the optic disc.

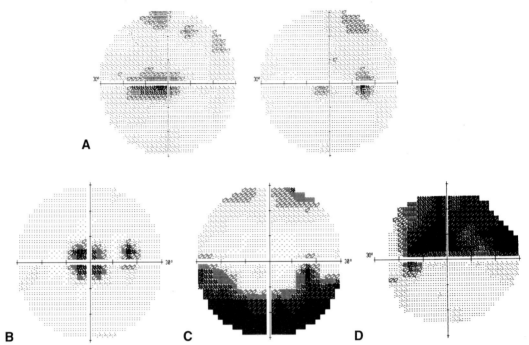

FIG III-12—A. Cecocentral scotomata in the left eye. Note inclusion of fixation, as well as the blind spot. The right eye of same patient shows a paracentral scotoma.

     B. Central scotoma in right eye. Note relatively intact peripheral field.

     C. Arcuate scotoma, right eye.

     D. Altitudinal defect, left eye of different patient.

Optic Chiasm

Lesions affecting the optic chiasm cause parasellar syndromes that may be grouped according to the site where chiasmal damage occurs and the visual field defect is produced (Fig III-13).

Fiber damage at the anterior chiasm Lesions that injure one optic nerve at its junction with the optic chiasm cause the anterior chiasmal syndrome. Diminished visual acuity and visual field loss in one eye accompany a superior temporal defect in the opposite eye (junctional scotoma) as a result of damage to one optic nerve combined with early compression of the optic chiasm (Fig III-13A). Rarely, a mass may compress the intracranial optic nerve, causing a temporal hemianopia with no involvement whatsoever of the visual field in the opposite eye. If a unilateral visual field defect respects the vertical meridian, neuroimaging should be considered to rule out the possibility of a prechiasmal compressive lesion.

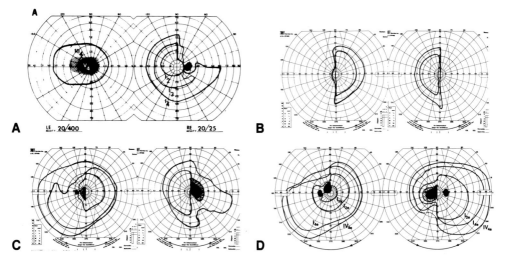

FIG III-13—A. Anterior chiasmal syndrome. Note severe loss of central vision in the left eye with constriction of the visual field. The right eye shows a superior temporal defect.

B. Complete bitemporal hemianopia caused by damage to fibers in the body of the optic chiasm.

C. Bitemporal scotomata resulting from damage to posterior macular fibers of the chiasm.

D. Incongruous homonymous hemianopic scotomata from lesion in right optic tract.

Fiber damage in the body of the chiasm   Lesions damaging the body of the chiasm produce relative or absolute bitemporal hemianopias, often without loss of visual acuity (Fig III-13B).

Fiber damage in the posterior chiasm   Lesions damaging fibers in this region destroy primarily posterior, macular-crossing fibers resulting in bitemporal hemianopic scotomata (Fig III-13C).

Fiber damage to the optic tract   Sellar or suprasellar lesions that expand posteriorly may compress fibers of the optic tract, resulting in a homonymous hemianopia.

Binasal hemianopia caused by lateral chiasmal compression   This condition is very rare. Binasal defects are most often the result of a disease process at the level of the optic disc, such as glaucoma. Infrequently, lesions anterior or posterior to the optic chiasm may compress and displace the chiasm or the intracranial optic nerves laterally against the internal carotid arteries, thus producing binasal field loss. True binasal hemianopia respecting the vertical midline is exceedingly rare and should rouse suspicion of a functional visual problem.

O'Connell JE, Du Boulay EP. Binasal hemianopia. *J Neurol Neurosurg Psychiatry.* 1973;36:697–709.

Pilley SJF, Thompson HS. Binasal field loss and prefixation blindness. In: Glaser JS, Smith JL, eds. *Neuro-Ophthalmology.* St Louis: Mosby; 1975:277–284.

The precise visual field defect produced by a lesion compressing the optic chiasm depends on the following:

☐ Location of the optic chiasm with respect to the sella turcica

☐ Direction in which growth of the lesion occurs

☐ Whether the lesion damages nerve fibers directly or compresses them against contiguous structures

Optic Tract

Retrochiasmal lesions produce *homonymous* visual field defects, i.e., matching, overlapping visual field loss in the temporal field of one eye and the nasal field of the other. Visual field defects from retrochiasmal lesions nearly always respect the vertical midline. If a homonymous visual field defect does not respect the vertical midline, the patient is probably not fixating well during testing. Alternatively, the patient may have bilateral prechiasmal visual field defects that are not truly homonymous.

Homonymous visual field defects may be absolute or incomplete. If incomplete, they can be either congruous or incongruous. *Congruous* visual field defects are identical in each eye. *Incongruous* field defects differ from one eye to the other. The degree of congruity is of some localizing value. Nerve fibers from corresponding retinal locations in each eye are not yet closely aligned while in the optic tract or lateral geniculate body, but they become increasingly aligned as they approach the occipital lobe. For this reason, a relatively anterior retrochiasmal lesion is likely to cause an incongruous partial homonymous hemianopia, whereas a posterior visual pathway lesion will produce a more congruous hemianopia.

The primary optic pathway is defined as the retinal nerve fiber layer, optic disc, optic nerve, optic chiasm, optic tract, and LGB. Any lesion of the primary optic pathway will eventually produce optic atrophy visible upon fundus examination. Lesions of the optic chiasm, optic tract, or LGB result in characteristic patterns of atrophy in the nerve fiber layer and optic disc (Figs III-14, III-15). Optic tract lesions are frequently accompanied by a slight relative afferent pupillary defect in the contralateral eye. This defect develops because the contralateral eye contributes slightly more fibers to each optic tract. Lesions of the LGB do not cause an afferent pupil defect because the pupillomotor fibers exit the optic tract anterior to the LGB.

Bell RA, Thompson HS. Relative afferent pupillary defect in optic tract hemianopias. *Am J Ophthalmol.* 1978;85:538–540.

Newman SA, Miller NR. Optic tract syndrome: Neuro-ophthalmologic considerations. *Arch Ophthalmol.* 1983;101:1241–1250.

Savino PJ, Paris M, Schatz NJ, et al. Optic tract syndrome. A review of 21 patients. *Arch Ophthalmol.* 1978;96:656–663.

Retrogeniculate Lesions

Lesions of the optic radiations in the temporal lobe produce superior homonymous hemianopic visual field defects. Lesions of the optic radiations in the parietal lobe cause inferior homonymous hemianopic visual field defects. Homonymous field defects from lesions of the optic radiations are often relatively incongruous. Other localizing neurologic symptoms or signs may accompany defect-producing lesions

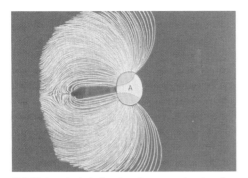

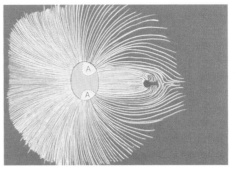

FIG III-14—Artist's drawing demonstrating band or bow-tie atrophy that occurs with loss of nasal macular and peripheral fibers in the contralateral eye of a patient with a pregeniculate homonymous hemianopia or a bitemporal hemianopia. A = atrophic optic disc regions. (Miller NR, Fine SL. *The Ocular Fundus in Neuro-Ophthalmologic Diagnosis.* St Louis: Mosby; 1977.)

FIG III-15—Artist's drawing showing pattern of nerve fiber loss and optic atrophy as a result of damage to fibers from ganglion cells temporal to the fovea in the ipsilateral eye of a patient with a pregeniculate homonymous hemianopia. A = atrophic optic disc regions. (Miller NR, Fine SL. *The Ocular Fundus in Neuro-Ophthalmologic Diagnosis.* St Louis: Mosby; 1977.)

in the temporal or parietal lobes. These symptoms and signs become particularly important in pinpointing a complete homonymous hemianopia, which is not localizing to any specific portion of the retrochiasmal visual pathway. Temporal lobe lesions often cause seizures and formed visual hallucinations. Parietal lobe lesions may be associated with hemiparesis, visual perceptual difficulty, agnosia, and apraxia. Lesions of the dominant parietal lobe are the cause of Gerstmann syndrome, a combination of acalculia, agraphia, finger agnosia, and left-right confusion.

Abnormalities in optokinetic nystagmus may occur if pursuit pathways that converge in the posterior cerebral hemisphere are damaged. If these pathways are affected, the OKN responses are abnormal when targets are rotated toward the lesion (opposite the hemianopia). The combination of a homonymous hemianopia and an OKN asymmetry or a smooth pursuit deficit suggests a deep posterior parietal lobe lesion. On rare occasions, occipital lobe lesions also may cause OKN.

As they draw closer to the primary visual cortex, fibers in the optic radiations that serve common retinal points in each eye come into more precise retinotopic alignment. For this reason, lesions of the distal optic radiations or the primary visual cortex produce more congruous homonymous field defects than do lesions of the proximal optic radiations. Lesions of the occipital cortex may cause a homonymous hemianopia with macular sparing. A macula-sparing homonymous hemianopia suggests a stroke involving the portion of the primary visual cortex supplied by the posterior cerebral artery. The tip of the occipital lobe receives a dual blood supply from both the middle cerebral artery and the posterior cerebral artery. After occlusion of the posterior cerebral artery, the primary visual cortex is destroyed, except for the region representing the macula at the posterior tip of the occipital lobe. This region remains perfused by the middle cerebral artery, thus sparing the macula. In some patients there is no collateral flow to the macular representation from the middle cerebral artery. In such individuals stroke involving the posterior cerebral artery causes a macula-splitting hemianopia.

In addition to macular sparing, several other characteristic patterns of visual field loss are classically associated with occipital lobe lesions.

Checkerboard field   This pattern is caused by bilateral, incomplete homonymous hemianopias, superior on one side and inferior on the opposite side; for example, a right upper homonymous quadrantic field defect combined with a left lower homonymous quadrantic field defect.

Bilateral homonymous hemianopia with bilateral macular sparing (keyhole field) Although the keyhole appears to be a true tubular field, careful visual field testing will show that it does expand when tested at different distances from a tangent screen. In addition, a step or notch can be found across the vertical midline at the upper and lower boundaries of the preserved central field, because the damage to each occipital lobe is not perfectly symmetrical.

Bilateral homonymous altitudinal defects   These defects are caused by infarction or trauma to both occipital lobes above or below the calcarine fissure; they can be either inferior or superior.

Cerebral blindness   This rare syndrome of blindness, also known as *cortical blindness,* results from bilateral occipital lobe destruction. Normal pupillary responses distinguish it from total blindness caused by bilateral prechiasmal lesions. Anton syndrome (denial of blindness) is classically associated with cerebral blindness, but it can occur from a lesion at any level of the visual system severe enough to cause blindness (e.g., bilateral, advanced cataracts). Patients with bilateral occipital lobe lesions occasionally have some residual visual function. Usually this preserved vision is a result of incomplete destruction of the primary visual cortex in each occipital lobe.

Another syndrome called *blindsight* refers to a rudimentary visual capacity that survives total bilateral destruction of primary visual cortex. This visual function may result from preservation of subcortical visual areas (e.g., the superior colliculus) or projections from the LGB and pulvinar that go directly to V2 without being processed first in V1. Unfortunately, blindsight is insufficient for any sustained or useful visual function after destruction of the primary visual cortex.

Lesions of the primary visual cortex may also produce *unformed visual hallucinations* from tumors, migraine, or drugs. *Formed hallucinations* are usually attributed to irritation of the extrastriate cortex.

Patients with cortical injury may sometimes perceive moving targets but not static ones; this *Riddoch phenomenon* may also occur with lesions in other parts of the visual pathway. The phenomenon probably reflects the fact that cells in the visual system respond better to moving stimuli than to static stimuli.

Riddoch G. Dissociation of visual perceptions due to occipital injuries, with especial reference to appreciation of movement. *Brain.* 1917;40:15–57.

Sanders MD, Warrington EK, Marshall J, et al. "Blindsight": Vision in a field defect. *Lancet.* 1974;1(860):707–708.

Summary

The previous sections have described visual field defects characteristic of lesions at different levels of the anterior and posterior visual systems. From these descriptions the following generalizations should be stressed:

☐ Retinal lesions, especially those involving the outer retina, cause visual field defects that correspond to the site of pathology visible upon fundus examination.

☐ Optic nerve lesions produce monocular field defects that generally do not respect the vertical midline. Optic disc lesions and retinal vascular occlusions often produce defects that respect the nasal horizontal meridian.

☐ Bitemporal hemianopias are produced by lesions involving the optic chiasm.

☐ Binasal defects occur from bilateral retinal or optic nerve lesions and, rarely, from compression of the lateral aspects of the optic chiasm.

☐ Lesions posterior to the optic chiasm cause homonymous visual field defects that respect the vertical midline. Temporal crescent syndrome is the only exception.

☐ A complete homonymous hemianopia is nonlocalizing. A CT scan or MRI should be obtained to pinpoint the locus and nature of the process responsible for the visual field defect.

☐ Visual acuity is never reduced by a unilateral lesion posterior to the optic chiasm (the patient can see 20/20 with a macula-splitting hemianopia).

☐ Visual field defects produced by lesions in the temporal lobe tend to be denser superiorly, while visual field defects produced by lesions in the parietal lobe tend to be denser inferiorly.

☐ Parietal lobe hemianopias may be associated with optokinetic nystagmus asymmetry.

☐ Occipital lobe hemianopias may be associated with macular sparing.

☐ Stroke causes 90% of isolated homonymous hemianopias.

> Trobe JD, Lorber ML, Schlezinger NS. Isolated homonymous hemianopia. A review of 104 cases. *Arch Ophthalmol.* 1973;89:377–381.

Pathology

Optic Disc Edema

Regardless of etiology, most forms of optic disc swelling share a similar pathophysiology. Histologically, the nerve fibers anterior to the lamina cribrosa become swollen from congestive peripapillary retinal changes and associated crowding in the optic disc and retina.

Obstruction of axoplasmic transport contributes to swelling of the optic disc. *Orthograde transport* takes place when axons in the optic nerve transport material from the somata of retinal ganglion cells to their terminals in the lateral geniculate body. *Retrograde transport* occurs from the LGB terminals back to the somata in the retina. Orthograde axoplasmic transport consists of both fast and slow components. The slow component transports axoplasm at about 2 mm/day, while the fast component moves at a rate of about 500 mm/day.

The following are among the mechanisms that may produce a blockage of axoplasmic flow in the optic nerve:

□ Ischemia

□ Inflammation

□ Raised intracranial pressure

□ Compression from a mass lesion

The blockage occurs usually at the level of the lamina choroidalis or lamina scleralis. The cessation of axoplasmic transport, particularly the rapid component, at the lamina cribrosa is a consistent finding in optic disc edema.

Venous obstruction with dilation of optic disc surface capillaries, distension and tortuosity of retinal veins, and superficial nerve fiber layer hemorrhages also develops with optic disc swelling. Table III-2 lists the mechanical and vascular clinical signs of optic disc edema that can be seen by direct ophthalmoscopy.

Hayreh SS. Pathogenesis of oedema of the optic disc. *Br J Ophthalmol.* 1964;48: 522–543.

Minckler DS, Tso MO, Zimmerman LE. A light microscopic, autoradiographic study of axoplasmic transport in the optic nerve head during ocular hypotony, increased intraocular pressure, and papilledema. *Am J Ophthalmol.* 1976;82:741–757.

Despite the common histopathologic and physiologic features shared by many forms of optic disc swelling, it is essential to identify the cause of optic disc swelling since the management differs greatly depending on the etiology. For all etiologies, optic disc edema may be early, fully developed, chronic, or late.

Frisen L. Swelling of the optic nerve head: a staging scheme. *J Neurol Neurosurg Psychiatry.* 1982;45:13–18.

TABLE III-2

SIGNS OF OPTIC DISC EDEMA

Mechanical signs

Elevation of the optic nerve head (3 diopters = 1 mm)
Blurring of the optic disc margins
Filling in of the physiological cup
Edema of the peripapillary nerve fiber layer
Retinal and/or choroidal folds

Vascular signs

Hyperemia of the optic disc
Venous dilation and tortuosity
Peripapillary hemorrhages
Exudates in the disc or peripapillary area
Nerve fiber layer infarcts

Papilledema The term *papilledema* should be used only when referring to disc swelling produced by increased intracranial pressure (Fig III-16). Early signs include the following:

◻ Swelling of the peripapillary nerve fiber layer

◻ Congestion of capillaries on the disc surface

◻ Dilated veins

◻ Loss of venous pulsations (however, 20% of normal patients have no spontaneous venous pulsations)

◻ Flame-shaped hemorrhages at the disc margin

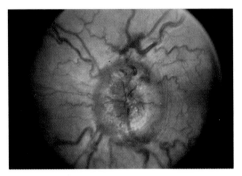

FIG III-16—Papilledema in a patient with pseudotumor cerebri.

The degree of disc swelling in papilledema is often asymmetric. Rarely, increased intracranial pressure causes papilledema in only one eye. As papilledema progresses, hemorrhages and cotton-wool spots on the disc become more prominent, the disc becomes more elevated, and swelling of the nerve fiber layer obscures the vessels at the disc margin. The peripapillary retina exhibits radial or concentric folds (Paton's lines) as it is pushed aside by swollen disc tissue. Venous dilation and tortuosity become prominent.

As papilledema becomes chronic, disc elevation persists, but hemorrhages and exudates resolve, and venous dilation decreases. Occasionally, chronic papilledema progresses to chronic atrophic papilledema, and the appearance of the disc changes. Disc elevation decreases; hyperemia gives way to pallor; small, glittering *pseudodrusen* appear on the surface of the disc; and retinal vessels become narrow. Loss of visual function often occurs and blindness may result.

In acute papilledema visual acuity is usually normal unless the macula is involved by exudate, edema, or hemorrhage. Color vision and pupillary responses are also normal. The visual field generally shows only an enlargement of the blind spot. Loss of visual field in severe or chronic papilledema may be peripheral, generalized, or sectorial. Occasionally, a superimposed ischemic optic neuropathy can cause sudden visual loss.

Other associated visual symptoms in patients with increased intracranial pressure include diplopia and transient visual obscurations. Diplopia occurs as a result of unilateral or bilateral sixth nerve paresis, probably caused by shifting of the brain stem with secondary stretching of the sixth nerve in the posterior fossa. Transient visual obscurations from disc edema are episodes of unilateral or bilateral visual loss lasting seconds that may occur many times daily. They occur more frequently with orthostatic changes. Increased intracranial pressure also causes headache, nausea, and vomiting.

All patients with suspected papilledema should be evaluated immediately for the underlying cause. After the history and physical examination, including blood pressure measurement to exclude hypertensive optic disc swelling, a contrast-enhanced MRI or CT scan of the head should be done. If neuroimaging shows no mass, a lumbar puncture should follow. Common causes of papilledema in adults are metastatic and primary intracranial tumors, infectious meningitis, carcinomatous meningitis, and pseudotumor cerebri; in children, posterior fossa tumors must be ruled out.

Sadun AA, Currie JN, Lessell S. Transient visual obscurations with elevated optic discs. *Ann Neurol.* 1984;16:489–494.

Pseudotumor cerebri (idiopathic intracranial hypertension) The diagnosis of pseudotumor cerebri is based on the following criteria:

☐ Normal head imaging scan, except for small ventricles in some patients

☐ Increased intracranial pressure as measured on lumbar puncture

☐ Normal cerebrospinal fluid composition

Although the age range of patients with this disease includes young children, the peak incidence occurs in the third decade of life. There is a strong female preponderance, and most patients are overweight. Presenting symptoms are severe headache and disturbances in vision such as diplopia, visual field loss, or transient obscurations. Some patients may complain of pulsatile tinnitus or dizziness. The headache may be worse when the patient is recumbent; nausea and vomiting may also occur.

The etiology of the increased intracranial pressure in patients with pseudotumor cerebri remains obscure. Although hormonal abnormalities have been implicated, no definite association between pseudotumor cerebri and a specific endocrinologic dysfunction has been established. The absorption of cerebrospinal fluid across the arachnoid granulations into the dural venous sinuses is probably impaired, but the mechanism for this defect is unknown. Raised intracranial pressure can also occur from chronic obstructive pulmonary disease; radical neck dissection; corticosteroid use or withdrawal; or use of medications such as vitamin A, tetracycline, and nalidixic acid.

Thrombosis of a dural venous sinus is an occasional cause of increased intracranial pressure. This process can occur following trauma, childbirth, spontaneous or induced abortion, or middle ear infection or in the context of a hypercoagulable state. If standard neuroimaging is negative in a patient with suspected papilledema, an MR venogram of the dural venous sinuses may be worthwhile to investigate the possibility of a clot, especially if the patient does not fit the profile of a typical pseudotumor cerebri patient (young obese female).

Pseudotumor cerebri may be either a short, self-limited process or a chronic disease. Treatment is required if the patient has headache or visual loss. No controlled studies have compared the various possible treatment modalities. The first step for the obese patient is to start a weight control program. Initial medical management generally consists of acetazolamide (Diamox) or furosemide (Lasix). Acetazolamide is probably more effective because it inhibits carbonic anhydrase, the enzyme responsible for production of cerebrospinal fluid. The use of corticosteroids is controversial. Although elevated intracranial pressure is frequently decreased with steroids, it may recur in many patients when the steroids are tapered. In addition, overweight patients with pseudotumor cerebri are poor candidates for chronic steroid use. However, a short course of high-dosage steroids can be useful in cases of acute visual loss from fulminant papilledema. In such cases surgery should be undertaken immediately to relieve the papilledema. Repeat lumbar punctures are theoretically effective in lowering intracranial pressure, but this approach is limited because it provides only temporary pressure reduction, technical difficulties arise in performing spinal taps in obese patients, and patients dislike multiple spinal taps.

If visual field loss occurs despite the patient's efforts to lose weight and treatment with acetazolamide, a surgical procedure is indicated. The alternatives are optic nerve sheath decompression and lumbar-peritoneal shunt. Both procedures have distinct advantages and disadvantages. Optic nerve sheath decompression carries a 1%–2% risk of blindness from optic nerve injury, central retinal artery occlusion, or central retinal vein occlusion during surgery. A lumbar-peritoneal shunt may occlude, become infected, or overshunt, causing low-pressure headaches. However, shunting entails no direct risk to the optic nerve, is probably more effective for headache relief, and will simultaneously treat a sixth nerve paresis, if present. The choice of procedure must be discussed with the patient.

The ophthalmologist must take an active role in following the patient with pseudotumor cerebri and in monitoring all parameters of optic nerve function. Quantitative perimetry should be done at regular intervals in order to detect any early signs of optic neuropathy. The frequency of visual field testing depends on the severity of papilledema and its response to treatment. Visual acuity, color vision, and contrast sensitivity functions are also useful monitoring tests (see chapter I). Fundus photographs can help the clinician document changes in disc appearance.

Remember that pseudotumor cerebri is a diagnosis of exclusion. All patients with papilledema should be considered to have an intracranial mass until proven otherwise.

Corbett JJ. Problems in the diagnosis and treatment of pseudotumor cerebri. *Can J Neurol Sci.* 1983;10:221–229.

Corbett JJ, Nerad JA, Tse DT, et al. Results of optic nerve sheath fenestration for pseudotumor cerebri: The lateral orbitotomy approach. *Arch Ophthalmol.* 1988;106:1391–1397.

Corbett JJ, Savino PJ, Thompson HS, et al. Visual loss in pseudotumor cerebri. Follow-up of 57 patients from five to 41 years and a profile of 14 patients with permanent severe visual loss. *Arch Neurol.* 1982;39:461–474.

Keltner JL. Optic nerve sheath decompression. How does it work? Has its time come? *Arch Ophthalmol.* 1988;106:1365–1369.

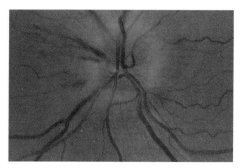

FIG III-17—Anterior ischemic optic neuropathy.

Keltner JL, Miller NR, Gittinger JW, et al. Pseudotumor cerebri. *Surv Ophthalmol.* 1979;23:315–322.

Pearson PA, Baker RS, Khorram D, et al. Evaluation of optic nerve sheath fenestration in pseudotumor cerebri using automated perimetry. *Ophthalmology.* 1991;98:99–105.

Wall M, George D. Idiopathic intracranial hypertension. A prospective study of 50 patients. *Brain.* 1991;114:155–180.

Anterior Ischemic Optic Neuropathy

Anterior ischemic optic neuropathy (AION) is an infarction of the optic nerve head caused by inadequate perfusion by the posterior ciliary arteries (Fig III-17). AION occurs in two forms: *arteritic* (related to giant cell arteritis) and *nonarteritic*. It is crucial to differentiate between these two forms of AION, because the management and implications are entirely different.

Onset of AION is sudden and usually painless. Vision loss is usually abrupt without further change, but deterioration may progress over several days or weeks. Visual acuity varies from 20/20 to no light perception, and altitudinal, arcuate, or central visual field defects are typical (Fig III-18). Examination shows an optic disc that is swollen, often with nerve fiber layer hemorrhages. Exudates can occur but are uncommon. In many cases, only part of the disc is swollen. The patient's relative age, lack of pain, and limited recovery of vision help to distinguish this condition from optic neuritis.

Arteritic anterior ischemic optic neuropathy   This condition occurs in *giant cell*, or *temporal*, *arteritis*, a generalized inflammatory disease of large and medium-sized arteries that develops almost exclusively in patients older than 55 and affects women about twice as often as men. The incidence of the disease rises rapidly with advancing age. Vessels of many organ systems may be involved, including renal, hepatic, mesenteric, coronary, and, rarely, intracranial arteries. Ocular involvement is generally associated with an inflammatory process of the posterior ciliary arteries. Histological examination shows a granulomatous inflammation with epithelioid cells, lymphocytes, giant cells, and disruption of the elastic lamina (Fig III-19). It has been postulated that giant cell arteritis is primarily a disease of smooth muscle cells of larger arteries, although the exact pathogenesis remains obscure.

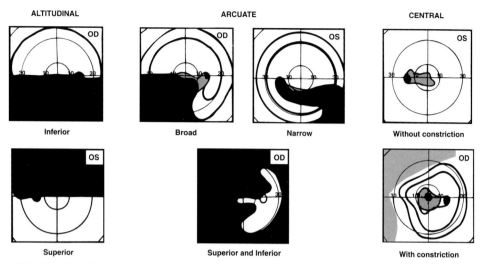

ALTITUDINAL	ARCUATE		CENTRAL

Inferior / Broad / Narrow / Without constriction

Superior / Superior and Inferior / With constriction

FIG III-18—Visual field defects in nonarteritic anterior ischemic optic neuropathy. (Reprinted from Miller NR, ed. *Walsh and Hoyt's Clinical Neuro-Ophthalmology.* 4th ed. Volume 1. Baltimore: Williams & Wilkins; 1995:213.)

Systemic features of the disease include the following:

□ Malaise

□ Weight loss

□ Fever

□ Scalp pain

□ Headache

□ Tenderness or aching of muscles and joints (polymyalgia rheumatica)

□ Tenderness over the temporal arteries

□ Ear pain

□ Jaw claudication

Occult giant cell arteritis (AION without systemic features) occurs occasionally. Therefore, the diagnosis of giant cell arteritis should be considered in all elderly patients with AION. Ocular symptoms include amaurosis fugax, sudden visual loss (either partial or complete), and diplopia. Visual loss is usually caused by AION; however, central retinal artery occlusion or ocular ischemic syndrome may also be present. Cerebral blindness has been reported. Diplopia may be a result of involvement of either the small arteries supplying the extraocular muscles within the orbit or of the vasa nervorum of the ocular motor nerves.

Patients with giant cell arteritis usually come to the attention of the ophthalmologist after the onset of visual loss in one eye. When one eye is involved by AION, the second eye is at great risk for visual loss in untreated patients. Involvement of the second eye usually occurs within 6 weeks, and often within a few days. Failure

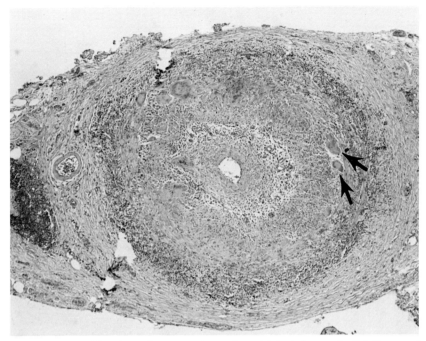

FIG III-19—Typical histologic changes in giant cell arteritis include round cell infiltrate and epithelioid cells in adventitia and media, loss of architecture in media, giant cells (arrows) lined up along the fractured internal elastic lamina at the junction between the media and intima, and thickened edematous intima with decreased size of lumen. (Reprinted from Cohen DN, Smith TR. Skip areas in temporal arteritis: Myth versus fact. *Trans Am Acad Ophthalmol Otolaryngol.* 1974;78:772–783.)

to diagnose and treat giant cell arteritis immediately after loss of vision in one eye is particularly tragic, since timely treatment with corticosteroids usually prevents an attack in the second eye. Giant cell arteritis should be managed as an ophthalmic emergency.

Giant cell arteritis may be suspected on the basis of clinical symptoms and signs and abnormal laboratory studies, but a temporal artery biopsy is necessary to firmly establish the diagnosis. Patients in the appropriate age group with AION should be questioned about the classic symptoms listed above. The temporal artery is examined for tenderness and a decreased pulse. A Westergren method erythrocyte sedimentation rate (ESR) should be obtained. It is often markedly elevated, but it may be normal in about 10% of patients. The ESR normally increases with age and is higher in women than in men. The normal value for this test can be approximated by dividing the age by 2 in men or adding 10 to the age before dividing by 2 in women. An extremely elevated ESR (e.g., greater than 80 mm/hr) should arouse a high degree of suspicion for giant cell arteritis. A second laboratory test of value is the hematocrit; patients with giant cell arteritis may have anemia of chronic illness. The lower the hematocrit, the higher the ESR; therefore, a patient with giant cell arteritis who is not yet anemic is likely to have a less elevated ESR.

The patient with AION who has no signs or symptoms suggesting giant cell arteritis and shows a normal ESR does not need a biopsy. However, if signs and symptoms of giant cell arteritis are present, or the ESR is elevated in an older patient, a temporal artery biopsy should be performed. In older patients presenting with bilateral, simultaneous AION, a temporal artery biopsy should be strongly considered, regardless of clinical symptoms and ESR.

Once the diagnosis of giant cell arteritis is suspected, therapy should be instituted immediately. A dosage of 60–120 mg of prednisone should be administered orally with consideration given to IV corticosteroid therapy for the first 48 hours. Corticosteroids should be given daily; an alternate-day regimen runs the risk of an infarction on the nontreatment day. Following institution of therapy, the patient should be followed for changes in ESR, symptoms, and signs. It is important to note that a temporal artery remains positive histopathologically for at least 2 weeks after corticosteroids are instituted. Therefore, in a patient with suspected giant cell arteritis, corticosteroids should be started immediately without waiting for the temporal artery biopsy, which can be done shortly after the start of therapy.

Because small segments of temporal artery may be normal in giant cell arteritis, the biopsy specimen should be at least 3 cm long. If the biopsy is negative (and serial sections have been examined) but corticosteroid therapy has resulted in marked improvement in symptoms and the ESR, the clinician should consider a biopsy of the opposite artery. If an adequate specimen of temporal artery is examined thoroughly on either side, and both biopsies are negative, the likelihood of giant cell arteritis is extremely low. Biopsy-negative cases do occur, but they are rare. The biopsy technique is described in the Brennan reference below.

Because of the severe systemic effects of giant cell arteritis, as well as the potential side effects of corticosteroid treatment, patients should be followed closely, not only by an ophthalmologist, but also by a primary care physician.

Brennan J, McCrary JA 3rd. Diagnosis of superficial temporal arteritis. *Ann Ophthalmol.* 1975;7:1125–1129.

Hayreh SS. Anterior ischaemic optic neuropathy: differentiation of arteritic from non-arteritic type and its management. *Eye.* 1990;4:25–41.

Hayreh SS, Podhajsky PA, Raman R, et al. Giant cell arteritis: validity and reliability of various diagnostic criteria. *Am J Ophthalmol.* 1997;123:285–296.

Hedges TR 3rd, Gieger GL, Albert DM. The clinical value of negative temporal artery biopsy specimens. *Arch Ophthalmol.* 1983;101:1251–1254.

Kansu T, Corbett JJ, Savino P, et al. Giant cell arteritis with normal sedimentation rate. *Arch Neurol.* 1977;34:624–625.

Keltner JL. Giant-cell arteritis. Signs and symptoms. *Ophthalmology.* 1982;89:1101–1110.

Nonarteritic anterior ischemic optic neuropathy   Patients with nonarteritic AION tend to be younger than those with giant cell arteritis, and they generally have less severe visual loss. Hypertension is present in approximately 50% of cases and diabetes mellitus in 25% of cases. Although incidence of cerebrovascular and cardiac disease is greater than expected, patients with this condition are generally in good health, and studies have not shown that life expectancy is shortened significantly. In contrast, patients with retinal artery disease (central retinal artery occlusion, branch retinal artery occlusion, and amaurosis fugax) have a high incidence of early death as well as cardiac and cerebrovascular disease.

Recurrence of ischemic optic neuropathy in the same eye is rare. The second eye, however, becomes involved in approximately 25% of cases over time. No treatment is known to be efficacious. Some studies have suggested that in the 5%–10% of cases showing further visual loss in a stepwise progression over the subsequent 2–3 weeks (progressive AION), optic nerve sheath decompression (ONSD) surgery may be beneficial. However, a masked, multicenter, prospective trial has shown that surgical treatment of AION is not effective. In 43% of untreated patients with nonarteritic AION, three lines or more of spontaneous improvement in vision occurred within 6 months of the event. This rate of spontaneous improvement was greater than anticipated and probably explains the initial reports that surgery might be efficacious. The etiology of nonarteritic AION remains unclear. Although vascular risk factors are important, crowding of the optic disc may also be a significant factor. Several studies have shown a smaller than normal cup/disc ratio in patients with nonarteritic AION.

Beck RW, Servais GE, Hayreh SS. Anterior ischemic optic neuropathy. IX. Cup-to-disc ratio and its role in pathogenesis. *Ophthalmology.* 1987;94:1503–1508.

Boghen DR, Glaser JS. Ischemic optic neuropathy. The clinical profile and history. *Brain.* 1975;98:689–708.

Doro S, Lessell S. Cup-disc ratio and ischemic optic neuropathy. *Arch Ophthalmol.* 1985;103:1143–1144.

Guyer DR, Miller NR, Auer CL, et al. The risk of cerebrovascular and cardiovascular disease in patients with anterior ischemic optic neuropathy. *Arch Ophthalmol.* 1985;103:1136–1142.

Hayreh SS, Sergott RC, Cohen MS, et al. The role of optic nerve sheath fenestration in management of anterior ischemic optic neuropathy. *Arch Ophthalmol.* 1990;108: 1063–1065.

The Ischemic Optic Neuropathy Decompression Trial Research Group. Optic nerve decompression surgery for nonarteritic anterior ischemic optic neuropathy (NAION) is not effective and may be harmful. *JAMA.* 1995;273:625–632.

The Ischemic Optic Neuropathy Decompression Trial Study Group. Characteristics of patients with nonarteritic anterior ischemic optic neuropathy eligible for the Ischemic Optic Neuropathy Decompression Trial. *Arch Ophthalmol.* 1996;114:1366–1374.

Repka MX, Savino PJ, Schatz NJ, et al. Clinical profile and long-term implications of anterior ischemic optic neuropathy. *Am J Ophthalmol.* 1983;96:478–483.

Sergott RC, Cohen MS, Bosley TM, et al. Optic nerve decompression may improve the progressive form of nonarteritic ischemic optic neuropathy. *Arch Ophthalmol.* 1989;107:1743–1754.

Posterior Ischemic Optic Neuropathy

Posterior ischemic optic neuropathy is a term that refers to ischemic damage to the retrobulbar optic nerve. It is a rare condition, occurring almost exclusively in the setting of severe anemia and hypotension. For example, cases have been reported after major blood loss from surgery, exsanguinating trauma, gastrointestinal bleeding, and renal dialysis. Under these circumstances, both eyes are often affected. The fundus usually appears normal, although optic disc edema may develop if the ischemic process extends far enough anteriorly. Treatment consists of prompt transfusion of blood and reversal of hypotension.

Optic Neuritis

Optic neuritis is characterized by acute or subacute visual loss, often associated with retrobulbar pain or pain with eye movement. It usually affects patients 15–45 years of age, predominately women. Generally the condition is unilateral and accompanied by loss of visual acuity, decreased color vision, and a central scotoma in the affected eye. Brightness sense is diminished, and paracentral scotomata, arcuate field defects, and altitudinal field loss can occur. An afferent pupillary defect almost invariably appears in the acute phase. In two thirds of patients the site of optic nerve inflammation is retrobulbar, and the optic disc appears normal on initial examination. In the remaining third of patients the inflammatory process is anterior, and optic nerve swelling (*papillitis*) is visible on fundus examination.

The clinical course is characterized by steadily worsening vision, which reaches its nadir by about 1 week before stabilizing. Acuity may vary from 20/20 to no light perception. Most patients recover vision gradually over several months. Recovery to 20/20 occurs in 71% of patients receiving no treatment beyond observation and to 20/40 or better in 95% of such patients within 1 year after an attack. Even with recovery to 20/20, however, patients may experience residual abnormalities in brightness sense, and abnormalities in pupillary reaction, optic disc appearance, color vision, contrast sensitivity, visually evoked cortical potential, and stereopsis may persist. *Uhthoff's phenomenon* (transient decrease in vision after exercise or elevation of body temperature) occurs in at least one half of patients after recovery.

Diagnosis   The diagnosis of optic neuritis rests principally upon the patient's history and clinical findings, despite the availability of neuroimaging and laboratory studies. Evaluation of optic neuritis should include a complete eye examination, including visual field testing of both eyes, with emphasis on optic nerve function (pupils, color and brightness sense). The history should include questions about recent viral illness, family history of visual loss or multiple sclerosis (MS), and past episodes of neurologic dysfunction. No laboratory evaluation is necessary in a typical case of optic neuritis. A CT scan or MRI of the head and orbits should be done if the history or examination is atypical of acute optic neuritis or if the clinician is contemplating treatment that may alter the natural history of the disease (see discussion below about corticosteroid therapy). Optic neuritis may cause thickening of the nerve on imaging studies; therefore, fat-suppressed gadolinium-enhanced MRI studies give the best results (see chapter II).

Other conditions that should be considered in the differential diagnosis of optic neuritis include the following:

- Retinal disorders, especially central serous retinopathy
- Big blind spot syndrome
- Multiple evanescent white dot syndrome
- Anterior ischemic optic neuropathy
- Syphilitic optic neuritis
- Postviral optic neuritis
- Leber hereditary optic neuropathy
- Nutritional optic neuropathy
- Toxic optic neuropathy
- Malignant optic glioma
- Other compressive lesions

Optic neuritis in children differs from the condition in adults. It is frequently bilateral and may be associated with meningoencephalitis. The etiology is usually postviral and not associated with multiple sclerosis.

Multiple sclerosis   Optic neuritis is associated with multiple sclerosis. Years ago it was thought that about one third of optic neuritis patients would go on to develop neurologic symptoms from MS. More recent long-term studies indicate that over decades the risk of developing MS is much higher, more than 60%. The likelihood of developing MS may be greater for women than men and greater when optic neuritis occurs at a younger age. Evidence of optic nerve disease appears in most patients with long-standing MS, but only 55% of these patients have clear-cut clinical episodes of optic neuritis. Isolated optic neuritis may represent a forme fruste of multiple sclerosis. MRI abnormalities in the brain are found in about half of patients with clinically isolated optic neuritis. There is, however, no definitive diagnostic laboratory test for MS, and many patients with plaques on MRI do not have neurologic signs or symptoms.

Treatment   The efficacy of corticosteroid therapy in optic neuritis has been controversial. The Optic Neuritis Treatment Trial, a large, multicenter prospective study conducted from 1988 to 1991 with yearly follow-up, has provided new data regarding this issue. Patients treated with oral prednisone did not have a better outcome than those treated with a placebo. Surprisingly, the patients who received oral prednisone appeared to have an increased rate of recurrent optic neuritis. These results show that treatment with oral prednisone is of no benefit for typical cases of optic neuritis and may even predispose patients to further attacks. Administration of high-dose IV methylprednisolone (250 mg qid for 3 days) followed by oral prednisone (1 mg/kg/day for 11 days) led to a slightly faster recovery of visual function, but the final visual acuity of these patients after 6 months did not differ significantly from that of placebo-treated patients.

Intravenous methylprednisolone treatment followed by oral prednisone was associated with a reduced rate of development of multiple sclerosis over a 2-year follow-up period, especially in the subgroup of patients with two or more foci of demyelination on MRI. However, by the end of a 3-year follow-up period, comparison of IV corticosteroid and placebo groups showed no significant difference in the rate of development of MS. Moreover, IV corticosteroids did not reduce the likelihood of subsequent attacks of optic neuritis.

On the basis of this study, an MRI in all patients with optic neuritis has been recommended by the Optic Neuritis Study Group. If two or more MRI foci of demyelination are found, or if visual loss is severe, IV corticosteroids are prescribed. The two potential benefits of IV corticosteroids are a slightly faster recovery of visual function and a reduction in the subsequent risk of neurologic events leading to a diagnosis of MS. Critics of the Optic Neuritis Treatment Trial have questioned this recommendation, pointing out that the conclusions pertaining to the risk of eventual MS are based upon the outcome in a rather small number of patients. In addition, the protective effects attributed to corticosteroids are no longer apparent by 3 years after treatment. Risks of corticosteroid treatment, although low, include acute psychosis, induced diabetes, and acute pancreatitis. The decision to obtain an MRI or to treat optic neuritis with IV corticosteroids must be shared by the clinician with the patient after a detailed discussion of these issues.

Corticosteroids can mask optic neuropathies that are caused by other etiologies. Steroid-responsive conditions that mimic optic neuritis include pituitary adenoma, craniopharyngioma, meningioma, medulloblastoma, plasmacytoma, optic nerve glioma, meningeal carcinomatosis, sarcoidosis, and photoreceptor degeneration as a remote effect of cancer.

Beck RW, Cleary PA, Anderson MM Jr, et al. A randomized, controlled trial of corticosteroids in the treatment of acute optic neuritis. The Optic Neuritis Study Group. *N Engl J Med.* 1992;326:581–588.

Beck RW, Cleary PA, Trobe JD, et al. The effect of corticosteroids for acute optic neuritis on the subsequent development of multiple sclerosis. The Optic Neuritis Study Group. *N Engl J Med.* 1993;329:1764–1769.

Optic Neuritis Study Group. The clinical profile of optic neuritis. Experience of the Optic Neuritis Treatment Trial. *Arch Ophthalmol.* 1991;109:1673–1678.

Perkin GD, Rose FC. *Optic Neuritis and its Differential Diagnosis.* New York: Oxford University Press; 1979.

Rizzo JF 3rd, Lessell S. Optic neuritis and ischemic optic neuropathy: Overlapping clinical profiles. *Arch Ophthalmol.* 1991;109:1668–1672.

Rizzo JF 3rd, Lessell S. Risk of developing multiple sclerosis after uncomplicated optic neuritis: a long-term prospective study. *Neurology.* 1988;38:185–190.

Slamovits TL, Rosen CE, Cheng KP, et al. Visual recovery in patients with optic neuritis and visual loss to no light perception. *Am J Ophthalmol.* 1991;111:209–214.

Trobe JD. Managing optic neuritis: results of the Optic Neuritis Treatment Trial. In: *Focal Points: Clinical Modules for Ophthalmologists.* San Francisco: American Academy of Ophthalmology. 1994;12:2.

Compressive Optic Neuropathy

Slowly progressive visual loss associated with a central scotoma and an afferent pupillary defect characterizes compressive optic neuropathy caused by a mass lesion. Sudden visual loss is most unusual, except in rare instances when sudden expansion of a tumor by hemorrhage can cause acute loss of nerve function. For example, pituitary apoplexy can produce sudden visual loss, headache, and diplopia. It is important for the clinician to be aware that a patient may inaccurately report acute visual loss upon accidentally discovering chronic decreased vision in one eye.

The optic disc in compressive optic neuropathy may appear swollen if an optic nerve tumor, orbital mass, or thyroid ophthalmopathy exists, but usually the nerve appears normal or pale. All patients with evidence of optic nerve dysfunction and progressive visual loss should be presumed to have a compressive lesion until proven otherwise. Likewise, all patients with incidentally discovered optic atrophy should be evaluated for compressive etiology. Optic neuropathies that are cortico-steroid-dependent require a work-up for optic nerve compression. Compression can occur anywhere along the intraorbital, intracanalicular, or intracranial course of the optic nerve and thus can be caused by a variety of orbital or intracranial mass lesions.

Optic nerve glioma   Most cases of optic nerve glioma present in the first decade of life. About 20% of all childhood orbital tumors are gliomas of the optic nerve. From 10% to 50% of patients with optic nerve gliomas have neurofibromatosis, and about 15% of patients with neurofibromatosis have optic nerve glioma. Visual loss is the most common initial symptom; strabismus and nystagmus result from loss of vision. Optic gliomas may be intraorbital (50%) or intracranial (50%). With intraorbital gliomas proptosis is common. The optic nerve may appear swollen or pale, and an ipsilateral afferent pupillary defect accompanies other findings typical of optic neuropathy. Chiasmal gliomas sometimes produce endocrine dysfunction from hypothalamic involvement. The glioma grossly appears as a fusiform swelling of the optic nerve. Pathologically, the tumor is a pilocytic astrocytoma of juvenile type with a benign cytologic appearance, although mixed gliomas have been reported. The diagnosis of optic nerve glioma is based on clinical and radiological findings. Neuroimaging shows a characteristic fusiform thickening and kinking of the nerve in the orbit.

Borit A, Richardson EP Jr. The biological and clinical behaviour of pilocytic astrocytomas of the optic pathways. *Brain.* 1982;105:161–187.

Feldon SE. Tumors of the anterior visual pathways. In: Jakobiec FA, Albert DM, eds. *Principles and Practice of Ophthalmology.* Philadelphia: Saunders; 1994.

Imes RK, Hoyt WF. Magnetic resonance imaging signs of optic nerve gliomas in neurofibromatosis 1. *Am J Ophthalmol.* 1991;111:729–734.

Jakobiec FA, Depot MJ, Kennerdell JS, et al. Combined clinical and computed tomographic diagnosis of orbital glioma and meningioma. *Ophthalmology.* 1984;91:137–155.

Lewis RA, Gerson LP, Axelson KA, et al. von Recklinghausen neurofibromatosis. II. Incidence of optic gliomata. *Ophthalmology.* 1984;91:929–935.

Most gliomas grow very slowly or cease growing after childhood. There are, however, reports of intracranial extension, chiasmal involvement, and subsequent involvement of the contralateral optic nerve. Hence, treatment is controversial. Some authorities feel that surgical therapy is not indicated for orbital optic gliomas unless a cosmetically unacceptable proptosis appears in a blind eye. Others advocate surgical resection involving removal of the affected nerve when the tumor is limited to one optic nerve. There is little support for surgical resection when the chiasm is involved. Radiation therapy has been advocated by some authorities, and favorable results have been achieved with chemotherapy. When a chiasmal tumor is large enough to cause hydrocephalus by occluding ventricular foramina, shunting procedures are necessary.

Alvord EC Jr, Lofton S. Gliomas of the optic nerve or chiasm. Outcome by patients' age, tumor site, and treatment. *J Neurosurg.* 1988;68:85–98.

Hoyt WF, Baghdassarian SA. Optic glioma of childhood: Natural history and rationale for conservative management. *Br J Ophthalmol.* 1969;53:793–798.

Imes RK, Hoyt WF. Childhood chiasmal gliomas: Update on the fate of patients in the 1969 San Francisco study. *Br J Ophthalmol.* 1986;70:179–182.

Wallace MR, Marchuk DA, Andersen LB, et al. Type 1 neurofibromatosis gene: identification of a large transcript disrupted in three NF1 patients. *Science.* 1990;249: 181–186.

Wright JE, McDonald WI, Call NB. Management of optic nerve gliomas. *Br J Ophthalmol.* 1980;64:545–552.

Wulc AE, Bergin DJ, Barnes D, et al. Orbital optic nerve glioma in adult life. *Arch Ophthalmol.* 1989;107:1013–1016.

Malignant optic glioma. This condition is a rare form of optic nerve glioma that occurs primarily in adults. These patients have malignant gliomas that originate in or near the anterior visual pathways. They present with pain and visual loss in one eye, followed by visual loss in the other eye, complete blindness in 2–4 months, and death in 3–9 months.

Hoyt WF, Meshel LG, Lessell S, et al. Malignant optic glioma of adulthood. *Brain.* 1973;96:121–132.

Slamovits TL, Burde RM, Miller NR, et al. Progressive visual loss with normal examination. A conundrum. *Surv Ophthalmol.* 1986;30:251–257.

Optic nerve meningiomas

Of all meningiomas only about 1% involve the optic nerve sheath. Optic nerve meningiomas make up about 5% of orbital tumors. Orbital meningiomas may arise from ectopic nests of meningeal cells that then compress the optic nerve from one side. Classically, patients present with decreased vision, and proptosis and optic disc edema are common. Three times as many women are affected as men. Adults, usually 40–50 years of age, are affected much more commonly than children.

Meningiomas derive from the outer arachnoid. Histologically, they have psammoma bodies and the characteristic whorls of concentrically packed spindle cells.

Examination may show the classic triad of visual loss, optic atrophy, and optociliary shunt vessels (Fig III-20). The optociliary shunt vessels develop because of chronic compression of the central retinal vein. Although optociliary vessels are associated with optic nerve sheath meningiomas, they are actually more commonly seen in patients with old central retinal vein occlusions. Sphenoid wing–orbital meningiomas often produce fullness of the temporal orbital fossa and orbit. Orbital scanning may reveal either a mass or diffuse thickening of the optic nerve. Following contrast, axial CT scans or MRI may show abnormal enhancement of the periphery of the nerve, the so-called railroad-track sign. Coronal scans may show a bull's-eye appearance. The optic canal may be enlarged.

Optic nerve meningiomas grow very slowly, but inexorably, and they sometimes lead to blindness. Since meningiomas of the optic nerve sheath usually cannot be removed without sacrificing visual acuity, many clinicians think that the lesions should merely be followed unless radiologic evidence shows intracranial involvement. Such intracranial extension is rare. Some success has been reported

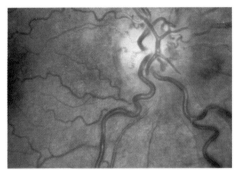

FIG III-20—Optic atrophy with numerous optociliary shunt veins. This patient has a long-standing
spheno-orbital meningioma.

from treating optic nerve meningiomas with radiation therapy. Meningiomas may
grow more rapidly during pregnancy and stabilize after delivery.

Frisen L, Hoyt WF, Tengroth BM. Optociliary veins, disc pallor and visual loss. A triad of
signs indicating spheno-orbital meningioma. *Acta Ophthalmol.* 1973;51:241–249.

Kennerdell JS, Maroon JC, Malton M, et al. The management of optic nerve sheath
meningiomas. *Am J Ophthalmol.* 1988;106:450–457.

Masuyama Y, Kodama Y, Matsuura Y, et al. Clinical studies on the occurrence and the
pathogenesis of optociliary veins. *J Clin Neuroophthalmol.* 1990;10:1–8.

Sibony PA, Krauss HR, Kennerdell JS, et al. Optic nerve sheath meningiomas. Clinical
manifestations. *Ophthalmology.* 1984;91:1313–1326.

Wilson WB. Meningiomas of the anterior visual system. *Surv Ophthalmol.* 1981;26:
109–127.

Infiltrative Optic Neuropathy

Disc swelling and visual loss may be caused by infiltration of the optic disc by
leukemias (monocytic, acute myelocytic, acute lymphocytic, chronic lymphocytic).
Lymphoma, plasmacytoma, and multiple myeloma may also infiltrate the optic
nerve. Infiltration of the nerve by metastatic carcinoma can produce visual
symptoms that antecede symptoms from the primary tumor. Infiltration of the optic
nerve head may also result from inflammatory and infectious conditions such as
sarcoidosis, tuberculosis, cryptococcosis, toxoplasmosis, toxocariasis, cytomegalovirus, or coccidioidomycosis. See chapter VIII for discussion of these conditions.

Following infiltration, the disc has an unusual appearance; it may appear
grayish white with associated hemorrhages, or a mass may be visible. Retrobulbar
infiltration can occur in lymphoreticular disease or meningeal carcinomatosis,
which represents metastasis to the meninges by cancer, usually originating from the
breast or lung. (See BCSC Section 4, *Ophthalmic Pathology and Intraocular Tumors,*
chapter V.) The optic nerve may be swollen as a consequence of several other

unusual primary tumors. For example, choristomas consisting of smooth muscle and fat and arachnoid cysts have been described within the optic nerve sheath.

Toxic/Nutritional Optic Neuropathy

Symmetrical bilateral optic neuropathies can occur from nutritional deficiency, tobacco-alcohol amblyopia, drugs, or toxins, or they may be a result of hereditary optic neuropathies. Specific etiologies include methanol, ethambutol, chloramphenicol, rifampin, and lead toxicity, as well as thiamine and vitamin B_{12} deficiency. Controversy remains concerning tobacco-alcohol amblyopia and whether it is a definite entity or represents a nutritional optic neuropathy. Generally, in all of these conditions the visual loss is gradually progressive and symmetrical. The classic field defect is a bilateral central or cecocentral scotoma. The optic disc may show subtle temporal pallor of the papillomacular bundle, and the nerve fiber layer may be thin or absent. If the cause is corrected, vision may recover to some extent.

Dominant Optic Neuropathy (Kjer Type)

Visual function in dominant optic neuropathy is moderately abnormal in both eyes, ranging from 20/25 to counting fingers but typically about 20/80. Onset is insidious and usually begins between 5 and 10 years of age. Slow progression of visual loss continues throughout life, but few patients deteriorate below a level of 20/800. Often a tritanopic color defect is demonstrable on the Farnsworth-Munsell 100-hue test. Central or cecocentral scotomata are the rule, but these may not be easy to find with routine testing. Striking temporal optic disc pallor is typical, often with focal excavation of the temporal disc.

Leber Hereditary Optic Neuropathy

This optic neuropathy affects men primarily. The age at onset of visual loss varies but is usually late teens to mid-20s; affected women tend to be older. Asymmetry of onset between the two eyes is usually days to weeks but may be months to years. Tobacco or alcohol use may trigger decompensation of an affected optic nerve. Cecocentral scotomata are the rule, and progression of visual loss is rapid. Vision improves months to years after onset of visual loss in 10%–20% of patients.

Ophthalmoscopic features help to make the diagnosis in the absence of a family history. In the acute phase the optic disc appears hyperemic, and the nerve fiber layer is prominent, giving the appearance of mild disc edema. Peripapillary telangiectasia occurs with dilation of small retinal capillaries. These vessels do not leak fluorescein but, rarely, can bleed. The large retinal vessels may appear tortuous. Optic atrophy develops later. When symptoms appear in the first eye, these ophthalmoscopic features may be noted in the still asymptomatic fellow eye.

Wallace has shown that Leber hereditary optic neuropathy is caused by a point mutation at codon 11778 in the mitochondrial gene encoding nicotinamide-adenine dinucleotide dehydrogenase (NADH), subunit 4 (see Singh reference on next page). Subsequently, additional mutations responsible for the disease have been identified, most in mitochondrial genes involved in oxidative phosphorylation. These findings suggest that the disease results from impairment of mitochrondrial enzymes involved in cellular energy metabolism.

The genetics of Leber hereditary optic neuropathy are peculiar. The defect is transmitted by mitochondrial DNA inherited from the mother, rather than from nuclear DNA. Men are predominantly affected, but no transmission takes place in the male line. Women transmit the disease to sons and the carrier state to daughters. It is not understood why female carriers infrequently develop visual symptoms from the disease. In some patients only a fraction of the mitochondria carry the mutation (heteroplasmy), and only when this fraction becomes high does the disease become clinically evident. No treatment has been shown to be effective.

The Cuba Neuropathy Field Investigation Team. Epidemic optic neuropathy in Cuba—clinical characterization and risk factors. *N Engl J Med.* 1995;333:1176–1182.

Johns DR. The molecular genetics of Leber's hereditary optic neuropathy. *Arch Ophthalmol.* 1990;108:1405–1407.

Kline LB, Glaser JS. Dominant optic atrophy. The clinical profile. *Arch Ophthalmol.* 1979;97:1680–1686.

Lott MT, Voljavec AS, Wallace DC. Variable genotype of Leber's hereditary optic neuropathy patients. *Am J Ophthalmol.* 1990;109:625–631.

Newman NJ, Wallace DC. Mitochondria and Leber's hereditary optic neuropathy. *Am J Ophthalmol.* 1990;109:726–730.

Nikoskelainen E, Hoyt WF, Nummelin K, et al. Fundus findings in Leber's hereditary optic neuroretinopathy. III. Fluorescein angiographic studies. *Arch Ophthalmol.* 1984;102:981–989.

Singh G, Lott MT, Wallace DC. A mitochondrial DNA mutation as a cause of Leber's hereditary optic neuropathy. *N Engl J Med.* 1989;320:1300–1305.

Smith JL, Hoyt WF, Susac JO. Ocular fundus in acute Leber optic neuropathy. *Arch Ophthalmol.* 1973;90:349–354.

Benign Papillophlebitis

This condition is characterized by unilateral disc swelling in young, otherwise healthy patients who generally have normal or nearly normal visual acuity, full visual field, and normal pupillary responses. There is often distension of retinal veins and nerve fiber layer hemorrhages. The etiology is unclear; it probably represents a partial or impending central retinal vein occlusion with disc swelling and congestion. Fluorescein angiography often shows impaired venous circulation. The optic disc edema either resolves without visual loss, or a frank central retinal vein occlusion may occur.

Optic Nerve Drusen

The word *drusen* comes from the German, meaning the crystals found in a geode. Optic nerve drusen are condensations of calcified hyaline-like material that develop within the substance of the optic nerve anterior to the lamina cribrosa. Their prevalence is 0.3%–1.0% clinically, 2.0% histopathologically, and they occur almost exclusively in whites. They are bilateral in 75%–80% of cases. The predisposition to drusen may be inherited as an autosomal dominant characteristic with incomplete penetrance. Optic disc drusen are associated with some forms of retinitis pigmentosa.

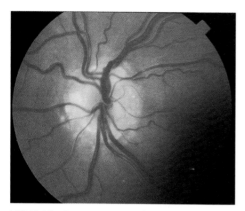

FIG III-21—Prominent optic disc drusen. Note the glistening crystal-like deposits bulging out from various parts of the optic disc. The disc is also raised, crowded, and lacks a physiologic cup.

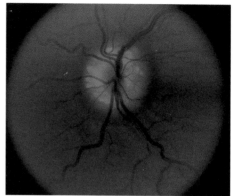

FIG III-22—"Fluorescein angiogram without fluorescein." When the standard barrier filters for a fluorescein angiogram are used, optic nerve drusen exhibit autofluorescence. However, this property is not of much diagnostic help, because buried drusen hidden within the optic disc substance do not exhibit autofluorescence, and exposed drusen can be seen simply with the ophthalmoscope. Compare to Figure III-21.

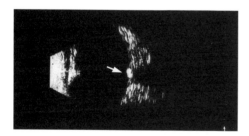

FIG III-23—B-scan ultrasound of the drusen (arrow) shown in Figure III-21. Drusen contain calcium and, therefore, appear bright on ultrasound, even with the gain turned low. This test is extremely useful for detecting buried drusen.

Superficial drusen appear as irregular, glistening yellow globules that may be isolated or clustered on or just below the surface of the optic nerve head. Superficial drusen are easily seen with the ophthalmoscope (Fig III-21), and they exhibit autofluorescence (Fig III-22). Deeper, buried drusen are not directly visible on ophthalmoscopy. Ultrasound or orbital CT scanning with thin cuts through the optic nervehead can demonstrate buried drusen (Fig III-23). With advancing age, buried drusen often become visible on the optic disc surface.

Histopathologically, drusen appear as concentric hyaline-like laminations. They stain positively for amino acids, acid mucopolysaccharides, calcium, and hemosiderin, and negatively for amyloid. They are insoluble in water, ether, and alcohol. The etiology of drusen is unknown, and they are generally asymptomatic. Visual loss may occur from progressive optic atrophy, acute AION, subretinal hemorrhage, or subretinal neovascularization. Visual field defects are common and include enlargement of the blind spot, nerve fiber bundle defects, and, occasionally, irregular constriction of the peripheral field (Fig III-24). Severe peripheral visual field loss eventually develops in some patients, but central field and acuity are almost always spared.

In some instances buried drusen may give rise to optic disc swelling that can mimic genuine papilledema. The ophthalmoscopic features of pseudopapilledema include the following:

□ Central cup absent but spontaneous venous pulsations often present

□ Anomalous branching of vessels on disc and increased number of major disc vessels

□ Disc margins showing irregular outline with derangement of peripapillary pigment epithelium

□ Absence of superficial capillary telangiectasia, hemorrhages, exudates, and cotton-wool spots

□ Absence of peripapillary retinal folds

□ Lack of fluorescein leakage from disc vessels

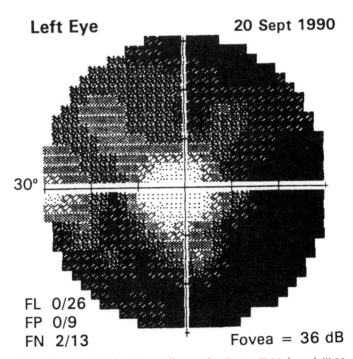

FIG III-24—Visual field of the eye illustrated in Figures III-21 through III-23. The central field is relatively preserved even with advanced peripheral visual field loss. The acuity was 20/20.

Optic discs with pseudopapilledema can also develop true papilledema, and chronic papilledema may demonstrate *pseudodrusen.*

Beck RW, Corbett JJ, Thompson HS, et al. Decreased visual acuity from optic disc drusen. *Arch Ophthalmol.* 1985;103:1155–1159.

Newman NJ, Lessell S, Brandt EM. Bilateral central retinal artery occlusions, disk drusen, and migraine. *Am J Ophthalmol.* 1989;107:236–240.

Reifler DM, Kaufman DI. Optic disk drusen and pseudotumor cerebri. *Am J Ophthalmol.* 1988;106:95–96.

Rosenberg MA, Savino PJ, Glaser JS. A clinical analysis of pseudopapilledema. I. Population, laterality, acuity, refractive error, ophthalmoscopic characteristics, and coincident disease. *Arch Ophthalmol.* 1979;97:65–70.

Savino PJ, Glaser JS, Rosenberg MA. A clinical analysis of pseudopapilledema. II. Visual field defects. *Arch Ophthalmol.* 1979;97:71–75.

Congenital Optic Disc Anomalies

There are a variety of congenital optic disc anomalies. Some are related and represent a continuum of cavitary optic disc anomalies.

Tilted optic disc   The tilted disc has the following features:

- An oval disc with one side displaced posteriorly, usually at the inferior margin, and the other side elevated anteriorly, usually at the superior margin
- A crescent on the side of the disc depression
- An oblique direction of retinal vessels

High myopia or moderate oblique myopic astigmatism is usually present. Pseudobitemporal field defects that do not respect the vertical midline may occur (Figs III-25, III-26).

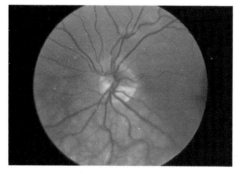

FIG III-25—Tilted optic disc.

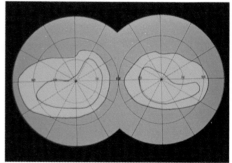

FIG III-26—Bitemporal visual field defects that do not respect the vertical midline caused by bilateral tilted optic discs. (Miller NR, Fine SL. *The Ocular Fundus in Neuro-Ophthalmologic Diagnosis.* St Louis: Mosby; 1977.)

Optic nerve dysplasia True optic nerve *aplasia* is rare. Typically, it occurs unilaterally in an otherwise healthy person, but it may be seen with anencephaly or major cerebral maldevelopment. Aplasia is not hereditary. A *coloboma* involving the optic nerve results from incomplete closure of fetal fissure and hence usually occurs inferiorly. It is often associated with chorioretinal defects, decreased visual acuity, and superior visual field defect. An *optic pit* is usually found in the inferior temporal portion of the disc. A pit may be associated with a serous macular detachment and a corresponding visual field defect. Fluid probably comes from the vitreous and enters the subretinal space through the pit. A *morning glory disc* is a funnel-shaped, enlarged, excavated disc with white connective tissue at the center, surrounded by a raised annulus of pigmented chorioretinal tissue. The optic disc appearance resembles the morning glory flower. This anomaly is usually unilateral and is twice as common in females. Visual acuity is usually 20/100 or worse. A nonrhegmatogenous retinal detachment around the disc may later develop. Morning glory disc is not hereditary.

Optic nerve hypoplasia The small disc of optic nerve hypoplasia (Fig III-27) may be unilateral or bilateral. The optic disc is underdeveloped but has relatively normal vessels. It is sometimes surrounded by a double ring sign caused by concentric choroidal-retinal pigment changes. The cause of optic nerve hypoplasia is often not identified, but this condition has been reported with increased incidence in children whose mothers have taken anti–epileptic seizure drugs, quinine, excessive alcohol, lysergic acid diethylamide (LSD), or other agents during pregnancy. Children born to mothers who have diabetes during pregnancy may have a special form of optic nerve hypoplasia called *superior segmental optic nerve hypoplasia,* with a matching inferior semialtitudinal visual field defect. Central acuity is normal.

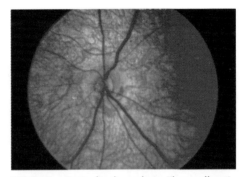

FIG III-27—Optic disc hypoplasia. The small optic disc is surrounded by a relatively hypopigmented ring of tissue (*double ring sign*). The retinal vessels are normal in appearance.

More important, hypoplasia may be a sign of congenital intracranial tumors such as craniopharyngioma or optic glioma. Many patients with optic nerve hypoplasia also have endocrine abnormalities and may develop hypoglycemic seizures or growth retardation if untreated. *Septo-optic dysplasia (de Morsier syndrome)* consists of optic nerve hypoplasia and the absence of the septum pellucidum with endocrine deficiencies.

Any of the above dysplasias may be associated with a basal encephalocele. Thus, the work-up should include neuroimaging and, in children with hypoplasia, a pediatric endocrinology evaluation.

Brown GC, Tasman W. *Congenital Anomalies of the Optic Disc.* New York: Grune & Stratton; 1983.

Nelson M, Lessell S, Sadun AA. Optic nerve hypoplasia and maternal diabetes mellitus. *Arch Neurol.* 1986;43:20–25.

Skarf B, Hoyt CS. Optic nerve hypoplasia in children: Association with anomalies of the endocrine and CNS. *Arch Ophthalmol.* 1984;102:62–67.

Stromland K. Ocular involvement in the fetal alcohol syndrome. *Surv Ophthalmol.* 1987;31:277–284.

Taylor D. Congenital tumours of the anterior visual system with dysplasia of the optic discs. *Br J Ophthalmol.* 1982;66:455–463.

Optic Nerve Trauma

Damage to one or both nerves may occur with blunt trauma to the head, often a frontal blow severe enough to cause loss of consciousness. Prognosis for recovery of vision is poor. Treatment with high-dose IV corticosteroids has been advocated. Surgical decompression of the optic canal in conjunction with corticosteroid use may be appropriate in selected cases.

Joseph MP, Lessell S, Rizzo J, et al. Extracranial optic nerve decompression for traumatic optic neuropathy. *Arch Ophthalmol.* 1990;108:1091–1093.

Kline LB, Morawetz RB, Swaid SN. Indirect injury of the optic nerve. *Neurosurgery.* 1984;14:756–764.

Seiff SR. High dose corticosteroids for treatment of vision loss due to indirect injury to the optic nerve. *Ophthalmic Surg.* 1990;21:389–395.

Spoor TC, Hartel WC, Lensink DB, et al. Treatment of traumatic optic neuropathy with corticosteroids. *Am J Ophthalmol.* 1990;110:665–669.

Steinsapir KD, Goldberg RA. Traumatic optic neuropathy. *Surv Ophthalmol.* 1994;38:487–518.

Warner JE, Lessell S. Traumatic optic neuropathy. *Int Ophthalmol Clin.* 1995;35:57–62.

Optic Atrophy

Optic atrophy is a general term used to describe the appearance of an optic disc that has lost its normal complement of healthy fibers. It is not a clinical diagnosis but a physical finding. Optic atrophy results from injury to any portion of the primary visual pathway: the retinal ganglion cell, nerve fiber layer, optic nerve, optic chiasm, optic tract, or lateral geniculate nucleus. Optic atrophy can be produced by any of the following diseases:

□ Ischemic optic neuropathy

□ Optic neuritis

□ Optic nerve sheath meningioma

□ Traumatic optic neuropathy

□ Leber hereditary optic neuropathy

□ Central retinal artery occlusion

If optic atrophy and enlargement of the optic cup are both present, the most likely diagnosis is glaucoma. However, with glaucoma the remaining neural rim usually has a normal color. Occasionally, compressive lesions or forms of optic neuropathy other than glaucoma can produce pathologic cupping and optic atrophy.

> Quigley HA, Anderson DR. The histological basis of optic disk pallor in experimental optic atrophy. *Am J Ophthalmol.* 1977;83:709–717.

> Sebag J, Delori FC, Feke GT, et al. Effects of optic atrophy on retinal blood flow and oxygen saturation in humans. *Arch Ophthalmol.* 1989;107:222–226.

> Trobe JD, Glaser JS, Cassady JC. Optic atrophy. Differential diagnosis by fundus observation alone. *Arch Ophthalmol.* 1980;98:1040–1045.

Lesions of the Optic Chiasm

Although many types of sellar and suprasellar tumors can produce chiasmal compression, tumors of the pituitary gland are the most common. Pituitary tumors can be divided into nonsecreting and secreting types. *Nonsecreting tumors* more often present with visual loss, and *secreting tumors* more often present with endocrine dysfunction. The exception is the prolactin-secreting tumor in male patients that usually presents with signs of chiasmal compression. Bromocriptine has been found to reduce the size of prolactin-secreting tumors.

> Burde RM. Pituitary tumors reassessed. *Am J Ophthalmol.* 1980;89:874–876.

> Lesser RL, Zheutlin JD, Boghen D, et al. Visual function improvement in patients with macroprolactinomas treated with bromocriptine. *Am J Ophthalmol.* 1990;109: 535–543.

Other extrinsic tumors causing chiasmal compression include meningiomas, generally seen in middle-aged women, and craniopharyngiomas, seen in children and adults. Aneurysms of the internal carotid or anterior cerebral arteries may also cause progressive loss of visual acuity and visual field, and may present as a chiasmal syndrome.

Intrinsic chiasmal tumors, such as gliomas, occur in children as well as adults. These tumors do not typically cause simple bitemporal field defects but often extend into both optic nerves, causing bilateral loss of visual acuity and complicated bilateral visual field defects.

Tumors that encroach upon the optic chiasm probably produce visual defects as a consequence of direct compression of the chiasmal nerve fibers. Interruption of the blood supply to the chiasm may also occur. Most visual field defects resulting from a chiasmal syndrome are relative rather than absolute.

On rare occasions, posterior fossa lesions may impinge on the aqueduct or produce hydrocephalus with dilation of the third ventricle, exerting pressure upon the chiasm and giving rise to visual defects suggestive of chiasmal compression. Since such patients also have papilledema, visual loss may be caused by combined mechanisms.

Rarely, severe frontal head trauma can damage the chiasm and cause bitemporal hemianopia. Often the visual loss is associated with diabetes insipidus, and a skull fracture is usually also present.

Disorders of Visual Integration

Visual information from the lateral geniculate bodies is conveyed to the primary visual cortex (V1) of both occipital lobes. Further visual processing occurs in V2, V3, V4, V5, and other adjacent areas in the occipital lobes. For a patient to read, information must travel from the occipital lobe to the angular gyrus in the parietal lobe of the dominant hemisphere (usually on the left side). Visual information from the right visual hemifield is transmitted directly from the left occipital cortex to the ipsilateral angular gyrus. Visual information from the left visual hemifield arrives in the right occipital cortex and must be transmitted through the splenium of the corpus callosum to reach the left angular gyrus.

The term *alexia* refers to the inability to read despite relatively normal vision. Pseudoalexia may be caused by illiteracy, developmental dyslexia, hemianopias that split fixation (especially right-sided), and expressive (Broca) or conduction aphasias in which comprehension is intact but verbal communication is impaired. Alexia with *agraphia,* the inability to write, occurs from left parietal lesions that involve the angular gyrus. Alexia without agraphia occurs from large left occipital lesions that also disrupt fibers crossing in the splenium of the corpus callosum from the right occipital cortex to the left angular gyrus. The patient is blind in the right visual field, and information from the left visual field cannot gain access to the left parietal lobe. As a result, the patient can see and write but cannot read. Reading ability should be checked in any patient with an occipital lesion.

Visual neglect occurs when the patient ignores one side of visual space. *Visual extinction* occurs when the patient ignores one side of visual space when presented with double simultaneous stimuli to both visual fields. These syndromes are usually associated with some degree of hemianopia, and they occur more often with right parietal lesions.

Lesions of the inferior occipitotemporal area cause a variety of syndromes. Visual *agnosia* occurs with bilateral lesions and is defined as the inability to recognize objects by sight, although the patient retains the ability to recognize them by touch, language, and intellect or in the presence of intact visual sensory processing. This condition should be distinguished from *anomia,* the inability to name objects. *Prosopagnosia,* the inability to recognize faces, occurs as a result of bilateral infero-occipital lesions. Often difficulty occurs in distinguishing members of other categories, such as automobiles, plants, or animals.

The inferior occipital area also subserves color sensation for the entire opposite visual field. A lesion here can cause loss of color sensation in the opposite hemifield; the visual world appears in shades of gray. This rare cerebral *achromatopsia* may be unilateral or bilateral; if bilateral, it is frequently associated with prosopagnosia. Superior homonymous visual field defects may also occur.

Visual hallucinations consist of two types. *Release hallucinations* (Charles Bonnet syndrome) occur in the setting of visual loss, usually recent, and are thought to occur from lack of input to visual association areas. The hallucinations may be formed (e.g., faces) or unformed (e.g., flashes of light), and they may occur in an area of blindness. They tend to be continuous and variable and can occur with lesions anywhere in the visual pathway. *Ictal hallucinations* are stereotyped and paroxysmal. Formed ictal hallucinations occur with temporal lobe disease. Unformed ictal hallucinations occur with occipital lobe disease.

Palinopsia is an abnormal perseveration of visual images. It is only rarely an isolated symptom and tends to occur with evolving lesions, more often in the right hemisphere. Other uncommon right parietal lobe syndromes exist, giving us a glimpse of the subtlety and complexity of cortical visual processing.

Brust JC, Behrens MM. Release hallucinations as the major symptom of posterior cerebral artery occlusion: a report of 2 cases. *Ann Neurol.* 1977;2:432–436.

Meadows JC. Disturbed perception of colours associated with localized cerebral lesions. *Brain.* 1974;97:615–632.

Siatkowski RM, Zimmer B, Rosenberg PR. The Charles Bonnet syndrome. Visual perceptive dysfunction in sensory deprivation. *J Clin Neuroophthalmol.* 1990;10: 215–218.

CHAPTER IV

Pupil

Pupillary size is determined by a number of factors, including age, level of alertness, level of retinal illumination, and the amount of accommodative effort. Activity in the parasympathetic and sympathetic efferent pathways mediates change in pupillary diameter.

Anatomy of Pupillary Pathways

Afferent Limb (Fig IV-1)

The pupil responds to light conveyed by a unique class of ganglion cells that send nerve fibers along the optic nerves to hemidecussate in the optic chiasm and enter the optic tracts. Afferent pupillary fibers exit the optic tracts just before the lateral geniculate bodies to enter the brain stem by way of the brachium of the superior colliculus. There they form synapses in the pretectal olivary and sublentiform nuclei. These pretectal nuclei then project to both ipsilateral and contralateral Edinger-Westphal nuclei in the oculomotor nuclear complex.

Parasympathetic Pathway

Efferent parasympathetic pupillary fibers exit the midbrain with cranial nerve III (oculomotor). Initially, these fibers are located on the dorsomedial surface of the nerve, where they are vulnerable to compression by aneurysms at the junction of the posterior communicating and internal carotid arteries, as well as by uncal herniation. As the third nerve courses forward in the subarachnoid space and cavernous sinus, the pupillary fibers move down around the outside of the nerve to enter the inferior oblique branch. The pupillary fibers finally synapse at the ciliary ganglion, which lies intraconally below the posterior orbital portion of the optic nerve. The short ciliary nerves then distribute the postganglionic fibers to the iris sphincter and ciliary body.

Sympathetic Pathway (Fig IV-2)

Efferent sympathetic pupillary output probably originates in the posterior hypothalamus. Fibers descend the brain stem predominantly in an uncrossed fashion, probably undergoing multiple synapses in the mesencephalon and pons. They coalesce in the lateral medulla oblongata and terminate in the intermediolateral cell column of the spinal cord at the eighth cervical to second thoracic levels (ciliospinal center of Budge). Pupillomotor fibers exit the spinal cord mainly at the first thoracic level and enter the cervical sympathetic chain at the level of the inferior cervical ganglion, the superior portion of the stellate ganglion. They ascend along the cervical sympathetic chain to synapse in the superior cervical ganglion.

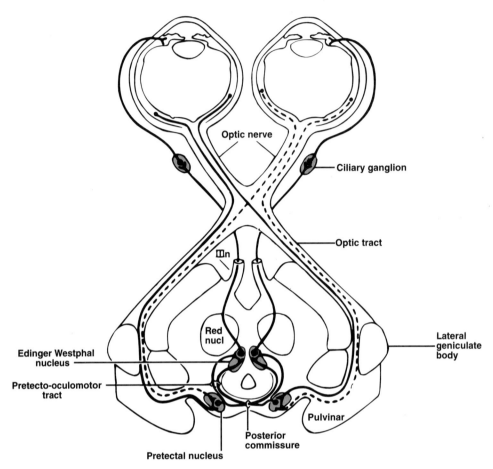

Labels on figure:
Optic nerve
Ciliary ganglion
Optic tract
IIIn
Red nucl
Lateral geniculate body
Edinger Westphal nucleus
Pretecto-oculomotor tract
Pulvinar
Posterior commissure
Pretectal nucleus

FIG IV-1—The pathway of the pupillary reaction to light.

Postganglionic fibers then travel with the internal carotid artery through the carotid canal to enter the cavernous sinus. These fibers leave the carotid plexus, briefly traveling with cranial nerve VI (abducens) in the cavernous sinus, and enter the orbit through the superior orbital fissure with the ophthalmic branch of cranial nerve V (trigeminal). They run parallel to fibers of the nasociliary nerve and travel with it through the ciliary body. The fibers then pass through the long ciliary nerves to terminate in the dilator muscle of the iris. Sympathetic efferent fibers to Müller's muscle of the upper eyelid and to similar muscle fibers in the lower eyelid diverge after passing through the superior orbital fissure, as shown in Figure IV-2.

Striph GG, Burde RM. Abducens nerve palsy and Horner's syndrome revisited. *J Clin Neuroophthalmol.* 1988;8:13–17.

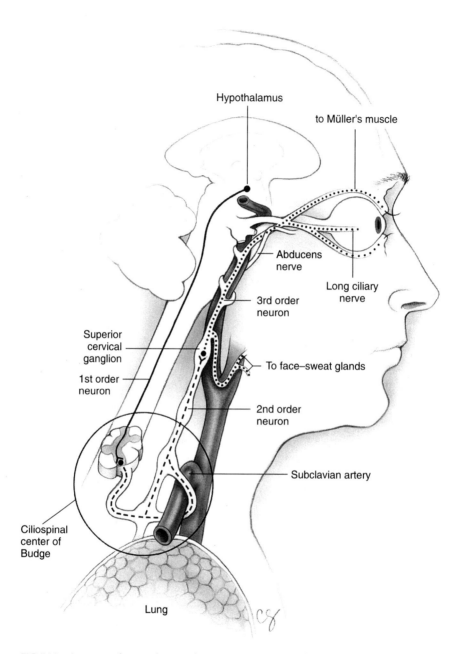

FIG IV-2—Anatomy of sympathetic pathway showing first order central neuron, second order intermediate neuron, and third order neuron pathways. Note the proximity of pulmonary apex to sympathetic chain. Note also the relationship of the intracavernous sympathetic fibers to the abducens nerve. (Illustration by Christine Gralapp.)

Near Response

The synkinetic near response consists of *accommodation* of the lens, *convergence,* and *pupillary miosis.* The anatomic pathway for pupillary constriction in response to near effort is less well defined than that for the light reflex, but it is clear that the two pathways are dissociated in the midbrain. Pupillary light–near dissociation is important in several clinical syndromes such as Parinaud, Argyll Robertson, Adie's, and amaurotic pupils (see discussion later in this chapter). Clinically, pupils that constrict well to light stimuli need not be tested for the near reflex. A poor near response in the presence of a good light response implies a lack of effort by the patient.

Loewenfeld IE. *The Pupil: Anatomy, Physiology, and Clinical Applications.* Detroit: Wayne State University Press; 1993.

Afferent Pupillary Defects

Shining a light in one eye of a normal subject causes both pupils to constrict equally. The pupillary reaction in the illuminated eye is called the *direct response,* and the reaction in the other eye is the *consensual response.* Because of the hemidecussation of afferent pupillomotor fibers in the chiasm, and because a second hemidecussation of the pupillomotor fibers takes place in the brain stem, the direct and consensual responses are equal. If one eye is blind, all input to the pupillary centers in the brain stem comes from the other eye, but the double hemidecussation ensures equal pupillary innervation and prevents inequality of the pupils, or *anisocoria.*

Shining a dim light in one eye of a normal subject will cause both pupils to constrict; a brighter light will cause more constriction. If a light is shone in one eye then quickly switched to the other eye, the response will be an initial constriction of both pupils followed by an equivalent, normal redilation. If the light is swung back to the first eye, the response will be the same.

If bright illumination of, say, the right pupil is alternated with dim illumination of the left pupil, the pupillary responses are more complex. Stimulation of the right eye causes a large pupillary constriction in both eyes followed by a small redilation. Switching to the dim light in the left eye causes a smaller initial constriction of both pupils followed by redilation to a diameter larger than that following the initial constriction.

Optic nerve disease causes light to appear dimmer in the affected eye than in the opposite eye. When light is shone in the normal eye, both pupils will constrict, then redilate slightly. When the same light is swung to the diseased eye, the initial constriction will be decreased or absent, and greater redilation will occur. The *alternating,* or *swinging, light test* indicates that the diseased eye has a *relative afferent pupillary defect* (RAPD), also called Marcus Gunn pupil (Figs IV-3 to IV-5).

RAPDs can be quantified by using neutral-density filters of increasing density to dim the light in front of the better eye. The measured degree of density can be used to follow a patient and to correlate pupil findings with the rest of the eye examination in order to make a diagnosis. If one pupil has an efferent defect and is unreactive, the alternating light test can still be done by observing the normally mobile pupil—its consensual response reflects afferent input from both eyes. A dim side light can be used to illuminate the functioning pupil when the swinging light is shone on the other eye; however, if the side light is too bright, it can create an RAPD in the illuminated eye.

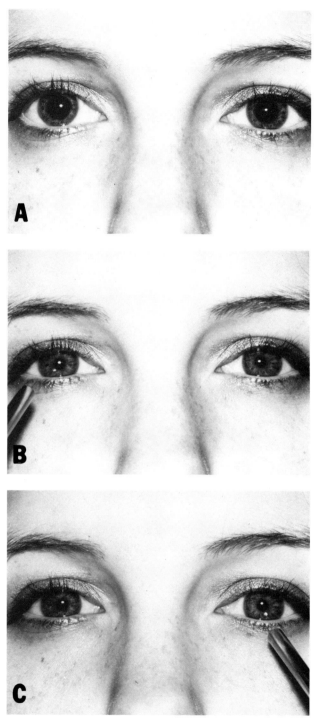

FIG IV-3—Testing for a relative afferent pupillary defect in a patient with a normal response. *A,* With diffuse illumination, pupils are of equal size. *B,* With light on right eye, both pupils constrict and remain constricted when light is swung to left eye in *C.* (Reprinted from Beck RW. The neuro-ophthalmic examination. In: *Neurologic Clinics.* Philadelphia: Saunders; 1983:1(4):811–813.)

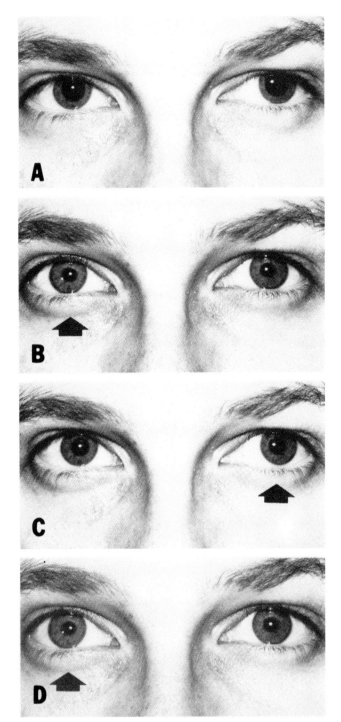

FIG IV-4—Testing for a relative afferent pupillary defect in a patient with a left optic neuropathy. (*Arrows* indicate which eye is being illuminated.) *A,* With diffuse illumination, pupils are of equal size. *B,* With light on right eye, pupils constrict briskly. *C,* Pupils dilate slightly when light is swung to left eye. *D,* When light is swung back to right eye, both pupils constrict to the size they were in *B.* (Reprinted from Beck RW. The neuro-ophthalmic examination. In: *Neurologic Clinics.* Philadelphia: Saunders; 1983:1(4):811–813.)

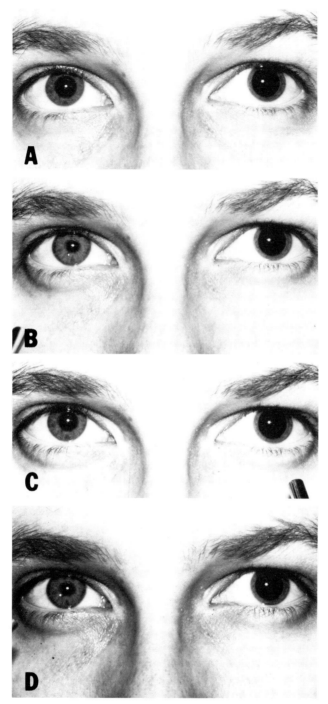

FIG IV-5—Testing for a relative afferent pupillary defect when one pupil is dilated. A left optic neuropathy is present. *A,* With diffuse illumination, left pupil is larger than right. *B,* With light on right eye, right pupil constricts but left does not. *C,* When light is swung to left eye, right pupil dilates slightly. *D,* Pupil again constricts when light is swung back to right eye. (Reprinted from Beck RW. The neuro-ophthalmic examination. In: *Neurologic Clinics.* Philadelphia: Saunders; 1983:1(4):811–813.)

The relative afferent pupillary defect is one of the most important signs in neuro-ophthalmology. It provides objective evidence of disease affecting the anterior visual system, particularly optic nerve disease. In general, the degree of pupillary reactivity to light is proportional to the amount of ganglion cell involvement. Unilateral optic nerve disease usually causes an RAPD, even if visual acuity is preserved. Bilateral optic nerve disease may cause an RAPD when one optic nerve is affected more than the other. Significant retinal disease causes an RAPD only when ganglion cell damage is significant. An RAPD is not seen in patients with media opacities, refractive errors, functional visual loss, or cortical lesions. Small RAPDs have been described in amblyopia, but these should always raise suspicion of underlying optic nerve pathology. Optic tract lesions cause RAPDs if visual field loss in one eye is greater than in the other. Because the temporal visual field is larger than the nasal field, complete tract lesions are associated with an RAPD in the eye contralateral to the lesion. RAPDs have been described in eyes contralateral to pretectal mesencephalic lesions despite the absence of visual field loss.

Bell RA, Thompson HS. Relative afferent pupillary defect in optic tract hemianopias. *Am J Ophthalmol.* 1978;84:538–540.

Forman S, Behrens MM, Odel JG, et al. Relative afferent pupillary defect with normal visual function. *Arch Ophthalmol.* 1990;108:1074–1075.

Kardon RH, Haupert CL, Thompson HS. The relationship between static perimetry and the relative afferent pupillary defect. *Am J Ophthalmol.* 1993;115:351–356.

Thompson HS, Corbett JJ, Cox TA. How to measure the relative afferent pupillary defect. *Surv Ophthalmol.* 1981;26:39–42.

Thompson HS, Montague P, Cox TA, et al. The relationship between visual acuity, pupillary defect, and visual field loss. *Am J Ophthalmol.* 1982;93:681–688.

Paradoxical Pupillary Phenomena

Rarely, paradoxical pupillary constriction in dim illumination after exposure to light can be observed in children with congenital abnormalities. It is seen in association with congenital stationary night blindness, congenital achromatopsia, and dominant optic atrophy.

Frank JW, Kushner BJ, France TD. Paradoxical pupillary phenomena. A review of patients with pupillary constriction to darkness. *Arch Ophthalmol.* 1988;106:1564–1566.

Lesions of the Midbrain

Efferent pupillary defects may occur with lesions involving the oculomotor nucleus or the fascicles of the third nerve coursing ventrally to exit the brain stem. Generally, other signs of brain stem involvement or third nerve palsy will also be apparent. Afferent pupillary defects occur when pupillomotor pathways are involved between the optic tract and the Edinger-Westphal nucleus. Three syndromes are clinically important: Argyll Robertson pupil, Parinaud dorsal midbrain syndrome, and pretectal afferent pupillary defects.

Argyll Robertson Pupil

This rare syndrome occurs in some patients with tertiary syphilis involving the central nervous system. Affected patients have small pupils (less than 2 mm) that are often irregular. The pupils do not react to light, but the near response is normal. This condition is one of the few in which a very miotic pupil reacts briskly. Iris atrophy frequently occurs; portions of the iris transilluminate, and dilation is poor after instillation of mydriatics. In the absence of optic atrophy and in the context of good visual acuity, this combination of findings is virtually pathognomonic of central nervous system syphilis. Argyll Robertson–like pupils are seen in diabetes, chronic alcoholism, encephalitis, and some degenerative disorders and following panretinal photocoagulation. Without special tests, this particular appearance cannot reliably be distinguished from conditions such as Adie's tonic pupil, which is discussed below. Furthermore, bilateral tonic pupils have been reported in neurosyphilis. Serologic tests for syphilis, such as serum FTA-ABS, should be considered in the evaluation of patients with bilateral pupillary light–near dissociation with miosis.

Fletcher WA, Sharpe JA. Tonic pupils in neurosyphilis. *Neurology.* 1986;36:188–192.

Parinaud Dorsal Midbrain Syndrome

Dorsal midbrain damage causes midposition pupils with poor light response and preserved near response, findings that would also occur in a patient who is blind. In Parinaud syndrome the lesions involve afferent pupillary pathways in the pretectum after the nerve fibers have left the optic tracts. Midbrain damage located more ventrally causes midposition pupils that are poorly reactive to both light and near stimuli.

Pretectal Afferent Pupillary Defects

Occasionally, a pretectal lesion will be predominantly unilateral or will involve one side more than the other. Such a lesion may cause an RAPD without an associated visual field defect (e.g., an isolated pretectal lesion on the right will cause a relative afferent pupillary defect on the left).

Ellis CJ. Afferent pupillary defect in pineal region tumour. *J Neurol Neurosurg Psychiatry.* 1984;47:739–741.

Anisocoria

Simple Anisocoria

Physiological anisocoria is the most common cause of a relative difference in pupillary size. About 20% of individuals have noticeable differences in pupillary diameter when one eye is compared to the other. Clinically, pupil differences of 0.2 mm can be detected, and anisocoria of 0.4 mm or more is readily visible. The condition is more common in older adults and is a source of concern when seen in children.

Usually, the pupils differ in size less than 1.0 mm. The amount of anisocoria in an individual can vary from day to day. In one study 41% of patients had anisocoria of 0.4 mm or more when observed over a period of 5 days. At any given examination 19% of patients showed 0.4 mm or more of anisocoria, although most of these individuals had anisocoria only part of the time. Anisocoria may be greater in dim light than in bright light, simulating Horner syndrome. Congenital or senile ptosis on the side of the smaller pupil can create problems in diagnosis. Pupils with simple anisocoria dilate normally after cocaine instillation without dilation lag.

The first step in determining the cause of anisocoria is a complete eye examination. Associated findings, such as ptosis or limitation of ocular motility, provide important clues. The evaluation of a patient with isolated anisocoria is much easier with the systematic approach illustrated in the flowchart (Fig IV-6).

Lam BL, Thompson HS, Corbett JJ. The prevalence of simple anisocoria. *Am J Ophthalmol.* 1987;104:69–73.

Loewenfeld IE. Simple central anisocoria: a common condition, seldom recognized. *Trans Am Acad Ophthalmol Otolaryngol.* 1977;83:832–839.

Roarty JD, Keltner JL. Normal pupil size and anisocoria in newborn infants. *Arch Ophthalmol.* 1990;108:94–95.

Thompson BM, Corbett JJ, Kline LB, et al. Pseudo-Horner's syndrome. *Arch Neurol.* 1982;39:108–111.

Lesions of the Parasympathetic System

Third nerve palsy   Pupillary involvement in third nerve palsy is almost always accompanied by ptosis and limitation of ocular motility. Pupillary dilation may be the only sign of third nerve palsy in two clinical situations: uncal herniation and basal meningitis (cryptococcosis, syphilis, tuberculosis, sarcoidosis). When the pupillary sphincter is completely paralyzed, pupil size depends on the level of sympathetic stimulation; it varies between 5 mm and 8 mm. Maximal anisocoria occurs in bright light.

Pupillary involvement helps the clinician to diagnose acute third nerve palsies. When the pupil is involved, an aneurysm at the junction of the internal carotid and posterior communicating arteries must be excluded. If the pupil is spared and all other functions of the third nerve are completely paretic, an aneurysm can likely be ruled out. Aberrant regeneration of cranial nerve III may cause a unique pupillary reaction. Portions of the pupillary sphincter contract with attempted movement of the eye medially. This phenomenon also appears with elevation or depression of the eye.

Czarnecki JS, Thompson HS. The iris sphincter in aberrant regeneration of the third nerve. *Arch Ophthalmol.* 1978;96:1606–1610.

Nadeau SE, Trobe JD. Pupil sparing in oculomotor palsy: a brief review. *Ann Neurol.* 1983;13:143–148.

Siatkowski RM. Third, fourth, and sixth nerve palsies. In: *Focal Points: Clinical Modules for Ophthalmologists.* San Francisco: American Academy of Ophthalmology; 1996;14:8.

Traumatic mydriasis   Blunt trauma to the eye can cause mydriasis by damaging the pupillary sphincter. The pupil may be relatively miotic after injury, but it soon becomes midsized and poorly responsive to bright light and dim illumination. Notches in the pupillary margin can be seen, and the iris may transilluminate near the sphincter muscle. Iris injury occurs frequently in patients with head trauma, and the dilated pupil may be mistakenly identified as a sign of uncal herniation.

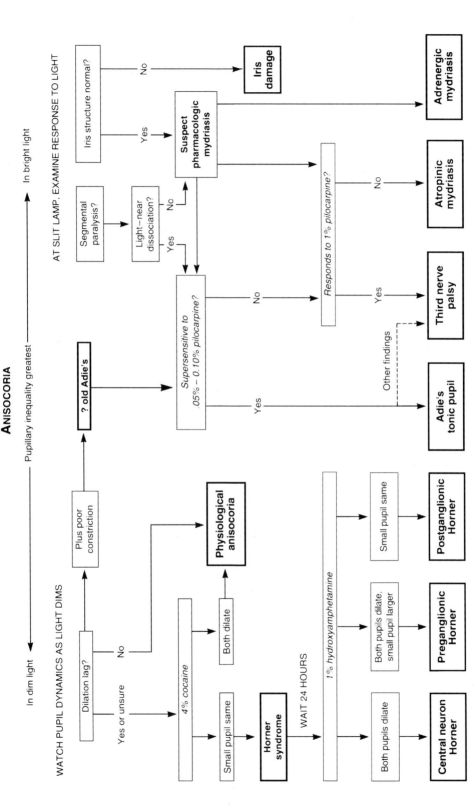

FIG IV-6—Flowchart for evaluation of anisocoria. (Modified with permission from Thompson HS, Kardon RH. Clinical importance of pupillary inequality. In: *Focal Points: Clinical Modules for Ophthalmologists.* San Francisco: American Academy of Ophthalmology; 1992;10:10.)

Prolonged or recurrent angle closure can also impair pupil function. Iris function is frequently abnormal following intraocular surgery, and interpretation of pupillary responses must be made with caution after careful slit-lamp examination.

Pharmacologic mydriasis When mydriatic medications are instilled in the eye, accidentally or intentionally, the pupil becomes dilated and reacts poorly to light and near reflex. In pharmacologic mydriasis, constriction is minimal. However, instilling pilocarpine 0.5% or 1.0% in an eye with mydriasis from third nerve palsy or Adie's syndrome causes marked pupillary constriction; in Adie's syndrome painful ciliary muscle spasm may be induced.

Pharmacologic agents, such as those used to treat glaucoma, may cause anisocoria if they are used to treat one eye or if absorption is asymmetrical. The anisocoria can be pronounced if a patient inadvertently injures the surface of one eye while instilling drops or if one eye is exposed, for example, from a Bell's palsy.

Tonic pupil (Adie's syndrome) Diagnostic features of tonic pupils include sluggish, segmental pupillary responses to light and better response to near effort followed by slow redilation. A tonic pupil is caused by postganglionic parasympathetic pupillomotor damage. *Holmes-Adie syndrome* includes other features such as diminished deep tendon reflexes in nearly 90% of patients and orthostatic hypotension. Seventy percent of patients are female. Tonic pupils are unilateral in 80% of cases, although the second pupil may later become involved.

In the initial stages a tonic pupil is dilated and poorly reactive. The examiner at the slit lamp can usually see segments of the sphincter constrict. The iris crypts stream toward the area of normal sphincter function, bunching up along the pupillary border in areas of normal function and thinning in the areas of paralysis, which also show entropion (Fig IV-7). A tonic pupil may appear relatively smaller after near effort, as it redilates slowly while the normal pupil redilates promptly. Tonic pupils may be associated with slow and tonic accommodation as well; after near effort, refocusing for distance may be delayed.

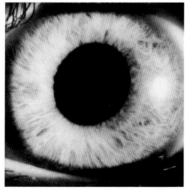

FIG IV-7—Iris abnormalities in a tonic pupil. Note streaming of iris crypts toward the normally constricting area where there is bunching of the pupillary border. (Reproduced by permission from Thompson HS. Segmental palsy of the iris sphincter in Adie's syndrome. *Arch Ophthalmol.* 1978;96:1615–1620. Copyright © 1978, American Medical Association.)

The tonic pupil is hypersensitive to topical parasympathomimetic solutions. Pilocarpine 0.05%–0.1% can be used to diagnose this condition, as the normal pupil will constrict slightly, confirming that the drug has been instilled in both eyes. Fifteen minutes after pilocarpine is instilled in both eyes, the pupils are examined to determine relative response. This strength of pilocarpine can be obtained by diluting commercial 1% solution with sterile saline for injection. Too strong a solution may cause painful ciliary spasm. In most cases, however, the clinical appearance of tonic pupil is so typical that pharmacologic testing is not necessary.

Patients with tonic pupils may have accommodative symptoms or photophobia, but just as often they have no symptoms and indicate that anisocoria was noticed by a friend or relative. Accommodative symptoms are difficult to treat. Fortunately, they usually resolve spontaneously within a few months of onset. When photophobia from a dilated pupil is a problem, topical dilute pilocarpine may be helpful. With time, the Adie's tonic pupil gets smaller.

Histopathologic examination of the ciliary ganglion in patients with Adie's tonic pupil has shown reduction in ganglion cells. Systemic conditions rarely associated with tonic pupils include herpes zoster and varicella, giant cell arteritis, syphilis, and orbital trauma. Bilateral tonic pupils may be seen in patients with diabetes, alcoholism, and dysautonomia associated with cancer and amyloidosis.

Harriman DG, Garland H. The pathology of Adie's syndrome. *Brain.* 1968;91:401–418.

Thompson HS. Adie's syndrome. Some new observations. *Trans Am Ophthalmol Soc.* 1977;75:587–626.

Thompson HS. Segmental palsy of the iris sphincter in Adie's syndrome. *Arch Ophthalmol.* 1978;96:1615–1620.

Episodic Pupillary Phenomena

Episodic unilateral mydriasis and episodic spasm of the pupillary sphincter have been described in young, healthy individuals who frequently have a history of headaches. Episodic mydriasis may last for hours and may be accompanied by headache and some blurring of vision. However, each episode is self-limited, and the condition has not been associated with any systemic or neurologic disease. Occasionally, patients who notice episodic pupillary dilation go on to develop sympathetic dysfunction with pupillary miosis and Horner syndrome. Patients with episodic, rhythmic constriction of the pupil without other neurologic or systemic abnormalities have been described.

Hallett M, Cogan DG. Episodic unilateral mydriasis in otherwise normal individuals. *Arch Ophthalmol.* 1970;84:130–136.

Thompson HS, Zackon DH, Czarnecki JSC. Tadpole-shaped pupils caused by segmental spasm of the iris dilator muscle. *Am J Ophthalmol.* 1983;96:467–477.

Lesions of the Sympathetic System

A lesion at any point along the sympathetic pathway results in Horner syndrome, which includes ptosis and miosis on the same side. Anisocoria is more apparent in dim illumination, and the affected pupil shows dilation lag: more anisocoria is seen 5 seconds after the lights are turned out than 15 or 20 seconds later. Light and near pupillary reactions are intact. The eyelid is ptotic because of paresis of Müller's muscle. There is apparent enophthalmos because the lower eyelid may be elevated;

exophthalmometry readings are equal. When the lesion is congenital, iris hetero-chromia will develop with the affected iris appearing lighter in color. Anhidrosis affects the entire ipsilateral side of the body with central, first-order neuron lesions. With lesions affecting the second-order neuron from the cervical spinal cord up to the superior cervical ganglion, anhidrosis affects the ipsilateral face. With post-ganglionic lesions from the superior cervical ganglion up to the eye, anhidrosis is either absent or limited to the forehead.

Confirmation of oculosympathetic dysfunction can be determined pharmaco-logically with topical cocaine 4%–10%. Cocaine blocks reuptake of norepinephrine released at neuromuscular junctions of the iris dilator muscle, thereby increasing the amount of norepinephrine available to stimulate the muscle. Following instillation of cocaine in a normal eye, the pupil will dilate, but in Horner syndrome the pupil dilates poorly, since little or no norepinephrine is being released into the synaptic cleft.

Localization of the lesion producing Horner syndrome can be further refined by the use of hydroxyamphetamine 1%, which acts by releasing norepinephrine from the presynaptic terminal. Hydroxyamphetamine in a normal eye will dilate the pupil, but in a postganglionic Horner syndrome, the nerve terminal has degenerated, and hydroxyamphetamine causes poor dilation. In a preganglionic Horner syn-drome, the postganglionic neuron is usually intact, and hydroxyamphetamine does dilate the pupil. Any pharmacologic test of pupillary function should not be done within 24 hours of instillation of other drops.

Localization of the lesion causing Horner syndrome is important. *First-order neuron lesions* are caused by central disorders of the nervous system such as vascular occlusion, particularly in the lateral medulla, as well as by tumors, cervical disc disease, and other disorders involving the upper cervical spinal cord. *Second-order neuron lesions* are caused by apical lung tumors (Pancoast syndrome), metas-tases, chest surgery, thoracic aortic aneurysms, or trauma to the brachial plexus. *Third-order neuron lesions* are caused by diseases of the neck such as tumors, surgery on the carotid artery or structures nearby, carotid artery dissection, and extension of tumors such as nasopharyngeal carcinoma into the cavernous sinus.

In addition to testing with cocaine and hydroxyamphetamine, careful history taking and examination are most useful in localizing Horner syndrome. Clues assist-ing in the localization of first-order neuron lesions include accompanying neurolog-ical symptoms and signs such as numbness, weakness, ataxia, and nystagmus. Second-order neuron lesions are associated with trauma and symptoms such as cough, hemoptosis, and swelling in the neck. Symptoms associated with third-order neuron lesions include numbness over the first as well as the second and/or third divisions of cranial nerve V, and double vision from sixth nerve palsy. Congenital Horner syndrome is usually caused by birth trauma to the brachial plexus. Horner syndrome acquired in early childhood indicates the possibility of neuroblastoma arising in the sympathetic chain of the chest.

Isolated postganglionic Horner syndrome is often benign but not always (see next paragraph). The clinician may find that examining old photographs for help in dating the lesion can aid the decision-making process in these cases. If the Horner syndrome has been present for several years, further examination will probably be unrewarding. However, Horner syndrome associated with pain deserves extra attention.

Postganglionic Horner syndrome with ipsilateral headache has several causes. Patients with typical cluster headaches may develop Horner syndrome on the ipsilateral side during an acute attack. The Horner syndrome often resolves, but it

TABLE IV-1

PHARMACOLOGIC TESTING FOR ABNORMAL PUPILS

CLINICAL PROBLEM	DRUG	ABNORMAL PUPIL	NORMAL PUPIL
Horner syndrome	Cocaine 4%–10%	Fails to dilate	Dilates
Preganglionic	Paremyd 1%	Dilates	Dilates
Postganglionic	Paremyd 1%	Fails to dilate	Dilates
Adie's tonic pupil	Pilocarpine 0.05%–0.1%	Constricts	No reaction
Pharmacologic	Pilocarpine 0.5%–1%	Fails to constrict	Constricts

may become permanent after repeated attacks. Patients with spontaneous dissection of the carotid artery may present with ipsilateral head pain and Horner syndrome. Such patients may also have amaurosis fugax and dysgeusia. This condition must be recognized, since stroke is a possible complication. MRI can show only intramural hemorrhage, which may not require treatment. Magnetic resonance angiography or arteriography can show true dissection of the carotid artery, which may require anticoagulation.

Some patients, usually middle-aged males, have Horner syndrome and daily unilateral headaches not characteristic of cluster, and no underlying pathology can be identified. The term *Raeder paratrigeminal syndrome* has been used to describe these patients. However, in the neurologic literature the term *Raeder syndrome* has been used to describe patients with painful oculosympathetic dysfunction caused by serious underlying disease. Risk factors for underlying disorders causing Horner syndrome include chronic pain, pulmonary or other systemic symptoms or signs suggesting malignancy, and additional cranial nerve abnormalities. In such patients the work-up should include MRI of the head including the cavernous sinus, neck, and apices of the lungs if localization of the condition is not obvious. If the level of the Horner syndrome can be determined by pharmacologic testing or identification of specific localizing signs or symptoms, more direct imaging with thinner sections on MRI should be obtained of the suspected area, such as the cavernous sinus, neck, nasopharynx, or lung (Table IV-1).

Cremer SA, Thompson HS, Digre KB, et al. Hydroxyamphetamine mydriasis in Horner's syndrome. *Am J Ophthalmol.* 1990;110:71–76.

Grimson BS, Thompson HS. Raeder's syndrome. A clinical review. *Surv Ophthalmol.* 1980;24:199–210.

Kardon RH, Denison CE, Brown CK, et al. Critical evaluation of the cocaine test in the diagnosis of Horner's syndrome. *Arch Ophthalmol.* 1990;108:384–387.

Kline LB, Vitek JJ, Raymon BC. Painful Horner's syndrome due to spontaneous carotid artery dissection. *Ophthalmology.* 1987;94:226–230.

Maloney WF, Younge BR, Moyer NJ. Evaluation of the causes and accuracy of pharmacologic location of Horner's syndrome. *Am J Ophthalmol.* 1980;90:394–402.

Woodruff G, Buncic JR, Morin JD. Horner's syndrome in children. *J Pediatr Ophthalmol Strabismus.* 1988;25:40–44.

CHAPTER V

Ocular Motor System

The *efferent visual complex* is responsible for movement of the eyes. Along with the afferent visual pathways, the pupillary system, and the adnexal orbital structures, it represents one of the basic components of the neuro-ophthalmic system as a whole. Problems with the ocular motor system leading to inability to align the fovea with an object of interest or instability of fixation may be perceived by the patient as a decrease in visual acuity, while malalignment of the visual axes leads to double vision. The clinician who wishes to assess the efferent visual systems requires an understanding of the neuroanatomic basis for ocular motility.

Teleology of Ocular Motility

Four basic physiologic principles underlie the importance of eye movements. Understanding the implications and requirements of these principles simplifies conceptualization of the different systems of ocular motility and is thus helpful to the clinician in recognizing pathologic involvement.

□ *An image projected constantly on the retina fades.* All sensory systems, including sight, sound, touch, taste, and smell, are sensitive to changes and perform poorly with constant stimulation.

□ *An image moving across the retina at greater than 4°/sec undergoes substantial reduction in resolution.* Maintenance of relative stability of images on the retina is critical for maximal acuity.

□ *Primates are foveate animals.* The specially adapted fovea has maximal resolution, and, therefore, aligning the fovea with the object of interest and maintaining alignment during both head and target movement optimizes visual acuity.

□ *The individual visual fields of the two eyes in primates overlap.* Bilateral simultaneous alignment of the two primary visual axes is, therefore, essential to avoid diplopia and visual confusion. In addition, as objects move closer or farther away, the relative inclination between the two visual axes must change.

The various eye movement control systems can be seen as being designed to respect these physiologic constraints. Microsaccadic *refixation movements* ensure retinal recovery through small continual square-wave refixation movements (conjugate saccades .1°–.2° off target with return movements following intersaccadic latency). The *pursuit system* and *optokinetic nystagmus* maintain stability of the object on the retina and the fovea in particular while the object moves, and the *vestibulo-ocular system* maintains stability during movement of the head. The *saccadic system* brings the object of interest into alignment with the fovea. The *vergence system* is responsible for bilateral simultaneous ocular alignment as the object moves closer to or farther from the subject. Abnormalities in these systems result in degradation of visual acuity.

Neuroanatomic and Physiologic Basis of Ocular Motility

The position of the eye in the orbit is ultimately a function of the static and dynamic forces created by all the tissues connected to the eye itself. These include the conjunctiva, Tenon's capsule, the optic nerve, the blood vessels feeding and draining the eye, and the six extraocular muscles. The purely elastic forces tend to align the eyes in a somewhat divergent pattern, as seen in a sedated or paralyzed patient. Continual tonic input to the extraocular muscles, however, brings the eyes closer to primary position alignment.

The four rectus muscles and the superior oblique muscle all originate in the area of the annulus of Zinn at the orbital apex. The inferior oblique muscle originates from the periorbita at the junction of the orbital floor with the posterior lacrimal crest. The posterior aspect of the sclera is the site of insertion for the inferior oblique muscle and the tendinous extension of the superior oblique muscle after it has passed through the trochlea. The rectus muscles insert directly on the anterior portion of the globe through tendon sheaths that penetrate posterior Tenon's capsule. The muscles themselves are held in position by intermuscular septae, posterior Tenon's capsule, and suspensory or pulley arrangements extending to the periorbita. These anatomic constraints limit our ability to transpose muscle positions.

The lateral rectus muscle moves the eye in abduction; the medial rectus in adduction. The superior rectus and inferior oblique muscles elevate the eye, while the inferior rectus and superior oblique muscles lower the eye (Fig V-1). The rectus muscles have their primary vertical action in abduction; the obliques have their

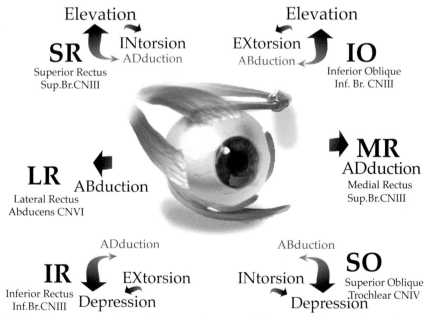

FIG V-1—Primary, secondary, and tertiary functions of the extraocular muscles, right eye. (Illustration by Craig A. Luce.)

primary vertical action in adduction. The vertical rectus muscles also act as adductors, while the obliques are abductors. The superior muscles (rectus and oblique) intort the eye; the inferior muscles extort the eye. (See also BCSC Section 2, *Fundamentals and Principles of Ophthalmology,* Part 1, Anatomy; and BCSC Section 7, *Orbit, Eyelids, and Lacrimal System,* chapter I, Orbital Anatomy.)

Ocular Motor Nerves

The six extraocular muscles are innervated by the three ocular motor nerves, cranial nerves III, IV, and VI. The innervation takes place one third of the way from the orbital apex in all but the inferior oblique, which is innervated just lateral to the edge of the inferior rectus muscle at its approximate midpoint.

Cranial Nerve III (Oculomotor)

The third nerve originates within the brain stem, follows a subarachnoid course, and exits the dura mater at the skull base in the posterior, superolateral aspect of the cavernous sinus. The nuclei of the third nerves are paired structures located along the midline of the dorsal brain stem in the midbrain. The blood supply to the medial aspect of the brain stem is from vessels directly off the basilar artery. Small perforators off circumflex arteries (posterior cerebral artery, superior cerebellar artery) may also supply the fascicular portion of the third nerve as it courses through the ventral midbrain.

Nucleus   The third nerve nucleus is located at the level of the superior colliculus, beneath the aqueduct in the periaqueductal gray matter of the rostral mesencephalon, or midbrain. It is complex and has subnuclei with crossed, combined, and uncrossed projections to the individual extraocular muscles. The subnuclei to inferior oblique, inferior rectus, and medial rectus muscles have uncrossed projections. The levator muscles share projections from the single midline central caudal nucleus. The superior rectus muscle subnucleus has a crossed projection; i.e., the right superior rectus subnucleus innervates the left superior rectus muscle (Fig V-2). The visceral Edinger-Westphal nucleus gives parasympathetic input to the ipsilateral pupil.

Lesions of the third nerve nucleus or its subnuclei are relatively rare. In nuclear lesions, ptosis should be bilateral or absent; the superior rectus muscle may be involved contralaterally and spared ipsilaterally, although it is more commonly affected bilaterally.

Büttner-Ennever JA, Akert K. Medial rectus subgroups of the oculomotor nucleus and their abducens internuclear input in the monkey. *J Comp Neurol.* 1981;197:17–27.

Ksiazek SM, Repka MX, Maguire A, et al. Divisional oculomotor nerve paresis caused by intrinsic brainstem disease. *Ann Neurol.* 1989;26:714–718.

Pusateri TJ, Sedwick LA, Margo CE. Isolated inferior rectus muscle palsy from a solitary metastasis to the oculomotor nucleus. *Arch Ophthalmol.* 1987;105:675–677.

Warwick R. Representation of the extraocular muscles in the oculomotor nuclei of the monkey. *J Comp Neurol.* 1953;98:449–503.

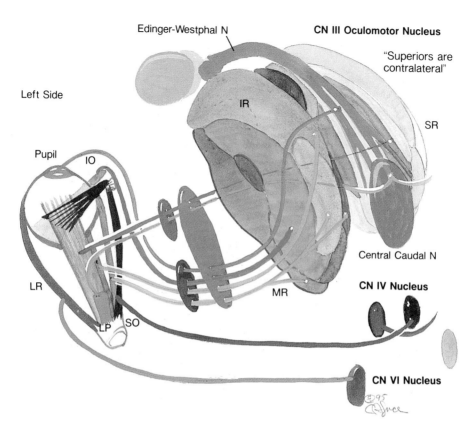

FIG V-2—Representation of left extraocular muscle subnuclei in CN III nucleus, CN IV nucleus, and CN VI nucleus. *IO,* inferior oblique; *IR,* inferior rectus; *LP,* levator palpebrae superioris; *LR,* lateral rectus; *MR,* medial rectus; *SO,* superior oblique; *SR,* superior rectus. (Illustration by Craig A. Luce.)

Fasciculus The oculomotor neurons leave the nuclear complex and pass ventrally through the red nucleus, exiting the brain stem through the medial portion of each cerebral peduncle to emerge in the interpeduncular space (Fig V-3). Partial third nerve palsies or even isolated complete third nerve palsies from fascicular lesions are usually of vascular or metastatic etiology. More often, however, a fascicular oculomotor palsy is accompanied by other neurologic symptoms. Most proximally, involvement of the superior cerebellar peduncle results in cerebellar ataxia (*Nothnagel syndrome*). Slightly more ventrally, involvement of the red nucleus and nearby medial lemniscus results in contralateral loss of sensation and rubral tremor (*Benedikt syndrome*). Distally (most ventrally), involvement of the fascicle compromises the cerebral peduncle, producing contralateral spastic paralysis (*Weber syndrome*).

Wolf JK. *The Classical Brain Stem Syndromes.* Springfield, IL: Charles C Thomas; 1971.

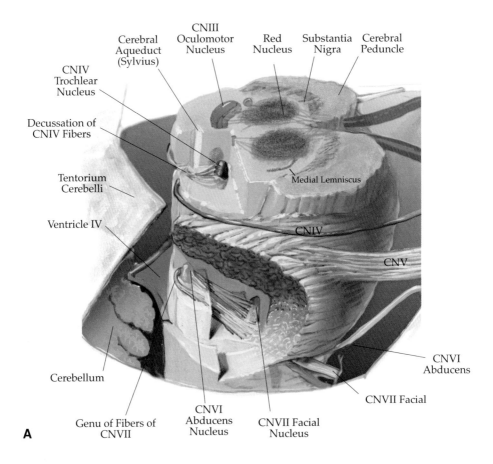

A

CNIV
Trochlear
Nucleus

Cerebral
Aqueduct
(Sylvius)

CNIII
Oculomotor
Nucleus

Red
Nucleus

Substantia
Nigra

Cerebral
Peduncle

Decussation of
CNIV Fibers

Tentorium
Cerebelli

Medial Lemniscus

Ventricle IV

CNIV

CNV

CNVI
Abducens

Cerebellum

CNVII Facial

Genu of Fibers of
CNVII

CNVI
Abducens
Nucleus

CNVII Facial
Nucleus

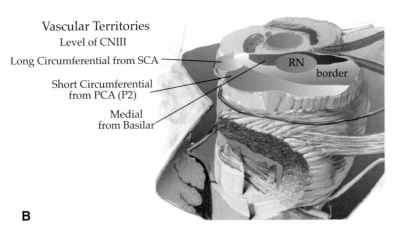

B

Vascular Territories
Level of CNIII

Long Circumferential from SCA

RN

border

Short Circumferential
from PCA (P2)

Medial
from Basilar

FIG V-3—*A,* Intra-axial course of the ocular motor nerves at the level of the pons (below) and midbrain (above). Note relation to the surrounding cerebellum and cranial nerves V and VII. *B,* Vascular territories of perforating branches off the vertebrobasilar arteries supplying portions of the third nerve within its intra-axial course in the midbrain. Compromise of these arteries produces classical intra-axial brain stem pathology. (Illustration by Craig A. Luce.)

Subarachnoid course (Fig V-4) The third nerve exits in the interpeduncular fossa and passes between the posterior cerebral and superior cerebellar arteries. It parallels the tentorial edge and the posterior communicating artery connecting the carotid artery with the P1 segment of the posterior cerebral artery. Cranial nerve III pierces the dura mater just lateral to the posterior clinoid process. Within the subarachnoid space, the nerve may be injured by an aneurysm of the posterior communicating artery or other mass lesions or from inflammation. A posterior communicating artery aneurysm, which typically arises at the junction of the posterior communicating artery and the internal carotid artery, is the most common cause of spontaneous, acute, complete third nerve palsy with pupil involvement. Injury to cranial nerve III may be produced by precipitous aneurysmal distension or blood extravasation, possibly producing intraneural hemorrhage. Because pupillary fibers are located peripherally (medially) in the third nerve, the pupil is involved in essentially all cases of aneurysm-induced third nerve palsy, and pain is a fairly constant feature.

Kerr FWL, Hollowell OW. Location of pupillomotor and accommodation fibers in the oculomotor nerve: experimental observations on paralytic mydriasis. *J Neurol Neurosurg Psychiatry.* 1964;27:473–481.

Acute elevation of supratentorial pressure, usually a result of mass lesion or hemorrhage, may force the medial aspect of the temporal lobe (the uncus) through the tentorial notch (*uncal herniation*). As a result, the third nerve may be stretched against the superior cerebellar artery or directly compressed. Pupillary involvement is an early sign, probably because of the superficial, dorsomedial location of the pupillomotor fibers at this level.

Intracavernous third nerve The lateral wall of the cavernous sinus is made up of two layers. The outer layer is the medial temporal dura mater, while the inner layer is a more diaphanous interconnection joining the sheaths of the third, fourth, and ophthalmic division of the fifth nerves. Once the third nerve enters the lateral wall of the cavernous sinus, it runs dorsal to the fourth nerve. Here it is susceptible to damage from carotid cavernous sinus fistula, aneurysm, tumors (particularly meningiomas, neurilemomas, cavernous hemangioma, and pituitary apoplexy) as well as infectious and granulomatous processes such as herpes zoster and Tolosa-Hunt syndrome. Within the cavernous sinus, third nerve palsy is often accompanied by signs related to the other ocular motor nerves and to cranial nerve V (trigeminal) and facial sensory loss.

An important exception is the nerve infarction associated with microvascular disease. Although often referred to as a diabetic third nerve palsy, this condition is not universally associated with glucose intolerance. This usually pupil-sparing palsy is most frequently seen in older patients and may be accompanied by intense periorbital pain. Significant pupillary involvement may occur in 10% of cases. Some presumed vasculopathic "peripheral" third nerve palsies may in fact be secondary to fascicular lesions with subtle evidence of involvement of other mesencephalic structures. Ischemic third nerve palsies spontaneously remit within about 12 weeks, although they may recur. Failure to completely resolve requires work-up for other than microvascular causes.

Hopf HC, Gutmann L. Diabetic 3rd nerve palsy: evidence for a mesencephalic lesion. *Neurology.* 1990;40:1041–1045.

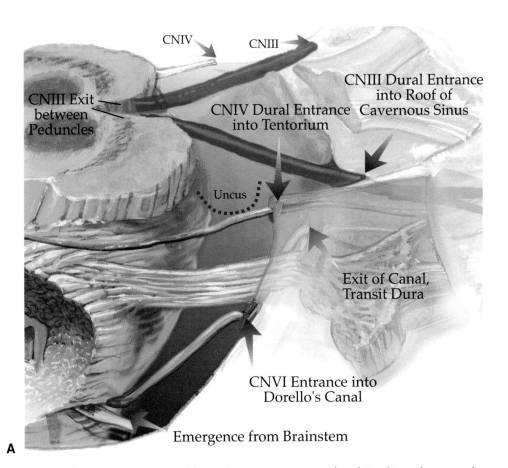

CNIV

CNIII

CNIII Exit between Peduncles

CNIII Dural Entrance into Roof of Cavernous Sinus

CNIV Dural Entrance into Tentorium

Uncus

Exit of Canal, Transit Dura

CNVI Entrance into Dorello's Canal

Emergence from Brainstem

A

FIG V-4—*A,* Subarachnoid course of the ocular motor nerves. Note the relationship to the surrounding dural structures, particularly the tentorium and the dura of the clivus. The nerves enter dural canals at the posterior aspect of the cavernous sinus for the third nerve, at the tentorial edge for the fourth nerve, and along the clivus for the sixth nerve. *B (facing page),* Major blood vessels and their relationships to the ocular motor nerves. Note the passage of the third nerve between the superior cerebellar artery below and posterior cerebral artery above. There is a vascular supply to the third nerve from branches off the posterior communicating artery, which is in close proximity. The sixth nerve also runs by the anterior inferior cerebellar artery, which is a major branch off the basilar artery.

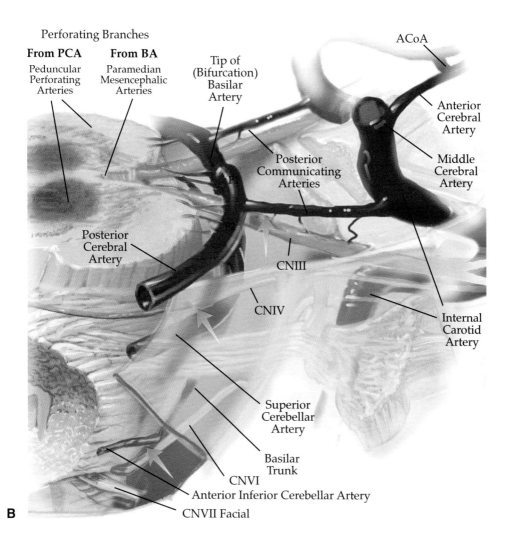

Perforating Branches

From PCA
Peduncular
Perforating
Arteries

From BA
Paramedian
Mesencephalic
Arteries

Tip of
(Bifurcation)
Basilar
Artery

ACoA

Anterior
Cerebral
Artery

Posterior
Communicating
Arteries

Middle
Cerebral
Artery

Posterior
Cerebral
Artery

CNIII

CNIV

Internal
Carotid
Artery

Superior
Cerebellar
Artery

Basilar
Trunk

CNVI

Anterior Inferior Cerebellar Artery

CNVII Facial

B

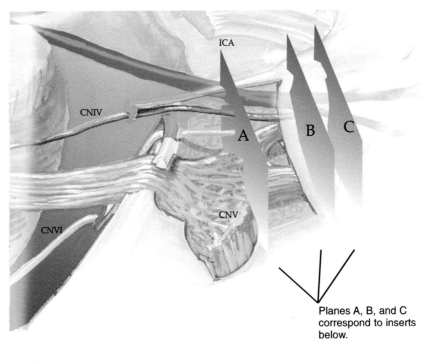

ICA

CNIV

A   B   C

CNV

CNVI

Planes A, B, and C
correspond to inserts
below.

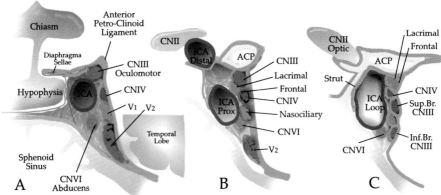

A

Chiasm

Anterior
Petro-Clinoid
Ligament

Diaphragma
Sellae

CNIII
Oculomotor

Hypophysis   ICA   CNIV

V_1 V_2

Temporal
Lobe

Sphenoid
Sinus

CNVI
Abducens

B

CNII

ICA
Distal   ACP   CNIII

Lacrimal

Frontal

ICA
Prox   CNIV

Nasociliary

CNVI

V_2

C

CNII
Optic   ACP

Lacrimal

Frontal

Strut

ICA
Loop   CNIV

Sup.Br.
CNIII

CNVI

Inf.Br.
CNIII

C

FIG V-4 cont.—*C,* Intracavernous course of the ocular motor nerves. The third and fourth nerves run in the lateral wall of the cavernous sinus along with the first and second divisions of the fifth cranial nerve. The sixth nerve runs in close approximation to the carotid artery within the cavernous sinus itself. As the nerves course toward the anterior aspect of the cavernous sinus and the superior orbital fissure, the first division of the fifth nerve (ophthalmic) divides into three branches: the lacrimal, frontal, and nasociliary. The first two of these cross over the top of the third and fourth nerves. The oculomotor nerve divides into a superior and inferior division, which crosses under the fourth nerve to enter the orbital apex through the annulus of Zinn. *D (facing page),* Intraorbital course of the ocular motor nerves. The fourth nerve crosses over the top of the optic nerve to innervate the superior oblique muscle in the supramedial portion of the orbit. The sixth cranial nerve innervates the lateral rectus muscle. The superior division of the third cranial nerve supplies the levator palpebrae and the superior rectus muscle from their underside. The inferior branch of the third nerve divides to supply the medial rectus muscle, the inferior rectus muscle, and a branch that travels along the lateral edge of the inferior rectus muscle to reach the inferior oblique muscle in the anterior orbit. *E,* Cross section of the superior orbital fissure showing the lacrimal frontal and trochlear nerves entering the orbit outside the annulus of Zinn and the superior and inferior divisions of the third nerve along with the abducens nerve and nasociliary nerve entering within the annulus of Zinn. (Illustrations by Craig A. Luce.)

120

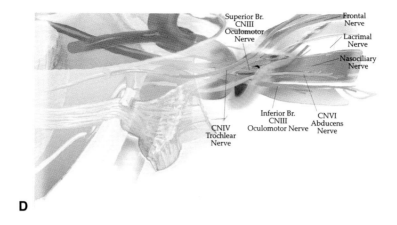

D

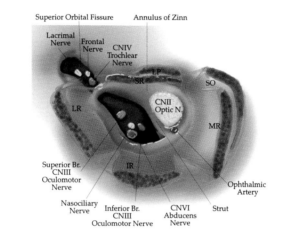

E

Orbital Just before the third nerve enters the orbit through the superior orbital fissure, it divides into superior and inferior branches. The superior division carries fibers innervating the superior rectus and the levator palpebrae superioris muscles; the inferior division carries fibers innervating the medial rectus, inferior oblique, and inferior rectus muscles as well as the parasympathetic fibers to the ciliary ganglion that will eventually innervate the iris sphincter and ciliary muscle. The most common cause of intraorbital damage to the third nerve is trauma with occasional involvement by viral infections and neoplastic processes.

Cranial Nerve IV (Trochlear)

Nucleus The fourth nerve arises in cells located in the periaqueductal gray matter beneath the aqueduct of Sylvius, caudal to and continuous with the third nerve nucleus within the midbrain. The medial longitudinal fasciculus passes inferolateral to the fourth nerve nucleus. Isolated fourth nerve palsy based in the nucleus is unusual, most often occurring with vascular disease, trauma, or demyelination. Contralateral nuclear fourth nerve palsy associated with ipsilateral Horner syndrome may result from involvement of descending sympathetic fibers in the mesencephalon.

Guy J, Day AL, Mickle JP, et al. Contralateral trochlear nerve paresis and ipsilateral Horner's syndrome. *Am J Ophthalmol.* 1989;107:73–76.

Fasciculus   The axons of the fourth cranial nerve curve dorsocaudally around the aqueduct, decussating completely in the anterior medullary velum and leaving the brain stem on its dorsal surface just caudal to the inferior colliculus. Cranial nerve IV is the only one to exit dorsally and to innervate contralaterally. Injury to the fasciculus is caused by lesions of the pineal region compressing the dorsal midbrain as well as processes similar to those affecting the nucleus. Fascicular involvement in the dorsal midbrain is esentially always bilateral.

Subarachnoid space   The fourth nerve curves around the brain stem, running just below the edge of the tentorium. It is often hidden beneath the edge and is prone to damage when the tentorial edge is sectioned neurosurgically. It pierces the dura mater just below cranial nerve III at the posterior end of the cavernous sinus. In its long intracranial course, cranial nerve IV is particularly susceptible to head trauma often mistakenly considered trivial.

Intracavernous   The fourth nerve courses within the lateral cavernous wall below the third nerve and above the first division of the fifth nerve. As the fourth nerve enters the superior orbital fissure, it first crosses over the third nerve to enter the orbital apex outside the annulus of Zinn. It then crosses over the optic nerve to innervate the superior oblique muscle. Surgery on the optic nerve in the canal and orbital apex can damage the fourth nerve.

Cranial Nerve VI (Abducens)

Nucleus   The sixth nerve arises in a collection of typical motor cells located in the floor of the fourth ventricle, beneath the facial colliculus in the caudal pontine paramedian tegmentum. The fasciculus of cranial nerve VII, the facial nerve, loops over the top of the sixth nerve nucleus, forming the genu of cranial nerve VII. The medial longitudinal fasciculus (MLF) passes medial to the sixth nerve nucleus. This nucleus contains both motor neurons and interneurons that project along the contralateral MLF to the contralateral medial rectus subnucleus, where they mediate conjugate gaze. Damage to the sixth nerve nucleus, therefore, results in a gaze palsy (conjugate inability to move either eye to the affected side) and not a unilateral abduction deficit. Ischemic, neoplastic, inflammatory, and, rarely, metabolic processes may affect the sixth nerve nucleus.

Leigh RJ, Zee DS. Diagnosis of central disorders of ocular motility and demyelination. In: *The Neurology of Eye Movements.* 2nd ed. Philadelphia: FA Davis; 1991:429.

Fasciculus   The fibers of the sixth nerve leave the nucleus and pass ventrally and laterally to exit the brain stem at the pontomedullary junction just lateral to the pyramidal prominence. Isolated sixth nerve palsy can result from a fascicular lesion, but more often associated neurologic deficits will be present as predicted by involvement of the nearby structures. If the damage to the fasciculus occurs in the ventral pons (Millard-Gubler syndrome), the pyramidal tract is involved, causing an ipsilateral abduction weakness associated with contralateral hemiplegia. These brain stem syndromes are almost always the result of brain stem vascular disease in the elderly. Demyelinating disease and tumors are occasionally the cause of damage to the fasciculus of the sixth nerve.

Johnson LN, Hepler RS. Isolated abducens nerve paresis from intrapontine, fascicular abducens nerve injury. *Am J Ophthalmol.* 1989;108:459–461.

Subarachnoid space After leaving the brain stem, the sixth nerve courses upward along the clivus. Within the prepontine basal cistern, the nerve is especially vulnerable to compression or infiltration by basilar tumors. Lesions arising laterally in the area of the cerebellopontine angle (most often acoustic neurinomas and meningiomas) may involve the sixth nerve as they enlarge. Each of these tumors can cause hearing loss and unsteadiness. Trauma may affect the sixth nerve as it ascends the clivus or as it crosses the petrous pyramid. Basilar skull fractures leading to sixth nerve palsies may also result in cerebrospinal fluid otorrhea as well as variable facial and auditory dysfunctions.

Increased intracranial pressure can cause downward displacement of the brain stem, producing a sixth nerve palsy by stretching the subarachnoid segment between its point of exit from the brain stem and its dural attachment on the clivus, especially where it is in contact with branches of the vertebrobasilar system. Along with headache, nausea, vomiting, and papilledema, sixth nerve paresis is a frequent finding in any condition, including pseudotumor cerebri, that causes increased intracranial pressure. Chapter VIII discusses these conditions in more detail.

Petrous pyramid The sixth nerve penetrates the dura mater just lateral to the superior clivus, passing through Dorello's canal. This canal is an enclosed space limited below by the petrous bone and above by the petroclinoid ligament connecting the petrous apex to the posterior clinoid. The inferior petrosal sinus exits through the same space, and it can compress the sixth nerve when dilated, as in a carotid cavernous fistula. Infectious or inflammatory processes originating in the middle ear (otitis media) or mastoid may affect the sixth nerve secondary to petrositis (Gradenigo syndrome). The sixth nerve passes lateral to the course of the carotid artery medial to Meckel's cave.

Intracavernous The sixth nerve is the only cranial nerve to run freely within the cavernous sinus. It is briefly joined inside the cavernous sinus by sympathetic branches from the paracarotid plexus; these subsequently pass to the iris dilator muscles along branches of the first division of the fifth nerve. This anatomy may account for the occasional association of postganglionic Horner syndrome with sixth nerve palsy as a result of an intracavernous lesion. The sixth nerve enters the orbit through the superior orbital fissure, passing within the annulus of Zinn to innervate the lateral rectus muscle.

Gutman I, Levartovski S, Goldhammer Y, et al. Sixth nerve palsy and unilateral Horner's syndrome. *Ophthalmology.* 1986;93:913–916.

Striph GG, Burde RM. Abducens nerve palsy and Horner's syndrome revisited. *J Clin Neuroophthalmol.* 1988;8:13–17.

Supranuclear Control (Fig V-5)

Horizontal Gaze Center

Signals resulting in conjugate horizontal movements of the two eyes are assembled within the dorsal pons. Burst cells within the pontine paramedian reticular formation (PPRF) provide the impetus for rapid movements to the side, but the horizontal gaze center itself is located within the sixth nerve nucleus. Lesions affecting this nucleus

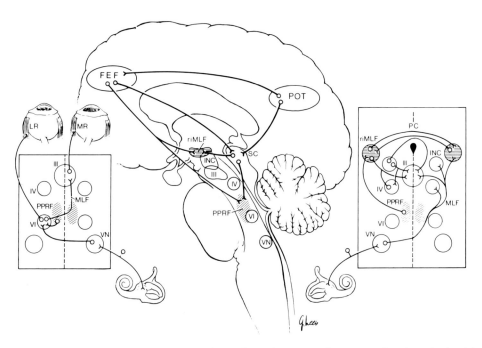

FIG V-5—Eye movement control. The center figure shows the supranuclear connections from the frontal eye fields (*FEF*) and the parieto-occipital-temporal junction region (*POT*) to the superior colliculus (*SC*), the rostral interstitial nucleus of the medial longitudinal fasciculus (*riMLF*), and the paramedian pontine reticular formation (*PPRF*). The FEF and SC are involved in the production of saccades, while the POT is thought to be important in the production of pursuit. Drawing on the left shows the brain stem pathways for horizontal gaze. Axons from the cell bodies located in the PPRF travel to the ipsilateral abducens nucleus (*VI*) where they synapse with abducens motoneurons, the axons of which travel to the ipsilateral lateral rectus muscle (*LR*), and with abducens internuclear neurons, the axons of which cross the midline and travel in the medial longitudinal fasciculus (*MLF*) to the portion(s) of the oculomotor nucleus (*III*) concerned with medial rectus (*MR*) function (in the contralateral eye). Drawing on the right shows the brain stem pathways for vertical gaze. Important structures include the riMLF, PPRF, the interstitial nucleus of Cajal (*INC*), and the posterior commissure (*PC*). Note that axons from cell bodies located in the vestibular nuclei (*VN*) travel directly to the abducens nuclei and, mostly by way of the MLF, to the oculomotor nuclei. *IV,* trochear nucleus. (Reproduced with permission from Miller NR. *Walsh and Hoyt's Clinical Neuro-Ophthalmology.* Baltimore: Williams & Wilkins; 1985.)

therefore result in an ipsilateral horizontal gaze palsy. These lesions may be vascular in origin. Obstruction of the perforating vessels affecting the blood supply to the sixth nerve nucleus also tends to affect the seventh nerve as well as a portion of the nucleus of the fifth nerve, resulting in a horizontal gaze palsy, an ipsilateral seventh nerve palsy, and facial sensory loss (Foville syndrome).

Vertical Gaze Centers

The vertical gaze centers are located within the midbrain just rostral to the third nerve nuclei. Here, they receive signals through the termination of the medial longitudinal fasciculus from below as well as direct signals from the supranuclear pathway. The burst cells in the rostral end of the PPRF provide important input. Thus, bilateral involvement of the MLF can create problems with vertical saccades. The primary vertical gaze center is within an area referred to as the *rostral interstitial nucleus* of the MLF, located dorsomedial to the anterior end of the red nucleus. The pathways for up and down movements are separated in the midbrain; the pathways for upgaze are more dorsal, crossing in the posterior commissure. The *interstitial nucleus of Cajal* located in the periaqueductal region also plays an active role in vertical gaze, sending interneurons to the contralateral superior rectus subnucleus in the third nerve nucleus.

Internuclear Connections

The medial longitudinal fasciculus provides the primary communication between the pontine horizontal gaze center and the vertical gaze centers within the midbrain. The MLF also carries information from the infranuclear centers below. They run as paired structures within the dorsal aspect of the median brain stem. This pathway is particularly important, as it conveys information from the contralateral horizontal gaze center to the ipsilateral third nerve subnucleus subtending the medial rectus muscle. Unilateral damage to an MLF produces an abnormality of adduction with horizontal gaze, an *internuclear ophthalmoplegia.* This damage may be caused by a mass lesion (neoplastic, infectious, arteriovenous malformation, etc.) but is usually related to an inflammatory plaque (demyelinating disease) in young patients or to microvascular disease in older patients. Demyelinating disease often produces bilateral involvement. Additional information is conveyed from the more caudal brain stem centers to the pons and midbrain along the brachium conjunctivum.

Infranuclear Input

Vestibular subnuclei located at the pontomedullary junction provide the fundamental tonic input to the horizontal and vertical gaze centers. The signal originating from the semicircular canals and passing through the vestibular nerves and their nuclei is the single most important determinant of the resting position of the eyes. Abnormalities of vestibular input result in *drift* of the eyes. The direction depends on which of the semicircular canals has been involved. Pathology is usually non–canal selective. The right vestibular system innervates the left horizontal gaze center and vice versa. Therefore, pathology within the right vestibular nerve or nucleus results in ipsilateral, or right, horizontal drift of the eyes secondary to corrective saccades (vestibular nystagmus) to the left. Other infranuclear input includes proprioceptive information conveyed from the extremities as well as from the neck.

Supranuclear Input

Volitional eye movements may be visually or nonvisually directed. Visually directed movements require target position information available from the occipital lobes and calcarine cortex or through the superior colliculus, which also contains retinotopic information. Nonvisually guided eye movements usually originate with activity in the premotor areas of the frontal lobes. Descending frontobulbar pathways act on the areas within the contralateral brain stem that contain the pause cells. *Pause cells* normally suppress the burst cells in the PPRF, and inhibition of the pause cells precedes conjugate saccadic eye movements. Information for visually guided saccades projects to the PPRF and the rostral interstitial nucleus of the MLF from the superior colliculi. Continuous visual feedback containing target position information passes through the posterior/superior temporal cortex to the ipsilateral gaze centers, probably mediated through the superior colliculi.

Cerebellar Gain

Gain in an engineering sense can be defined as the ratio of the output of a system to the input. For example, when the head rotates to the right, the vestibulo-ocular reflex should move the eyes in an equal and opposite direction to the left. Maintenance of this gain of "one" is the responsibility of connections to the cerebellum. Pathology affecting the cerebellum–brain stem connections may result in abnormalities of vestibular gain or inability to adjust gain. The cerebellum and its connections are also responsible for controlling the gain in the saccadic and pursuit systems.

Saccadic System

Saccades are rapid conjugate eye movements (up to 400°–500°/sec) initiated by burst cells lying within the PPRF (Fig V-6). Their activation requires suppression of pause cell activity. Pause cells are inhibited by corticobulbar projections from the frontal eye fields (voluntary eye movements) or by neurons within the superior colliculus responding to a visual target. The pause cells are located in the nucleus raphe interpositus midline between the rootlets of the sixth nerve. Abnormalities in these pause cells permit continuous burst cell firing, leading to *saccadomania,* which is seen clinically as *opsoclonus,* or *flutter* (see chapter VI).

There are three clinical characteristics of saccades: latency, velocity, and accuracy. *Latency,* the time it takes to initiate a saccadic movement, varies between 200 and 250 msec. Saccadic *velocity* is determined by the size of the saccade; the larger the saccade, the faster the peak velocity. Slow eye movements in pathologic conditions may be demonstrated to be saccadic if they maintain an appropriate relationship between the velocity and the size of the movement. *Accuracy* refers to the eyes arriving at the desired position. Failure to do so (*saccadic dysmetria*) may result from saccades being either too small (hypometria) or too large (hypermetria). Dysmetria may be found with abnormalities in gain related to cerebellar disease.

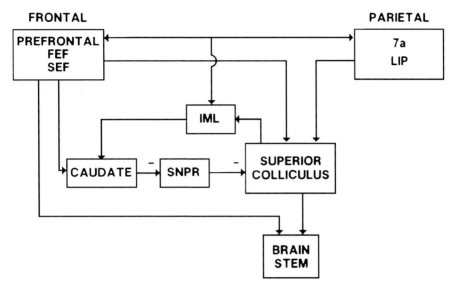

FIG V-6—A block diagram of the major structures that participate in the control of saccades. *FEF,* frontal eye fields; *SEF,* supplementary eye fields; *IML,* intramedullary lamina of thalamus; *LIP,* lateral intraparietal area; *SNPR,* substantia nigra, pars reticulata. Negative signs indicate inhibitory projections. Not shown here is the pulvinar because of its uncertain role in saccade generation. The pulvinar does, however, have connections with the superior colliculus and both the frontal and parietal lobes; it may be important for directing visual attention. (Reproduced with permission from Leigh RJ, Zee DS. *The Neurology of Eye Movements.* Philadelphia: Davis; 1991.)

Neural Integrator

Moving the eyes away from primary position is opposed by elastic restoring force ready to bring the eyes back to center. To maintain the eyes in an eccentric position requires increased input. Thus, saccadic movements to an eccentric position must bring the eyes into position and then maintain them once they have arrived. The *neural integrator* automatically converts the *velocity command* that determines the size of the saccade into a *position command* that indicates how much additional tonus is necessary to maintain the eye in that eccentric position (Fig V-7). The integration of these signals has been isolated to the area of the nucleus prepositus hypoglossi in the area of the medial vestibular nucleus at the level of rostral medulla.

The neural integrator may be affected by metabolic abnormalities including alcohol and antiseizure medications (phenytoin). A "leaky" neural integrator may not maintain eccentric position, and the eyes will drift back toward center with correcting saccades attempting to keep them eccentric. Gaze paretic nystagmus is characteristic of an abnormality in the neural integrator. Nystagmus takes place with the fast phase in the direction of the eccentric gaze.

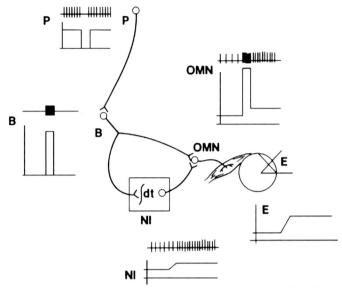

FIG V-7—The relationship between pause cells (*P*), burst cells (*B*), and the cells of the neural integrator (*NI*) in the generation of the saccadic pulse and step. Pause cells cease discharging just before each saccade, allowing the burst cells to generate the pulse. The pulse is integrated by the neural integrator to produce the step. The pulse and step combine to produce the innervational change on the ocular motoneurons (*OMN*) that produces the saccadic eye movements (*E*). Vertical lines represent individual discharges of neurons. Underneath the schematized neural (spike) discharge is a plot of discharge rate versus time. (Reproduced with permission from Leigh RJ, Zee DS. *The Neurology of Eye Movements.* Philadelphia: Davis; 1991.)

Smooth Pursuit

The pursuit system is a semivoluntary pathway responsible for maintaining fixation on a moving target (Fig V-8). Pursuit latency is shorter than that for saccades (approximately 125 msec), but maximal peak velocity is limited to 30°–60°/sec. Pursuit movements may not be made spontaneously but require a target. This target does not have to be visual; it may be proprioceptive or in rare cases produced by visual imagination. Recent work indicates the importance of the middle temporal visual area as well as the adjacent medial superior temporal cortical area. Both of these regions receive inputs from the primary visual cortical centers and in turn project ipsilaterally to the dorsolateral pontine nuclei. A double decussation has been postulated but not proven. These projections eventually change the tonus through the vestibular nuclei, probably through the vestibulocerebellar connections involving the flocculus and dorsal vermis (lobule VI–VII). Thus, lesions of the cerebellar flocculus may affect pursuit movements.

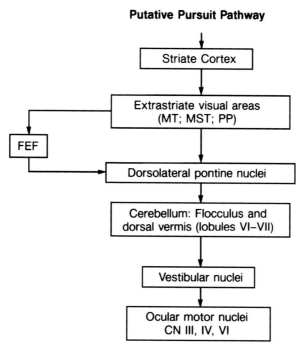

Putative Pursuit Pathway

Striate Cortex

Extrastriate visual areas
(MT; MST; PP)

FEF

Dorsolateral pontine nuclei

Cerebellum: Flocculus and
dorsal vermis (lobules VI–VII)

Vestibular nuclei

Ocular motor nuclei
CN III, IV, VI

FIG V-8—A hypothetical anatomic scheme for smooth pursuit eye movements. The pathway starts with striate cortex, which receives inputs from the lateral geniculate nuclei (indicated by topmost arrow). *MT,* middle temporal visual area; *MST,* medial superior temporal visual area; *PP,* posterior parietal cortex; *FEF,* frontal eye fields. (Reproduced with permission from Leigh RJ, Zee DS. *The Neurology of Eye Movements.* Philadelphia: Davis; 1991.)

Vestibulo-Ocular Reflex

Teleologically, the oldest eye movement is that associated with the vestibulo-ocular reflex (VOR). The pathway is a three-neuron connection from the vestibular neuron through the vestibular nucleus directly to the contralateral horizontal gaze center, resulting in the shortest latency (16 msec) of all eye movements. Vestibular eye movements have a high peak velocity (up to 300°/sec). The distinction between the relatively limited pursuit system and the rapid vestibulo-ocular reflex may easily be seen clinically: a paper cannot be read when it is shaken at more than approximately 60°/sec, while it can easily be read when the head is moved at far greater velocities from side to side. In the first case, the pursuit system breaks down at relatively low velocities; in the second, the vestibulo-ocular reflex maintains stability over a much greater range of velocities. Damage to the vestibular pathway results in an initial ocular position bias, which can be compensated for by cerebellar change in the gain. Improvement occurs with time, but subtle abnormalities may persist (see chapter VI).

Vergence System

The vergence system keeps the image of the target on corresponding elements of the two retinas by controlling the relative alignment of the visual axes. There are two primary stimuli to vergence eye movements: *blur* (accommodative vergence) and *diplopia* (disparity vergence). Vergence is a component of the *near triad,* which also includes accommodation and pupillary constriction (see chapter IV). These disconjugate movements are slow relative to saccades. Latency between stimulation of vergence and the eye movement is about 160 msec.

Supranuclear control of vergence movements is not yet fully understood. Experimentally, stimulation of frontal and occipital eye fields both produce convergence. Neurons in areas of the middle temporal region and parietal cortex discharge in response to retinal disparity and objects moving in depth. The immediate premotor initiation of vergence probably resides in neurons near the oculomotor nuclei that project to the medial rectus subnucleus. A subgroup of cells in the medial rectus subnucleus may have a selective function in vergence movements.

Leigh RJ, Zee DS. Vergence eye movements. In: *The Neurology of Eye Movements.* 2nd ed. Philadelphia: FA Davis; 1991:280–283.

Mays LE, Porter JD, Gamlin PD, et al. Neural control of vergence eye movements: neurons encoding vergence velocity. *J Neurophysiol.* 1986;56:1007–1021.

Clinical Abnormalities of the Ocular Motor System

Abnormalities in the ocular motor system may be manifest as blurring of vision, double vision, or sensation of movement of the environment. Another rare symptom is tilt of the environment, seen in lateral medullary disease.

Often the patient may be asymptomatic in spite of abnormalities in ocular motility. The five basic ocular motor pathways can be tested individually. They are

- Vestibulo-ocular reflex (VOR)
- Optokinetic system
- Saccades
- Pursuit
- Convergence

Gross abnormalities may be picked up during duction and version testing (see chapter I). Subtle defects require concentration on the characteristics of each individual ocular motor system.

Duncan GW, Parker SW, Fisher CM. Acute cerebellar infarction in the PICA territory. *Arch Neurol.* 1975;32:364–368.

Testing for Central Abnormalities of the Ocular Motor System

Ocular Stability

Abnormalities of ocular stability may occur with pathology affecting the vestibular pathways and also with abnormalities in the cerebellar connections responsible for gain. While gross abnormalities can be seen immediately, subtle ones are most easily detected by fixating on the optic disc with a direct ophthalmoscope. Patients should have dilated pupils and no fixation target (in the dark). Normal microsaccadic refixation movements may be seen as small square-wave movements of the disc. Macrosaccadic square-wave jerks (larger movements of the disc) may indicate cerebellar pathology. In addition, a tendency to drift with subtle primary position nystagmus may be obvious. Subtle abnormalities in the neural integrator may be found by moving the eye into eccentric gaze and looking for failure to maintain eccentric gaze with drift back toward midline.

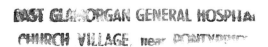

Vestibulo-Ocular Reflex (VOR)

Assessment of the gain of the VOR is most easily accomplished with a direct ophthalmoscope. The examiner fixates the disc while rotating the patient's head horizontally. This test should be performed in the dark with no fixation clues. Failure to maintain the disc in direct view of the ophthalmoscope indicates an abnormality of the gain. A drift of the disc in the direction opposite to head rotation indicates a gain of less than 1. This simple test described by David Zee can pick up very subtle abnormalities in vestibular gain.

> Zee DS. Ophthalmoscopy in examination of patients with vestibular disorders. *Ann Neurol.* 1978;3:373–374.

An even more subtle test described by Zee involves having the patient spontaneously shake his or her head from side to side with eyes closed. With 20–30 seconds of head shaking, the vestibular systems are maximally stimulated. The patient is then instructed to open the eyes, again in a darkened environment, and the disc is re-examined with the direct ophthalmoscope. While the eyes may well have been stable prior to stimulation, induced drift indicates a subtle asymmetry in the vestibular input, indicating a greater reserve in the side away from which the disc is drifting. If these clinical observations are inadequate, detailed recordings of eye movement can be made with electro-oculogram (EOG), infrared tracking, or magnetic scleral coil.

Optokinetic Nystagmus

The importance of asymmetric optokinetic nystagmus (OKN) in the past was substantial. "Cogan's rule" held that abnormalities of the optokinetic system that appeared when the OKN drum was rotated toward the side of pathology in the setting of homonymous hemianopia indicated a greater likelihood of neoplastic as opposed to vascular phenomena. As vascular pathophysiology is far more common than tumors, this conclusion frequently is not true. In addition, modern neuroimaging has reduced the value of asymmetric OKN as a means of distinguishing vascular from neoplastic processes. However, asymmetry in the optokinetic system does indicate the likelihood of more extensive involvement of the descending pathways through the middle temporal (MT) and medial superior temporal (MST) areas.

Pursuit

In clinically assessing pursuit, it is important not to move the stimulus too rapidly. Inability to maintain fixation on a target can be judged relatively easily. *Cogwheel pursuit* indicates that saccadic correction movements are present to make up for abnormalities within the pursuit system. A subtle way of looking for abnormalities in the pursuit system is *pursuit at zero velocity.* The patient is told to fixate on his or her thumb while being rotated in a chair. This so-called suppression of the vestibulo-ocular reflex requires an intact pursuit system. Drift of the eyes with correcting saccades indicates abnormalities somewhere along the connection from the MT and MST areas to the brain stem nuclear centers located from the pontomedullary junction to the midbrain. Subtle pursuit abnormalities are commonly a result of demyelinating disease in young patients and may indicate microvascular disease in the elderly. Inflammatory, infectious, and neoplastic processes and intra-axial arteriovenous malformations may also lead to abnormalities in pursuit.

Saccades

As discussed in chapter V, evaluation of saccades should specifically include the three key features: latency, velocity, and accuracy. While detailed velocity measurements require sophisticated quantitative evaluation, gross abnormalities in saccadic velocity are easy to see. Failure of the saccade to reach the target appropriately is indicated by a secondary correcting saccade or by a slow eye movement (*glissade*). Failure to initiate a saccade to a voluntary command suggests a diagnosis of ocular motor apraxia. Abnormalities in the nuclear gaze center must be excluded, usually by the use of infranuclear stimuli through the vestibulo-ocular reflex to elicit both slow and fast movements.

Convergence

Convergence can be tested with an accommodative target, which should not be a penlight but rather an object with enough detail to require attempts at accommodation. Thus, the entire three-part reflex (convergence, accommodation, and pupillary miosis) can be checked. Vergence movements are slow. Relative abnormalities of convergence may be seen with change in alignment from a distant target to a near one (increased exophoria at near).

Pathology of Ocular Motility

Ocular Motor System Abnormalities Without Symptoms

Supranuclear disturbances are frequently discovered without visual symptoms or complaints. Occasionally, patients may note difficulty with reading or blurred vision.

Ocular motor apraxia   Ocular motor apraxia is characterized by an inability to initiate normal voluntary horizontal saccades. *Congenital ocular motor apraxia* is an impairment of voluntary horizontal eye movements resulting in extreme contraversive ocular deviation on body or head rotation (i.e., an involuntary deviation of the eyes to one side on head rotation) with conspicuous compensatory head thrusts on attempted horizontal gaze to either side. Random saccadic movements are fully retained, and vertical eye movements are normal, but the fast phase of OKN is absent. Over a period of years, the head thrusts become less apparent so that only the slightest rotation is necessary to initiate horizontal refixational eye movements. The location of the lesion in congenital ocular motor apraxia is unknown, although abnormalities in the corpus callosum have been reported.

    Acquired ocular motor apraxia results from bilateral lesions of the supranuclear gaze pathways, which are usually localized to the frontoparietal cortex. A defect in bidirectional saccadic initiation occurs without affecting either smooth pursuit or responses to oculocephalic stimulation, although the fast phases of vestibular (caloric) nystagmus are impaired. Patients with acquired ocular motor apraxia blink to break the fixation reflex and then turn toward the new fixation point while the fixation reflex is disrupted.

Cogan DG. A type of congenital ocular motor apraxia presenting jerky head movements. *Am J Ophthalmol.* 1953;36:433–441.

Zee DS, Yee RD, Singer HS. Congenital ocular motor apraxia. *Brain.* 1977;100:581–599.

Gaze palsy and preference Acute damage to the frontal lobe from ischemia, trauma, or infection can result in the inability to generate a voluntary saccade in the direction away from the lesion. Similar findings may be seen with damage to the descending frontobulbar pathways. Following a parietotemporal lesion, an acute gaze preference toward the side of the lesion may occur. These deficits may be overcome by the vestibulo-ocular reflex (doll's head phenomenon) and may gradually improve following acute, usually vascular, injury. MRI can be used to localize involvement. Most commonly, parietotemporal lesions are vascular in origin, but they can also be seen with neoplastic, inflammatory (demyelinating), and infectious processes.

Horizontal gaze palsies may be congenital with aplasia of both sixth nerve nuclei. This condition is invariably accompanied by bilateral seventh nerve palsies and occasionally associated with problems with other lower cranial nerves (Möbius syndrome). Affected patients often use their vergence systems to move the eyes medially. Ocular malalignment may result, but early onset and adaptive suppression usually obviate diplopia (Fig VI-1).

Towfighi J, Marks K, Palmer E, et al. Möbius syndrome: neuropathologic observations. *Acta Neuropathol.* 1979;48:11–17.

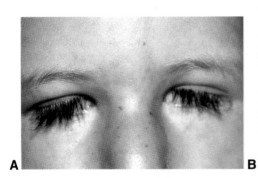

A

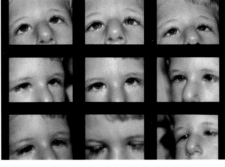

B

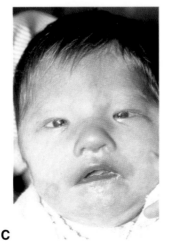

C

FIG VI-1—*A,* A 4-year-old with facial diplegia and bilateral sixth nerve palsies, diagnostic of Möbius syndrome. *B,* Adduction is possible with convergence, but neither eye would abduct. *C,* Facial appearance is often characteristic in Möbius syndrome with flattening of the nasolabial folds and droop of the corner of the mouth.

Vertical gaze palsies may be caused by pathology within the rostral midbrain. This pathology can be neoplastic, inflammatory, traumatic, or ischemic. Often both sides of the rostral midbrain and overlying diencephalon are supplied by a single artery, the artery of Percheron, arising from the proximal segment of one of the posterior cerebral arteries. Pathologic conditions at the termination of the basilar artery such as embolus, thrombosis, aneurysm, or surgical trauma can result in difficulty with vertical eye movements. Extrinsic and, less commonly, intrinsic (glioma) mass lesions may produce problems with vertical gaze by compressing the dorsal midbrain. These lesions are usually situated at or near the pineal gland and include pinealomas, teratomas, and germ cell tumors. Less common causes include demyelinating disease, neurosyphilis, or trauma. In addition to impaired upgaze, affected patients usually demonstrate eyelid retraction (Collier's sign), light–near dissociation (constriction of pupil to a near target but not to light), and convergence-retraction nystagmus (cofiring of the four horizontal rectus muscles induced by attempted up saccades that is best elicited with a downwardly rotating OKN drum). Accommodation may be variably affected (Fig VI-2).

> Collier J. Nuclear ophthalmoplegia, with special reference to retraction of the lids and ptosis and to lesions of the posterior commissure. *Brain*. 1927;50:488–498.

If only the descending frontobulbar pathways are affected, vestibulo-ocular reflex movements may be maintained. Commonly, these patients have complaints of double vision caused by an associated skew deviation. They may also complain of blurry vision, especially when reading.

Saccadic slowing Saccadic slowing that is independent of hypometria or abnormalities in latency may be seen with the following:

- Muscle disease (progressive external ophthalmoplegia)
- Neuromuscular defects (myasthenia, which is more commonly associated with small hypervelocity saccades)
- Ophthalmoplegia (usually disconjugate)
- Intra-axial pathology
- Wilson disease
- Huntington disease
- Cerebellar degeneration
- Ataxia-telangiectasia
- Progressive supranuclear palsy (PSP; Steele-Richardson-Olszewski syndrome)

In the case of PSP, vertical gaze is preferentially affected in early stages with particular impairment of downgaze, leading to the "dirty tie syndrome." A form of basal ganglion disease, PSP is marked by increasing rigidity, dysarthria, and dementia. Patients may be diagnosed initially as having Parkinson disease. Other possible ocular findings include decreased blink frequency, blepharitis, blepharospasm, and occasionally apraxia of eye opening. Ocular movements gradually deteriorate to include loss of vestibularly induced movements as well.

Many diseases characterized by saccadic slowing are associated with inability to suppress spontaneous saccades to a visual target. Huntington disease, Wilson disease, and other disorders that affect the frontobulbar pathways including PSP are particularly likely to be associated with this condition.

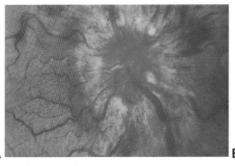

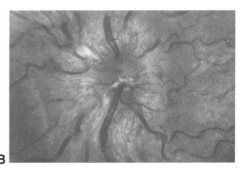

A

B

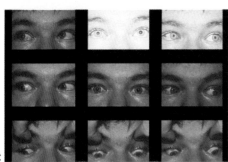

C

FIG VI-2—A 24-year-old with a 2-week history of headache and double vision. *A and B,* Funduscopic examination reveals bilateral disc elevation characteristic of papilledema. *C,* Patient shows evidence of weakness in upgaze and convergence-retraction nystagmus. *D,* Patient's pupils demonstrate failure to react to a direct light stimulus, but do react to a near target (*E*). *F and G,* MRI confirms the presence of a lesion involving the dorsal midbrain, which is subsequently demonstrated to be a dysgerminoma.

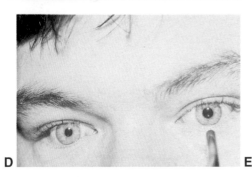

D

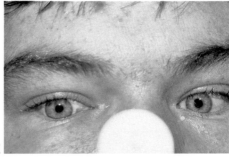

E

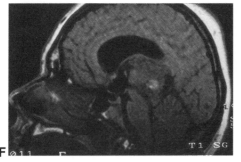

F

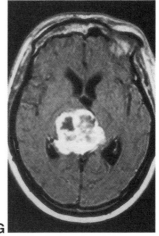

G

Olivopontocerebellar atrophy may occur on a hereditary or sporadic basis. Its onset occurs in early adulthood with unsteadiness of station and gait. Speech becomes slurred, and dementia may be apparent. Optic atrophy and pigmentary degeneration of the retina may also occur. Eye movements become progressively slowed in all directions, finally resulting in complete external ophthalmoplegia. Histopathologically, there is atrophy of the cerebellar cortex, the olives, and the gray matter of the pons along with degeneration of the middle cerebellar peduncles and the restiform bodies.

Leigh RJ, Newman SA, Folstein SE, et al. Abnormal ocular motor control in Huntington's disease. *Neurology.* 1983;33:1268–1275.

Lennox G, Jones R. Gaze distractibility in Wilson's disease. *Ann Neurol.* 1989;25:415–417.

Steele JC, Richardson JC, Olszewski J. Progressive supranuclear palsy: a heterogeneous degeneration involving the brain stem, basal ganglia and cerebellum with vertical gaze and pseudobulbar palsy, nuchal dystonia and dementia. *Arch Neurol.* 1964;10:333–359.

Pursuit deficits   While patients with abnormalities affecting the pursuit system may complain of blurred or decreased vision, they are often unaware of any problem. Gross abnormalities in smooth pursuit are usually obvious on testing versions, but subtle changes may be best appreciated by testing pursuit at zero velocity. Induced saccadic movements, especially when asymmetric, indicate pathology affecting the pursuit pathways. These changes are most commonly seen with vascular disease but may also occur with mass lesions. Reduction in gain, resulting in catch-up saccades even with relatively slow-moving targets, may occur with Parkinson disease or progressive supranuclear palsy and may also be seen in patients taking a variety of medications. In young patients demyelinating disease is a frequent cause of abnormalities in smooth pursuit. It is difficult to define the exact site of pathologic involvement.

Ocular Instability: Nystagmoid Movements

Ocular instability may be present only in eccentric gaze, which suggests the neural integrator as the area of primary pathology, or in primary position. Abnormalities in ocular motor stability may be congenital or acquired. Instability usually appears as nystagmus, but a subset of abnormalities in ocular stability have nonrhythmic components and are defined separately. Chief among these abnormalities are pathologic processes that affect the pause cells, leading to continuous saccadic activity. The resulting movements may be recognized by reduction in intersaccadic latency with immediate movement in the opposite direction. When solely horizontal, this response is referred to as *ocular flutter.* When both horizontal and vertical components exist, it is called *opsoclonus.* In both cases the pathophysiology of abnormalities in the pause cells may be related to vascular or neoplastic processes, but these abnormalities often have an underlying immune mechanism, frequently a paraneoplastic syndrome that is presumed to cause direct damage to the pause cells. This mechanism may be associated with neuroblastoma in children or small cell carcinoma of the lung or cancer of the breast or ovaries in adults.

Digre KB. Opsoclonus in adults. Report of three cases and review of the literature. *Arch Neurol.* 1986;43:1165–1175.

Kilgo GR, Schwartze GM. Opsoclonus. Update on clinical and pathologic associations. *J Clin Neuroophthalmol.* 1984;4:109–113.

Wolpow ER, Richardson EP Jr. Case records of the Massachusetts General Hospital (case 9-1988). *N Engl J Med.* 1988;318:563–570.

Damage to the connections between the inferior olive, the red nucleus, and the dentate nucleus within the vestibular cerebellum, usually caused by vascular events, results in *oculopalatal myoclonus.* Continuous slow vertical eye movements are associated with coincident movement of the palate. An additional association between vertical eye movements and facial activity is *oculomasticatory myorhythmia,* seen in Whipple disease, an infectious disease of the bowel. *Ocular bobbing* consists of intermittent, usually conjugate rapid downward movements of the eyes followed by a slower return to primary position. This abnormality is classically seen with intrinsic pontine lesions, often secondary to hemorrhage, and is most frequently seen in comatose patients. When this movement is reversed (a slow downward movement and rapid correction upward), it is referred to as *ocular dipping.*

Schwartz MA, Selhorst JB, Ochs AL, et al. Oculomasticatory myorhythmia: a unique movement disorder occurring in Whipple's disease. *Ann Neurol.* 1986;20:677–683.

Susac JO, Hoyt WF, Daroff RB, et al. Clinical spectrum of ocular bobbing. *J Neurol Neurosurg Psychiatry.* 1970;33:771–775.

Tahmoush AJ, Brooks JE, Keltner JL. Palatal myoclonus associated with abnormal ocular and extremity movements. A polygraphic study. *Arch Neurol.* 1972;27:431–440.

Ocular Instability: Nystagmus

Most nystagmus is conjugate. Exceptions include convergence-retraction nystagmus and see-saw nystagmus. *Convergence-retraction nystagmus* involves cocontraction of all four horizontal muscles induced by attempts at up saccades. It is classically seen as part of the dorsal midbrain syndrome along with limited upgaze, light–near dissociation, and eyelid retraction (Collier's sign). *See-saw nystagmus,* usually seen with pathology affecting the parasellar region, involves one eye rising and usually intorting while the other eye falls and extorts.

Daroff RB. See-saw nystagmus. *Neurology.* 1965;15:874–877.

Druckman R, Ellis P, Kleinfeld J, et al. Seesaw nystagmus. *Arch Ophthalmol.* 1966;76: 668–675.

Smith JL, Zieper I, Gay AJ, et al. Nystagmus retractorius. *Arch Ophthalmol.* 1959;62: 864–867.

Relatively *unilateral nystagmus* can also occur, which may be entirely unilateral but is more often simply asymmetric. Often vision is extremely poor in one eye, but this condition may also occur in patients with spasmus nutans associated with torticollis and head oscillations that usually appear within the first year of life and spontaneously resolve. Characteristically, the nystagmus is very rapid and of small amplitude. Signs including head nodding and torticollis disappear during sleep, and patients should be otherwise neurologically and ophthalmologically normal. If other ocular abnormalities are detected on examination (e.g., subnormal visual function or optic atrophy), or if other neurologic symptoms are present, MRI is advisable to rule out suprasellar/hypothalamic pathology, usually glioma. Even children who are initially considered normal except for their spasmus nutans can be found to harbor such a lesion; thus, careful follow-up is mandatory.

Newman SA, Hedges TR III, Wall M, et al. Spasmus nutans—or is it? *Surv Ophthalmol.* 1990;34:453–456.

Weissman BM, Dell'Osso LF, Abel LA, et al. Spasmus nutans. A quantitative prospective study. *Arch Ophthalmol.* 1987;105:525–528.

Yee RD, Jelks GW, Baloh RW, et al. Uniocular nystagmus in monocular visual loss. *Ophthalmology.* 1979;86:511–518.

Although *congenital nystagmus* is classically horizontal, maintaining its horizontal aspect even in vertical gaze, it can occasionally be vertical or torsional. It tends to be accentuated by visual attention, diminished by convergence, and minimal at a null point. There may be associated inversion of optokinetic nystagmus. When the OKN drum rotates in the direction of the slow phase, the nystagmus decreases or may even reverse. This reaction may occur in almost two thirds of patients with congenital nystagmus. Congenital nystagmus can arise from abnormalities of the afferent system if occurrence is early. Abnormal ocular bias therefore cannot be corrected. Latent nystagmus is a form of congenital nystagmus brought out by covering one eye; the uncovered eye drifts toward midline with corrective saccades into abduction, and the slow phase exponentially decays. Acquired nystagmus that is present only in eccentric gaze is a result of pathology affecting the neural integrator.

Gelbart SS, Hoyt CS. Congenital nystagmus: a clinical perspective in infancy. *Graefes Arch Clin Exp Ophthalmol.* 1988;226:178–180.

Acquired nystagmus in primary position is most often caused by abnormalities in vestibular input (Table VI-1). Specific lesions affecting the pathway from the vestibular system to the central coordinating centers may also produce drift with rhythmic corrections. Horizontal jerk nystagmus is the most common result. Much has been written about distinguishing peripheral from central vestibular involvement, but the advent of neuroimaging has made this distinction less critical. The two most useful distinguishing features are hearing, which is always involved with peripheral pathology, and the ability to damp the nystagmus with fixation, which is usually not possible with central lesions.

Asymmetric vertical drift is also possible with pathology affecting the central vestibular projections. Lesions that have compressed the cervical medullary junction, preferentially affecting the crossing pathways responsible for downgaze, are particularly likely to result in a drift of the eyes upward and, therefore, downbeat nystagmus. This condition is classically seen with an Arnold-Chiari malformation but may appear with any lesion that compresses the brain stem in the area of the foramen magnum (tumors and basilar invagination). Other etiologies include microvascular disease associated with vertebrobasilar insufficiency; multiple sclerosis; encephalitis; and various metabolic disorders including abnormalities of magnesium depletion, Wernicke's encephalopathy, and lithium intoxication.

Upbeat nystagmus is somewhat less localizing, possibly caused by midline cerebellar (vermis) pathology. Pathophysiology includes microvascular disease, multiple sclerosis, cerebellar degeneration, and various metabolic abnormalities. Up-

TABLE VI-1

VESTIBULAR NYSTAGMUS

SYMPTOM OR SIGN	PERIPHERAL (END-ORGAN)	CENTRAL (NUCLEAR)
Direction of nystagmus	Unidirectional; fast phase opposite lesion	Bidirectional or unidirectional
Purely horizontal nystagmus without torsional component	Uncommon	Common
Vertical or purely torsional nystagmus	Never present	May be present
Visual fixation	Inhibits nystagmus and vertigo	No inhibition
Severity of vertigo	Marked	Mild
Direction of spin	Toward fast phase	Variable
Direction of pastpointing	Toward slow phase	Variable
Direction of Romberg fall	Toward slow phase	Variable
Effect of head turning	Changes Romberg fall	No effect
Duration of symptoms	Finite (minutes, days, weeks) but recurrent	May be chronic
Tinnitus or deafness	Often present	Usually absent
Common causes	Infection (labyrinthitis), Meniere's disease, neuronitis, vascular disorders, trauma, toxicity	Vascular, demyelinating, and neoplastic disorders

Reprinted with permission from Daroff RB, Troost BT, Dell'Osso LF. Nystagmus and saccadic intrusions and oscillations. In: Tasman W, Jaeger EA, eds. *Duane's Clinical Ophthalmology.* Philadelphia: JB Lippincott Co; 1990; vol 2, chap 11, p 12.

beat nystagmus can be induced in smokers from nicotine. Usually this response is seen only in the dark.

> Sibony PA, Evinger C, Manning KA. The effects of tobacco smoking on smooth pursuit eye movements. *Ann Neurol.* 1988;23:238–241.

Horizontal and vertical nystagmus may occur simultaneously. If they are out of phase, the resulting elliptical or rotary movements are often associated with oscillopsia. While multiple pathologic processes are possible, demyelinating disease is the most common cause.

> Aschoff JC, Conrad B, Kornhuber HH. Acquired pendular nystagmus with oscillopsia in multiple sclerosis: a sign of cerebellar nuclei disease. *J Neurol Neurosurg Psychiatry.* 1974;37:570–577.

Periodic alternating nystagmus characteristically shows a cycle: the nystagmus reverses its direction approximately every 2 minutes. This form of nystagmus may be congenital but can also be acquired and related to Arnold-Chiari malformation, demyelinating disease, cerebellar degeneration, and other posterior fossa pathology.

Baclofen tends to eliminate periodic alternating nystagmus in most patients with acquired disease.

Daroff RB, Dell'Osso LF. Periodic alternating nystagmus and the shifting null. *Can J Otolaryngol.* 1974;3:367–371.

Halmagyi GM, Rudge P, Gresty MA, et al. Treatment of periodic alternating nystagmus. *Ann Neurol.* 1980;8:609–611.

Ocular Misalignment: Diplopia

As mentioned in chapter I, it is extremely important to determine whether diplopia is abolished by covering one eye before initiating an extensive ocular motor system work-up. Monocular diplopia is commonly related to media abnormalities (high astigmatism, corneal irregularity including keratoconus, or lens opacities) or, rarely, retinal pathology. Binocular diplopia results from malalignment of the visual axes. Deviations that are the same in all fields of gaze are *comitant.* These deviations are traditionally considered related to congenital strabismus. Since most strabismus is associated with adaptive mechanisms, including facultative suppression, double vision is not usually a manifestation. It is possible, however, that the patient's eye position has drifted so that fixation falls outside of the patient's suppression scotoma, or that a previously compensated heterophoria may have decompensated. Another cause of a comitant deviation, divergence insufficiency (esodeviation at distance greater than near) has been considered a benign syndrome that may spontaneously resolve. Bilateral sixth nerve palsies, particularly those caused by demyelinating disease, and myasthenia should be considered in the differential diagnosis of a comitant horizontal deviation. An apparently comitant deviation may not neces-sarily be congenital and can, in fact, represent a relatively long-standing acquired deviation with spread of comitance.

When the separation between the visual axes varies with gaze direction, the deviation is said to be *incomitant.* This type of deviation is particularly well seen with a Hess-Lees screen, which demonstrates unequal size boxes with an incomitant deviation. Incomitant deviations may be explained by Hering's law, which holds that innervation to pairs of yoke muscles is equal. Thus, in the setting of either a paretic or restrictive phenomenon, the deviation should be greater when the eyes are moved into the field of the paretic muscle or away from the field of the restrictive muscle. With time, however, individual muscle gain is reset, and uniformity of the deviation across the ocular motor positions increases.

Skew deviation is a result of asymmetric involvement of the vertical inputs from the vestibular system anywhere between the pontomedullary junction to the vertical gaze centers in the midbrain (Fig VI-3). While most skew deviations are incomitant, they occasionally may be relatively comitant and thus masquerade as congenital strabismus. Skew deviations are discussed in further detail below.

Restrictive syndromes   Incomitant deviations, while most commonly caused by paretic syndromes, may also be the result of restrictive pathology or primary over-action (see below). As mentioned in chapter I, the distinction between restrictive and paretic syndromes is made definitively by forced duction testing, although suspicion is often raised by failure to fit the pattern of an individual nerve palsy (Fig VI-4). One problem, however, is that subtle restrictive findings may be difficult to appreciate. Elevation of intraocular pressure of more than 4 mm Hg when the eye is directed into

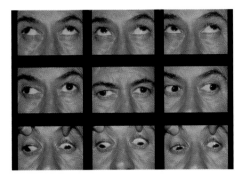

FIG VI-3—A 53-year old man complaining of double vision following cardiac catheterization. Motility examination reveals mild limitation in adduction bilaterally, worse on the left than the right, with a left hypertropia on downgaze. The adducting delay is a result of bilateral involvement of the medial longitudinal fasciculus (INO). The vertical deviation represents a skew deviation caused by asymmetric involvement of the vertical pathways.

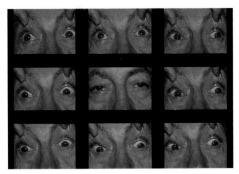

FIG VI-4—A 68-year-old man with a 60-year history of intermittent horizontal diplopia and a long history of mild bilateral ptosis. On examination his afferent system is entirely normal, but he demonstrates marked limitation in ductions in all directions, slightly more in vertical than horizontal. Saccades are markedly slowed, and moderate orbicularis weakness and mild bilateral ptosis are evident. CPEO can be distinguished from restrictive disease by forced duction testing and from ophthalmoplegia by its failure to fit a pattern and its almost universal associated ptosis and orbicularis weakness.

eccentric gaze is strongly suggestive of a restrictive component in the opposite muscle. Failure to elevate the pressure does not exclude the possibility of restrictive phenomena, as the patient may not be trying or a combined paretic and restrictive etiology may exist. The other particularly useful diagnostic clue for restrictive phenomena is a history of trauma or prior surgery and evidence of local orbital pathology. While paretic phenomena can occur anywhere along the course of the ocular motor pathways, restrictive phenomena must be a result of pathology within the orbit itself. Thus, the finding of enophthalmos, proptosis, globe dystopia, ptosis, sensory loss, injection, or other local orbital phenomena may suggest a restrictive problem. The most common restrictive etiologies are thyroid ophthalmopathy, trauma, idiopathic inflammatory disease of the orbit, and neoplastic processes. Tumors may directly extend to involve the extraocular muscles or may, rarely, infiltrate or metastasize to the muscles themselves.

Zappia RJ, Winkelman JZ, Gay AJ. Intraocular pressure changes in normal subjects and the adhesive muscle syndrome. *Am J Ophthalmol.* 1971;71:880–883.

Primary overaction syndromes Fortunately, primary overaction syndromes are rare. They include primary oblique overaction, convergence spasm, superior oblique myokymia, and ocular neuromyotonia. Convergence spasm can mimic a sixth nerve palsy or other cause of abduction deficit. Miosis with increasing esodeviation usually confirms the diagnosis. While convergence spasm is occasionally seen with prolonged reading, it often has a psychogenic component and may be associated with malingering. Patients may respond to periodic relaxation of accommodation and reading glasses, or they may require cycloplegia.

Intermittent repetitive firing of the superior oblique muscle thought to be related to ephaptic transmission within the fourth nerve produces superior oblique myokymia. Patients may report intermittent double vision but also vertical or torsional oscillopsia. This syndrome is best diagnosed if the clinician can see the patient during one of the episodes. The fine amplitude vertical and torsional movements are often best seen at the slit lamp. Acquired myokymia usually responds to carbamazepine (Tegretol).

Ocular neuromyotonia may affect either the third or sixth cranial nerves (Fig VI-5). It is usually seen in patients with a history of radiation therapy to parasellar lesions. The clinician can often detect this condition by having the patient look in the direction of the affected muscle (into abduction in the case of sixth nerve ocular neuromyotonia or into adduction, elevation, and depression in the case of third nerve ocular neuromyotonia). Failure of the muscle to subsequently relax results in a transient induced deviation. These patients may also respond to treatment with carbamazepine.

Another rare overaction syndrome is oculogyric crisis. It was first described associated with postinfectious parkinsonism but is most frequently seen currently as an acute effect of phenothiazine overdose. These patients demonstrate bilateral tonic supraduction associated with neck hyperextension, usually without visual complaints.

Lessell S, Lessell IM, Rizzo JF 3rd. Ocular neuromyotonia after radiation therapy. *Am J Ophthalmol.* 1986;102:766–770.

Shults WT, Hoyt WF, Behrens M, et al. Ocular neuromyotonia. A clinical description of six patients. *Arch Ophthalmol.* 1986;104:1028–1034.

Tyler TD, Ruiz RS. Propranolol in the treatment of superior oblique myokymia. *Arch Ophthalmol.* 1990;108:175–176.

Paretic syndromes   The majority of abnormalities of ocular motility are the result of weakness. While the ocular motor nerve innervating the extraocular muscles has traditionally been the assumed culprit, it is critical to remember that a paretic syndrome may also be caused by pathology involving the muscle itself, the myoneural junction, or even the internuclear or supranuclear pathways. Inflammation involving the extraocular muscles can produce transient weakness within a single muscle. Usually, other signs appear including pain, proptosis, and possibly numbness. MRI or CT scan can help the clinician make the appropriate diagnosis.

Myopathies

Mitochondrial abnormalities of the extraocular muscles can produce a slowly progressive weakness. Initially, slowed saccades are associated with bilateral ptosis. Involvement may be asymmetric with variable ocular malalignment. In spite of this malalignment, patients do not usually complain of diplopia. Associated facial weakness may cause problems with eyelid closure and secondary corneal exposure, especially following ptosis surgery. Chronic progressive external ophthalmoplegia (CPEO) may also be associated with systemic abnormalities including cardiac conduction defects (Kearns-Sayre syndrome), variable retinal pigmentary changes,

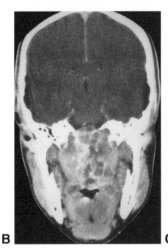

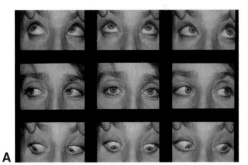

FIG VI-5—A 35-year-old woman who has been followed for an embryonal chordoma, two surgical resections, and radiation therapy. She has noted double vision on attempts to look to the left. *A,* Nine cardinal positions reveal a mild abduction deficit on the left side. *B and C,* MRI demonstrates the presence of the residual chordoma affecting the brain stem and parasellar region. *D,* Patient is instructed to look to the left. *E and F,* When she attempts to look back straight and then to the right, the left eye does not come back to the right side. The persistence of firing of the left sixth nerve, as seen in ocular neuromyotonia, is responsible.

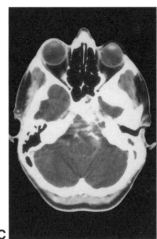

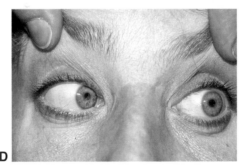

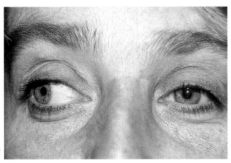

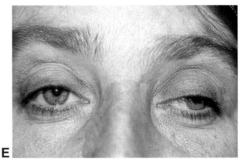

and hearing impairment. The potential for heart block makes cardiac evaluation essential. Deletions of the mitochondrial genome may be seen in more than 50% of these patients. Abnormalities of the mitochondria themselves are seen as "ragged red fibers" on special histologic staining and as inclusion body abnormalities on electron microscopic (EM) studies of muscle biopsy (Fig VI-6).

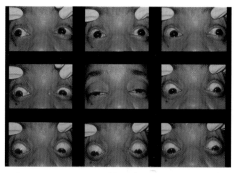

FIG VI-6—A 42-year-old with a 2-year history of progressive ptosis and significant problems with ocular motility. She was unaware of problems with double vision. Extraocular muscle examination confirms slowed and limited saccades in all directions, and a biopsy of her deltoid demonstrates ragged red fibers consistent with her clinical diagnosis of CPEO.

Moraes CT, DiMauro S, Zeviani M, et al. Mitochondrial DNA deletions in progressive external ophthalmoplegia and Kearns-Sayre syndrome. *N Engl J Med.* 1989;320: 1293–1299.

Myotonic dystrophy may be associated with a mild form of CPEO. Patients may be somewhat more likely to complain of double vision. Red and green polychromatic cataractous dots can be seen.

Lessell S, Coppeto J, Samet S. Ophthalmoplegia in myotonic dystrophy. *Am J Ophthalmol.* 1971;71:1231–1235.

Myoneural Junction Disease

Myoneural junction abnormalities are usually the result of the induction of antibodies against the acetylcholine receptors on the extraocular muscles as in myasthenia gravis, but they may be paraneoplastic as in Lambert-Eaton syndrome (most frequently associated with small cell carcinoma of the lung). While the hallmark of myasthenia is fatigability and variability, it is possible for myasthenia to present as any ocular motor abnormality. Myasthenia does not, however, produce abnormalities of the pupil, pain, or numbness. Classically, myasthenia affects the eyelid and produces ptosis, but not invariably.

When ptosis is not present, the diagnosis of myasthenia gravis requires a high degree of suspicion. A positive Tensilon test, the presence of acetylcholine receptor antibodies (present in approximately 50% of patients with isolated ocular involvement), or single-fiber EMG studies showing a decremental response can confirm the diagnosis. While false-positive Tensilon tests have been reported, the finding of a marked change in the ocular motor pattern with the administration of Tensilon is extremely suggestive of myasthenia gravis. One additional means of establishing the diagnosis is to examine the patient after prolonged rest (sleep test). Myasthenia remains the great masquerader of ocular motor abnormalities, and it should always be considered. This caution is particularly true in the setting of an apparent internuclear ophthalmoplegia (INO), but myasthenia has been reported to resemble almost any other ocular motor abnormality.

Odel JG, Winterkorn JM, Behrens MM. The sleep test for myasthenia gravis. A safe alternative to Tensilon. *J Clin Neuro-Ophthalmol.* 1991;11:288–292.

Internuclear Ophthalmoplegia

Pathologic involvement of the medial longitudinal fasciculus results in an adducting delay or paresis of the ipsilateral eye with attempt at contralateral gaze. Frequently, but not always, nystagmus of the abducting contralateral eye is associated. Because of the induced exodeviation, these patients most commonly note horizontal diplopia. Residual adducting activity can usually be demonstrated by using the vergence system and stimulating the eyes with an accommodative target.

Age is a far better predictor than unilateral or bilateral involvement in establishing a differential diagnosis (Fig VI-7). Most INOs in adolescents and adults younger than 50 are caused by demyelinating disease. In the older population microvascular compromise associated with vertebrobasilar insufficiency is the most common diagnosis. Arteriovenous malformations, neoplasia (metastatic or intrinsic glioma), and other inflammatory causes are far less common. With more rostral involvement at the level of the midbrain third nerve nucleus, bilateral INOs are often associated with a large-angle exodeviation, wall-eyed bilateral INO (WEBINO) (Fig VI-8).

Bogousslavsky J, Fox AJ, Carey LS, et al. Correlates of brain-stem oculomotor disorders in multiple sclerosis. Magnetic resonance imaging. *Arch Neurol.* 1986;43:460–463.

Gonyea EF. Bilateral internuclear ophthalmoplegia. Association with occlusive cerebrovascular disease. *Arch Neurol.* 1974;31:168–173.

McGettrick P, Eustace P. The W.E.B.I.N.O. syndrome. *Neuroophthalmology.* 1985;5: 109–115.

Skew deviation   Asymmetric involvement of the internuclear connections subserving vertical gaze produces a skew deviation. As previously noted, this deviation may be comitant but is more frequently incomitant with the hyperdeviation characteristically increasing on ipsilateral downgaze. Skew deviations have been traditionally considered rare outside the neuro intensive care unit. Subtle abnormalities of vertical alignment and movement are not uncommon following ischemic, inflammatory, traumatic, and neoplastic involvement of the brain stem in any location from the

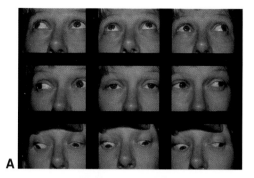

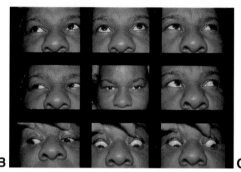

FIG VI-7—Two patients with evidence of internuclear ophthalmoplegia with adducting delay, increasing exodeviation on contralateral gaze, and some abducting nystagmus of the contralateral eye. A, A 35-year-old with a history of optic neuritis whose INO is a result of a demyelinating plaque. B, A 50-year-old hypertensive, diabetic patient with a presumed microvascular etiology. C, Hess screen of patient shown in B.

A

B

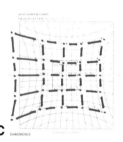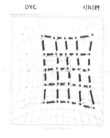

C

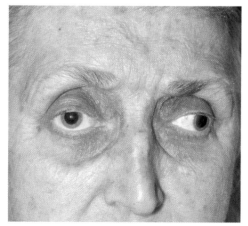

FIG VI-8—A 73-year-old hypertensive woman who suffered a parietal intracerebral hemorrhage with additional microvascular involvement of the midbrain. She has bilateral ptosis and a 50Δ–60Δ exotropia and cannot adduct either eye past the midline. Rostral involvement of the medial longitudinal fasciculus has bilaterally produced this WEBINO syndrome.

pontomedullary junction to the rostral midbrain. When there is an associated INO, the pathology is found more frequently on the side of the higher eye. It has been suggested that torsional deviation does not occur, although this may not be true universally.

Keane JR. Ocular skew deviation. Analysis of 100 cases. *Arch Neurol.* 1975;32: 185–190.

Ophthalmoplegia

The diagnosis of ophthalmoplegia rests on the recognition of patterns of abnormality. The single most important piece of information in determining the appropriate diagnosis and work-up of a patient with presumed ophthalmoplegia is the presence of an *isolated* cranial nerve palsy. It is therefore imperative that patients be examined with extreme care for signs of other cranial nerve pathology; other neurologic long tract, motor, or sensory abnormalities; or other brain stem pathology. The second most helpful determinant of the differential diagnosis is the age of the patient. The following three sections discuss in detail palsies of the sixth, fourth, and third cranial nerves.

Harley RD. Paralytic strabismus in children. Etiologic incidence and management of the third, fourth, and sixth nerve palsies. *Ophthalmology.* 1980;87:24–43.

Richards BW, Jones FR Jr, Younge BR. Causes and prognosis in 4,278 cases of paralysis of the oculomotor, trochlear, and abducens cranial nerves. *Am J Ophthalmol.* 1992; 113:489–496.

Rucker CW. Paralysis of the third, fourth and sixth cranial nerves. *Am J Ophthalmol.* 1958;46:787–794.

Rucker CW. The causes of paralysis of the third, fourth and sixth cranial nerves. *Am J Ophthalmol.* 1966;61:1293–1298.

Rush JA, Younge BR. Paralysis of cranial nerves III, IV, and VI. Cause and prognosis in 1,000 cases. *Arch Ophthalmol.* 1981;99:76–79.

Siatkowski RM. Third, fourth, and sixth nerve palsies. In: *Focal Points: Clinical Modules for Ophthalmologists.* San Francisco: American Academy of Ophthalmology; 1996;14:8.

Sixth Nerve Palsy

A sixth nerve palsy is suspected on the finding of an isolated abduction deficit. This deficit need not be complete and may, in fact, be indicated only as an esodeviation increasing on ipsilateral gaze. Strongly supportive of a sixth nerve etiology is the finding of slowed ipsilateral saccades. The sixth nerve may be affected within the brain stem by inflammatory lesions (postviral, demyelinating, etc.), particularly in the young patient, and by vascular lesions, especially in the older patient. Other pathology includes metabolic diseases such as vitamin B deficiencies and Wernicke-Korsakoff syndrome. In children a pontine glioma may present as unilateral or bilateral sixth nerve palsy. Intra-axial lesions usually result in other neurologic findings, including involvement of the seventh cranial nerve and facial sensation. If the ventral brain stem is involved, associated abnormalities of the corticospinal tract lead to contralateral hemiparesis (Millard-Gubler syndrome). As described in chapter

V, involvement of the sixth nerve nucleus means the patient will show a gaze palsy, usually without associated diplopia. Often as the gaze palsy begins to clear, additional involvement of the fascicle will lead to more rapid improvement in the adducting eye, causing the appearance of a relative ipsilateral sixth nerve palsy and possibly diplopia.

Within the subarachnoid space, the sixth nerve is subject to the following types of pathology:

☐ Inflammatory (sarcoid)

☐ Infectious (meningitis, particularly basilar meningitis such as tuberculosis or fungus)

☐ Infiltrative (including lymphoproliferative abnormalities)

☐ Compressive (usually arising from the clivus: meningioma, chordoma, chondrosarcoma, metastatic disease)

In addition, lesions of the cerebellar pontine angle may get large enough to affect the sixth nerve (neurilemoma of cranial nerve VIII, the auditory nerve, or meningiomas). These lesions are usually associated with decreased hearing and vestibular findings as well as seventh nerve dysfunction and facial sensory loss. Finally, the subarachnoid sixth nerve may be affected by shifts in position of the brain stem that cause tugging on the nerve itself. Changes in intracranial pressure as with acute hydrocephalus, following lumbar puncture, and associated with pseudotumor cerebri are particularly likely to affect the sixth nerve.

As cranial nerve VI passes over the petrous pyramid, it may be affected by trauma, enlargement of the inferior petrosal sinus associated with a direct or dural cavernous fistula, inflammatory lesions within the petrous pyramid (Gradenigo syndrome), or neoplastic processes. Meningiomas or neurilemomas may affect the sixth nerve within the posterior cavernous sinus or as it crosses the petrous pyramid (Fig VI-9). In addition, nasopharyngeal carcinoma invading the skull base through the foramen lacerum may produce sixth nerve palsy as well as pain and decreased hearing. Aneurysms of the intracavernous carotid artery often present with sixth nerve palsy but may also have sensory changes and a Horner syndrome.

Congenital sixth nerve palsies almost never occur in isolation. Congenital absence of the sixth nerve is seen in *Duane syndrome* (Fig VI-10). The lateral rectus muscle in these patients is innervated by various branches from the third nerve, which results in narrowing of the palpebral fissure with attempted adduction. Cocontraction commonly causes upshoot and downshoot. Variable abnormalities in adduction often appear as well. Patients are frequently unaware of the abnormality and usually do not have trouble with double vision. Bilateral involvement of the sixth and seventh nerves is characteristic of *Möbius syndrome.* Other lower cranial nerves may also be involved. Patients with both Duane and Möbius syndromes usually cross-fixate, using their intact adduction.

Miller NR, Kiel SM, Green WR, et al. Unilateral Duane's retraction syndrome (Type 1). *Arch Ophthalmol.* 1982;100:1468–1472.

Work-up of presumed sixth nerve palsy As mentioned above, the most important feature to determine is whether the nontraumatic sixth nerve palsy is isolated. Any evidence of associated dysfunction of the third, fourth, fifth, seventh, or eighth cranial nerves or of sympathetic abnormalities is an indication for a work-up including at least an MRI with and without gadolinium. Evidence of increased intracranial

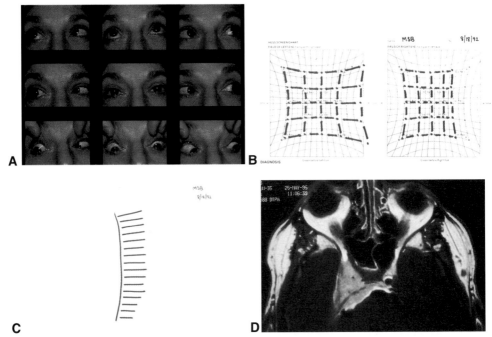

FIG VI-9—*A,* This 55-year-old woman first complained of double vision, which she noticed was worse on right gaze. *B,* Hess screen confirms the presence of an abduction deficit on the right. *C,* Binocular single-vision field demonstrates double vision on right gaze, quantitating the relative movement of the two eyes and helping clinician determine whether patient is worsening with time. *D,* Gadolinium-enhanced MRI demonstrates a clival and cavernous sinus meningioma on the right side, resulting in sixth nerve palsy.

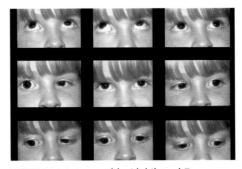

FIG VI-10—A 4-year-old with bilateral Duane syndrome with limitation in abduction bilaterally and palpebral fissure narrowing on adduction.

pressure, such as a history of headaches or findings of papilledema and obesity, might indicate that the sixth nerve dysfunction is nonlocalizing. While an acute inflammatory or microvascular sixth nerve palsy may have some associated pain, significant pain is an indication for a work-up.

In the older patient in the vasculopathic age group the presumptive diagnosis of a microvascular sixth nerve palsy anticipates that it should clear within a period of 2–3 months. Failure to resolve or any evidence of progression is an indication for MRI. In children postviral inflammatory lesions are possible, but these should also clear. Acute onset of a sixth nerve palsy associated with trauma might also call for a limited work-up that checks the other cranial nerves, especially the seventh and the eighth.

In adolescents and young adults demyelinating disease may be an under-recognized cause of sixth nerve palsy. In the absence of other findings, the yield of neuroimaging (MRI) is low. Failure to resolve or development of any other long tract signs or brain stem findings suggests the presence of a pontine or cerebellar glioma, ependymoma, or medulloblastoma. All patients must be seen in follow-up, and persistence of sixth nerve dysfunction is always an indication for MRI. Metabolic syndromes as etiologies of sixth nerve palsies are rare. Cerebrospinal fluid analysis may be indicated in the setting of a negative MRI.

Fourth Nerve Palsy

A fourth nerve palsy is the presumptive diagnosis in a patient presenting with vertical double vision and no signs or history suggestive of restrictive phenomena. Finding a hyperdeviation also raises suspicion of a fourth nerve palsy. The hyperdeviation should increase on contralateral gaze and with ipsilateral head tilt. This response is most expeditiously checked with a Maddox rod and penlight moved into the nine cardinal positions and held in primary position as the patient's head is tilted. The lines of the Maddox rod are tilted with the patient, and the testing must be done with the patient upright. If the deviation does not follow the expected pattern, subtle restrictive problems or a skew deviation must be reconsidered. Double Maddox rod testing should show evidence of between 3° and 10° of excyclotorsion. Results that show greater than 10° of excyclotorsion raise the possibility of a bilateral fourth nerve palsy.

Fourth nerve palsies are either congenital or acquired. The presence of a head tilt in old photographs ("biopsying the family album") or a vertical fusional range of greater than 3Δ is strongly suggestive of a long-standing or congenital fourth nerve paresis. It is remarkable how often patients are unaware of a previous head tilt until old photographs, including driver licenses, are examined (Fig VI-11). The most common cause of an acquired fourth nerve palsy is head trauma, which may have been so trivial the patient was never aware of its significance and has forgotten it. In older patients microvascular causes are the leading diagnosis of fourth nerve palsies.

Nuclear involvement of the fourth nerve is extremely uncommon, although it has been reported with vascular disease (including arteriovenous malformation), trauma, and demyelination. The fourth nerve may be involved as it exits the brain stem, crossing in the superior medullary velum. Lesions of the pineal gland (pine-aloma, pinealoblastoma, teratoma, dysgerminoma, or choriocarcinoma) may all affect the fourth nerve, usually bilaterally and frequently with other signs of the dorsal midbrain syndrome.

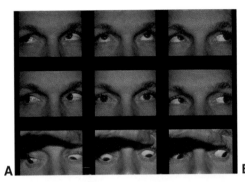
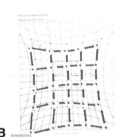
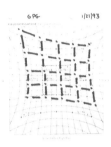

A

B

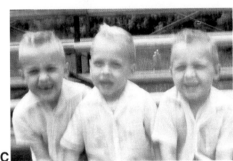

C

FIG VI-11—A 34-year-old man complaining of vertical double vision with a remote history of a bicycle accident. *A,* His nine cardinal positions demonstrate a right hypertropia increasing on left gaze and with right head tilt. *B,* Hess screen confirms the presence of a right hypertropia increasing on left gaze. *C,* Patient has 14Δ of right hypertropia in primary position. Normally, vertical fusion ranges are only 3Δ. The ability to fuse more than normal led to review of childhood photographs, which show a long-standing head tilt suggestive of a congenital or extremely long-standing fourth nerve dysfunction.

The fourth nerve in the subarachnoid space may be affected most commonly by microvascular abnormalities. Other inflammatory pathology (including meningitis) and vascular phenomena (including a carotid cavernous fistula) can impair trochlear function within the area of the cavernous sinus. Iatrogenic fourth nerve pathology following a neurosurgical procedure is not rare, occurring most frequently when the tentorial edge is cut.

Clinical approach to fourth nerve palsy   The yield of an isolated fourth nerve palsy work-up is very low (tumor and aneurysm rarely cause isolated fourth nerve palsy), even in the absence of a history of head trauma. Older patients should be seen in follow-up to make sure that the fourth nerve palsy is clearing. The possibility of a restrictive syndrome, such as thyroid ophthalmopathy, or old trauma should always be considered, and myasthenia gravis should never be forgotten.

Third Nerve Palsy

The diagnosis of a third nerve palsy is suggested by abnormalities in the function of the superior rectus, inferior rectus, inferior oblique, and medial rectus muscles. In addition, as the third nerve innervates the levator palpebrae superioris and pupil, involvement of the eyelid with induced ptosis would be expected. The eye is often deviated out and slightly down with associated ptosis.

Isolated extraocular muscle palsies are unlikely to represent a third nerve palsy, especially in the following cases: an apparent superior rectus weakness without ptosis; an inferior oblique "weakness" without medial and inferior rectus weakness, which is possibly Brown syndrome; or an isolated medial rectus weakness, most likely an INO. Myasthenia may involve the extraocular muscles and levator but spares the pupil and is never associated with pain.

Abnormalities of the pupil such as mydriasis and failure to react may be signs of third nerve involvement. However, because of the peripheral location of the pupillary fibers in the extra-axial portion of the third nerve, it is possible for sparing of the pupil to coexist with even complete involvement of the extraocular muscles and levator. It is very rare for an acute third nerve palsy to be caused by a mass lesion when the pupil is completely spared, which is not true for progressive oculomotor dysfunction. Up to 50% of slowly progressive third nerve palsies resulting from a slowly expanding parasellar lesion (carotid cavernous aneurysm, meningioma, pituitary adenoma, etc.) may be unassociated with pupillary compromise. In addition, sympathetic dysfunction, which is common with cavernous sinus lesions, may partially mask pupillary involvement by reducing mydriasis.

Acute onset of third nerve palsy associated with a dilated, nonreactive pupil is presumed to represent an aneurysm, usually of the posterior communicating artery. When associated with headache and stiff neck, it may represent an aneurysmal subarachnoid hemorrhage. Neoplastic, inflammatory, and even microvascular causes may also result in a pupil-involving third nerve palsy. Pain is an almost constant finding with an aneurysmal third nerve palsy, but it is also frequent with a microvascular paresis. Third nerve dysfunction associated with ophthalmoplegic migraine can mimic that caused by an aneurysm. This rare syndrome is usually preceded by a headache, and initial onset essentially always occurs in childhood.

Congenital third nerve palsies often represent perinatal trauma. Pupil involvement is variable, aberrant regeneration is common, and divisional palsies may occur. Congenital abnormalities account for almost 50% of third nerve palsies in children. Slowly progressive oculomotor palsy is an indication for repeat MRI in spite of previous negative studies, as neurilemomas can remain cryptic.

Abdul-Rahim AS, Savino PJ, Zimmerman RA, et al. Cryptogenic oculomotor nerve palsy. The need for repeated neuroimaging studies. *Arch Ophthalmol.* 1989;107:387–390.

One rare congenital syndrome is cyclical oculomotor palsy. An eye with an underlying third nerve palsy develops intermittent spasms during which the paretic eye turns from its exotropic position toward midline, the ptotic eyelid elevates, and the dilated pupil constricts.

Loewenfeld IE, Thompson HS. Oculomotor paresis with cyclic spasms. A critical review of the literature and a new case. *Surv Ophthalmol.* 1975;20:81–124.

Clinical approach to third nerve palsy   An acute isolated pupil-sparing third nerve palsy in a vasculopathic patient over 40 does not require work-up other than blood pressure and fasting blood sugar tests. It is important, however, to follow these patients for expected recovery within 3 months. The patient must be instructed in the importance of seeking medical attention for any additional findings such as facial palsy, weakness, or numbness. In particular, the patient should be instructed to check pupil size in a mirror and to report any pupillary enlargement. In the setting of third nerve palsy associated with trauma, the work-up may include only a careful check for evidence of an associated carotid cavernous fistula, including orbital bruit, arterialized episcleral vessels, or elevated intraocular pressure with an increase in pulse pressure.

When the pupil is enlarged or the third nerve dysfunction is progressive, a work-up is indicated. MRI with gadolinium is the primary diagnostic study. When combined with MRA, it can show aneurysms larger than 4 mm and neoplastic, inflammatory, and infectious processes. While symptomatic aneurysms smaller than 4 mm are uncommon, traditional angiography remains the standard for excluding the presence of an aneurysm. Inflammatory lesions and even some infiltrative processes (lymphoma) may not show up on MRI. Analysis of the cerebrospinal fluid for cells (high-volume cytology) as well as serology and protein may be helpful. Often serial MRIs over a period of years are required to uncover the etiology in cases of cryptogenic third nerve palsies. Chapter II discusses the various neuroimaging studies in detail.

Huston J 3rd, Nichols DA, Luetmer PH, et al. Blinded prospective evaluation of sensitivity of MR angiography to known intracranial aneurysms: importance of aneurysm size. *Am J Neuroradiol.* 1994;15:1607–1614.

Tomsak RL, Masaryk TJ, Bates JH. Magnetic resonance angiography (MRA) of isolated aneurysmal third nerve palsy. *J Clin Neuroophthalmol.* 1991;11:16–18.

Children may have transient ophthalmoplegia following viral infection or vaccination. If an immediate work-up is deferred, follow-up should be scheduled to make sure recovery is complete. As aneurysms are rare in children, arteriography is almost never indicated in patients younger than 10 years. In adolescents and young adults, pupil involvement, progressive third nerve paresis, or association with other neurologic signs or symptoms necessitates a work-up. In patients older than 70 years, an erythrocyte sedimentation rate may be used to screen for giant cell arteritis. Although the diplopia that results from giant cell arteritis is most likely a result of orbital hypoperfusion that leads to extraocular muscle ischemia, it is still important to consider giant cell arteritis as a cause of ophthalmoplegia in the elderly.

Barricks ME, Traviesa DB, Glaser JS, et al. Ophthalmoplegia in cranial arteritis. *Brain.* 1977;100:209–221.

An incomplete third nerve palsy presents a more difficult diagnostic situation. Divisional palsies (superior rectus and levator, or medial rectus, inferior rectus, and inferior oblique) were previously thought to indicate pathology within the cavernous sinus or orbital apex. It is now clear that divisional palsies also occur with pathology that is located more proximally, including within the midbrain. While it is possible for microvascular disease to cause divisional involvement, these patients should be carefully worked up with an MRI with gadolinium. Superior division palsies may represent ophthalmic artery aneurysms.

Guy JR, Day AL. Intracranial aneurysms with superior division paresis of the oculomotor nerve. *Ophthalmology.* 1989;96:1071–1076.

Relative pupil sparing also presents diagnostic difficulties. In the setting of significant motility impairment, slight dilation of the pupil may occur with microvascular disease. Progressive pupillary enlargement is always an indication for work-up.

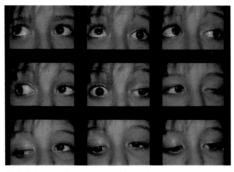

FIG VI-12—A 12-year-old with acute traumatic third nerve palsy following a bicycle accident. The eyelid gradually opened on its own, but patient has been left with double vision. Nine cardinal positions demonstrate residual problems with vertical gaze and hang-up of the left eyelid with attempted adduction and depression. In addition, patient's pupil becomes miotic with attempted adduction, elevation, or depression, characteristic of aberrant regeneration.

As a damaged third nerve recovers, misdirection of fiber regrowth can result in *aberrant regeneration*. The three classical findings in aberrant regeneration are

□ Eyelid elevation or hang-up with adduction and depression

□ Miosis with elevation (miosis also appears with adduction and depression but is more expected as part of the near reflex)

□ Persistent vertical gaze limitation caused by cocontraction of the superior and inferior recti (Fig VI-12)

Aberrant regeneration is common after trauma or compression by an aneurysm or tumor, but it does not occur after microvascular compromise. The development of aberrant regeneration in the setting of a diagnosed diabetic third nerve palsy requires reevaluation including an MRI. Evidence of aberrant regeneration without a history of third nerve palsy, *primary aberrant regeneration,* is presumptive evidence of a slowly expanding lesion, most commonly a meningioma or carotid cavernous aneurysm.

Cox TA, Wurster JB, Godfrey WA. Primary aberrant oculomotor regeneration due to intracranial aneurysm. *Arch Neurol.* 1979;36:570–571.

Schatz NJ, Savino PJ, Corbett JJ. Primary aberrant oculomotor regeneration. A sign of intracavernous meningioma. *Arch Neurol.* 1977;34:29–32.

Multiple Cranial Nerve Palsies

Just as recognition of associated neurologic signs or symptoms is important in assessing cranial nerve palsies, diagnosing involvement of more than a single ocular motor nerve paresis is critical. Recognizing the presence of a sixth nerve palsy in the setting of a known third or fourth nerve palsy is usually easy. It is more difficult to detect involvement of the fourth nerve in the presence of a third nerve palsy. This involvement is suggested by failure of intorsion with attempted downgaze with the eye in abduction.

While microvascular disease rarely causes simultaneous involvement of more than one cranial nerve, paresis of extraocular muscles innervated by two or more ocular motor nerves requires work-up. Pain or facial sensory loss suggests pathology in the area of the cavernous sinus that may be neoplastic (meningioma, neurilemoma, pituitary adenoma, metastatic disease), vascular (carotid cavernous fistula or aneurysm), or inflammatory (sarcoid, Tolosa-Hunt syndrome). MRI can visualize the pathology in the majority of cases. Cerebrospinal fluid analysis for evidence of neoplastic or inflammatory cells should be considered if the MRI is negative. Evidence of elevated protein and pleocytosis may appear in the cerebrospinal fluid in the setting of postinfectious polyradiculoneuropathy (Fisher syndrome). Multiple cranial nerve palsies associated with diffuse weakness, particularly respiratory, may be caused by botulism, usually from ingestion of contaminated food.

Blau I, Casson I, Lieberman A, et al. The not-so-benign Miller Fisher syndrome: a variant of the Guillain-Barré syndrome. *Arch Neurol.* 1980;37:384–385.

Terranova W, Palumbo JN, Breman JG. Ocular findings in botulism type B. *JAMA.* 1979;241:475–477.

Painful ophthalmoplegia of Tolosa-Hunt syndrome will respond to corticosteroid therapy. This response has been suggested as a diagnostic criterion. Unfortunately, mass lesions (particularly lymphoproliferative) may also respond to a course of corticosteroids, and Tolosa-Hunt syndrome should be considered a diagnosis of exclusion following MRI with gadolinium. Failure to fit the pattern of a single cranial nerve palsy should always stimulate reconsideration of myasthenia, skew deviation, or restrictive strabismus.

Kline LB. The Tolosa-Hunt syndrome. *Surv Ophthalmol.* 1982;27:79–95.

Bilateral cranial nerve involvement is always an indication for work-up. Bilateral sixth nerve palsies are only rarely caused by microvascular disease. MRI should be the first step in approaching diagnosis in this setting.

Keane JR. Bilateral sixth nerve palsy. Analysis of 125 cases. *Arch Neurol.* 1976;33: 681–683.

Sergott RC, Glaser JS, Berger LJ. Simultaneous, bilateral diabetic ophthalmoplegia. Report of two cases and discussion of differential diagnosis. *Ophthalmology.* 1984; 91:18–22.

Treatment of Diplopia

Acute ocular malalignment of any etiology is often best treated with occlusion therapy. In the case of a comitant deviation, prisms (either ground into the patient's glasses or applied as a stick-on Fresnel) may provide realignment. Ground-in prisms are usually limited to 7–8Δ per lens depending on the amount of refractive correction. Fresnel prisms can correct much greater deviations but cause blurring of the image.

Diplopia from incomitant deviations is more difficult to relieve. Prisms may be useful in giving the patient at least some area of binocular single vision. Botulinum toxin type A (Botox) injections may be used to temporarily weaken the secondarily overacting contralateral agonist. The effect may last from 6 to 12 weeks. Injection of the ipsilateral antagonist offers the secondary advantage of decreasing muscle contracture.

When the deviation has stabilized for a minimum of 3–6 months, strabismus surgery can realign the eyes. Surgery should be designed to achieve alignment in primary position and down reading gaze with fusion in horizontal gaze as a secondary goal. Gaze positions above the midline are far less important. Operations that weaken overacting muscles are usually more successful in increasing the area of binocular single vision than attempts at strengthening underacting muscles. A Faden procedure to limit the excursion of the normal eye may also be helpful in maximizing the area of binocular single vision. Incomplete cranial nerve palsies often do very well with surgery. A complete fourth nerve palsy can usually be entirely realigned. The response of a complete sixth nerve palsy is less satisfactory, usually achieving alignment only in a limited area. When a third nerve palsy is complete, surgery is rarely useful.

The work-up of patients with ocular motor complaints is a common challenge faced by ophthalmologists as well as neurologists. Several excellent texts provide more detail on the clinical approach.

Beck RW, Smith CH. *Neuro-Ophthalmology: A Problem-Oriented Approach.* Boston: Little, Brown & Co; 1988:153–227.

Burde RM, Savino PJ, Trobe JD. *Clinical Decisions in Neuro-Ophthalmology.* 2nd ed. St Louis: Mosby–Year Book; 1992:200–320.

Leigh RJ, Zee DS. *The Neurology of Eye Movements.* 2nd ed. Philadelphia: FA Davis; 1991.

CHAPTER VII

Cranial Nerve VII, the Facial Nerve

Neuroanatomy

An understanding of disorders of cranial nerve VII, the facial nerve, starts with knowledge of the applicable anatomy. The seventh nerve pathway can be divided into four segments: supranuclear, nuclear, fascicular, and peripheral.

Supranuclear Pathways

Volitional facial movement is primarily controlled by the precentral motor cortex of the frontal lobe. Fibers descend in the internal capsule and cerebral peduncle within the corticobulbar tract to the seventh nerve nuclei in the pons. The fibers subserving the upper facial musculature are derived from both seventh nerve nuclei, whereas fibers subserving only the lower face arise from the contralateral nucleus (Fig VII-1). As a result, unilateral upper motor neuron lesions spare the forehead and usually leave voluntary eyelid closure intact.

Periodic and emotional blinking and related facial movements are under the control of extrapyramidal pathways with interconnections between the basal ganglia, thalamus, and brain stem tegmentum. Lesions in the basal ganglia may impair emotional or periodic blinking while sparing volitional eyelid movements. This distinction is seen in parkinsonism, a disorder of basal ganglial connections with a markedly reduced rate of periodic blinking.

Nucleus and Fasciculus

The motor portion of the seventh nerve nucleus is located ventrolateral and slightly caudal to the sixth nerve nucleus in the pons. Fibers leave the nucleus dorsally and arch around the sixth nerve nucleus along the genu of the seventh nerve. Parasympathetic fibers for lacrimation and salivation from the superior salivatory nucleus join with sensory fibers for taste and other visceral and somatic sensory functions heading toward the solitary nucleus to form the intermediary nerve. The intermediary nerve joins the motor fibers of the seventh nerve before they exit the brain stem at the pontomedullary junction.

Peripheral (Infranuclear) Segment (Fig VII-2)

The motor portions of the seventh nerve and the intermediary nerve traverse the lateral pontine cistern and enter the internal auditory canal with cranial nerve VIII, the vestibulocochlear nerve, then depart from the eighth nerve to enter the fallopian canal. At the level of the geniculate ganglion, the fibers destined for the lacrimal

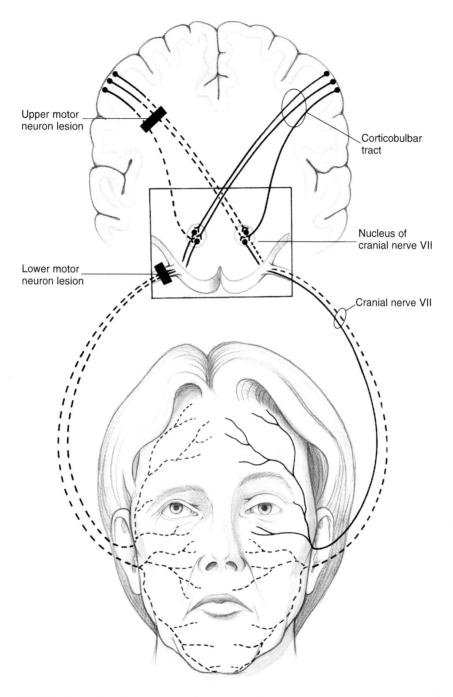

Upper motor neuron lesion

Corticobulbar tract

Nucleus of cranial nerve VII

Lower motor neuron lesion

Cranial nerve VII

FIG VII-1—The dashed lines show the distribution of facial muscles paralyzed after a supranuclear lesion of the corticobulbar tract and after a lower motor neuron lesion of the facial nerve. (Illustration by Christine Gralapp.)

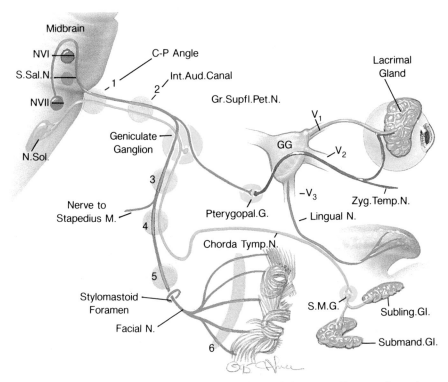

FIG VII-2—Distribution of peripheral seventh nerve and topical diagnosis of lesions. Blue indicates location of lesion; numbers are keyed to text below. (Illustration by Craig A. Luce.)

Peripheral lesions almost always result in a facial monoplegia including the orbicularis oculi muscle (lagophthalmos) and frontalis muscle, plus

1. Cerebellopontine angle: decreased tearing, dysacusis, loss of salivary secretion, loss of taste from anterior two thirds of tongue, hearing impairment, nystagmus, vertigo, ataxia, and adjacent brain stem and other cranial nerve findings (see text).

2. Internal auditory canal: same as from cerebellopontine angle except without brain stem and other cranial nerve findings.

3. Between the geniculate ganglion and the branch to the stapedius: loss of taste from anterior two thirds of tongue, impaired salivary secretion.

4. Between the branch to the stapedius and the chorda tympani: loss of taste from anterior two thirds of tongue, impaired salivary secretion.

5. Distal to chorda tympani nerve: isolated paralysis of facial muscles.

6. Distal to branching of seventh nerve after it leaves the stylomastoid foramen: smaller groups of facial muscles weakened, e.g., orbicularis oculi, brow with sparing of lower facial muscles.

Abbreviations used in diagram:

Grt.Supfl.Pet. N. = greater superficial petrosal nerve
Zyg.Temp.N. = zygomaticotemporal nerve
GG = Gasserian ganglion
N.Sol. = solitary nucleus
S.M.G. = submandibular ganglion
C-P Angle = cerebellopontine angle
S.Sal.N. = superior salivary nucleus

gland leave the seventh nerve and traverse the greater superficial petrosal nerve and vidian nerves to reach the postganglionic neurons in the sphenopalatine ganglion. Postganglionic fibers originating in this ganglion send parasympathetic innervation to the lacrimal gland along the maxillary division of the fifth nerve and the lacrimal nerve.

Within the fallopian canal, the seventh nerve gives off the motor nerve to the stapedius muscle and the chorda tympani nerve. The chorda tympani carries taste fibers from the anterior two thirds of the tongue and provides secretory input to the submandibular and sublingual glands. The seventh nerve exits the skull through the stylomastoid foramen and divides within the parotid gland into temporofacial and cervicofacial trunks. The terminal branching of these divisions is quite variable.

Clinical Evaluation of Seventh Nerve Function

Although evaluation of the seventh nerve is frequently limited to its motor functions, testing of sensory and autonomic functions is at times useful. Motor function can be readily assessed by observation. At rest, any asymmetry of facial expression or eyelid blink is noted. The palpebral fissure on the side of seventh nerve paresis is wider as a result of the relaxed tone of the orbicularis oculi nerve. The clinician can test the various muscle groups by asking the patient to smile, to forcibly close the eyes, and to wrinkle the forehead. The degree to which the eyelashes become buried on each side can reveal subtle orbicularis oculi weakness. The corneal blink reflex provides an assessment of both seventh and fifth nerve function. The clinician can whisper or use a quiet watch to test hearing and assess simultaneous involvement of the eighth nerve as a result of cerebellopontine angle tumors.

Any aberrant facial movements at rest or during volitional movement should be noted. Synkinetic movements that result from regenerating axons reinnervating muscles different from those originally served may follow any facial neuropathy. In this situation the involved facial muscles may remain weak. When axons originally destined for the orbicularis oculi reinnervate the lower facial muscles, each blink may cause a twitch of the corner of the mouth or a dimpling of the chin. Conversely, movements of the lower face, such as pursing the lips, smiling, or chewing with the mouth closed, may evoke involuntary eyelid closure.

Other disorders of aberrant facial innervation include lacrimation evoked by chewing (crocodile tears), in which fibers originally supplying mandibular and sublingual glands reinnervate the lacrimal gland by way of the greater petrosal nerve. This syndrome usually follows severe proximal seventh nerve injury and may be accompanied by decreased reflex tearing and decreased taste from the anterior two thirds of the tongue. The Marcus Gunn jaw-winking syndrome, characterized by eyelid elevation with jaw movement, is caused by anomalous communication between the trigeminal (pterygoid) and oculomotor (levator) nerves.

Frueh BR. Associated facial contractions after seventh nerve palsy mimicking jaw-winking. *Ophthalmology.* 1983;90:1105–1109.

May M, Galetta S. The facial nerve. In: Tasman W, Jaeger EA, eds. *Duane's Clinical Ophthalmology.* Philadelphia: JB Lippincott Co; 1994; vol 2; chap 8:30–31.

The localization of a seventh nerve palsy can be guided by monitoring of autonomic functions such as salivation and lacrimation and testing of sensation. Sugar or vinegar placed on the anterior two thirds of the tongue can be used to test taste. Cutaneous sensation can be tested along the posterior aspect of the external auditory canal and tympanic membrane. Lesions of the seventh nerve from the cerebellopontine angle to the geniculate ganglion typically impair all functions of the nerve, whereas lesions distal to the geniculate ganglion affect only certain functions depending on their location, as shown in Figure VII-2. A dissociation of motor, sensory, and autonomic functions is also possible with pontine lesions proximal to the joining of the motor portion of the seventh nerve with the intermediary nerve. Testing should include functions of the sixth and fifth as well as eighth nerves, which, if abnormal, may help localize the cause of a seventh nerve palsy.

Seventh Nerve Disorders

It is useful to divide seventh nerve problems into disorders of underactivity and disorders of overactivity.

Disorders of Underactivity

Facial weakness may occur with supranuclear, nuclear, or infranuclear lesions.

Supranuclear lesions A lesion in the facial portion of the precentral gyrus results in a contralateral paralysis of volitional facial movement, which involves the lower face more severely than the upper face. Emotional and reflex facial movements such as smiling and spontaneous blinking are usually preserved because they are controlled through extrapyramidal pathways.

With extrapyramidal disorders, such as parkinsonism or progressive supranuclear palsy, spontaneous facial expression is minimal, and the spontaneous blink rate is usually reduced. Volitional facial movements generally remain intact.

> May M, Galetta S. The facial nerve. In: Tasman W, Jaeger EA, eds. *Duane's Clinical Ophthalmology.* Philadelphia: JB Lippincott Co; 1994; vol 2; chap 8:2–3.

Brain stem lesions Ipsilateral facial weakness involving both the upper and lower face may occur with a pontine disorder. Vascular lesions and intraparenchymal tumors are the most common causes. Other evidence of a pontine disturbance is to be expected, such as ipsilateral corneal and facial anesthesia, sixth nerve palsy, lateral gaze palsy, cerebellar ataxia, and contralateral hemiparesis. A dissociation between the autonomic, sensory, and motor functions of the seventh nerve may be present. Large lesions of the pons may produce facial diplegia, which is also seen in Möbius syndrome, a congenital disorder involving bilateral sixth nerve palsies.

> May M, Galetta S. The facial nerve. In: Tasman W, Jaeger EA, eds. *Duane's Clinical Ophthalmology.* Philadelphia: JB Lippincott Co; 1994; vol 2; chap 8:27.

Peripheral lesions Seventh nerve lesions may occur from a multitude of causes (Table VII-1). Testing of the sensory and autonomic functions of the seventh nerve help pinpoint the responsible lesion. Concomitant impairment of the fifth, sixth, or eighth cranial nerves or cerebellar signs may indicate tumors in the cerebellopontine angle.

Bell's palsy represents the most common type of facial neuropathy, but it must remain a diagnosis of exclusion. It is typically a disease of adults that is characterized by the sudden onset of facial paresis. Pain may either precede the palsy or occur concurrently. Facial numbness may be reported, although cutaneous sensation is usually intact. Decreased tearing, diminished taste, and dysacusis also may be noted.

TABLE VII-1

Idiopathic Bell's palsy

Infections

Herpes zoster

Lyme disease

Acute or chronic otitis media

Other: syphilis, meningitis, infectious mononucleosis, varicella, enterovirus, rubella, mumps, leprosy, tuberculosis, mucormycosis, tetanus, diphtheria, human immuno-deficiency virus

Pontine infarct or hemorrhage

Pontine demyelination

Neoplasms

Pontine glioma

Cerebellopontine angle
  Acoustic neuroma
  Meningioma
  Metastatic carcinoma
  Cerebellar tumors
  Cholesteatoma
  Glomus jugulare tumor

Intratemporal bone
  Squamous cell carcinoma
  Facial nerve neurinoma
  Cholesteatoma
  Glomus jugulare tumor

Parotid gland
  Mucoepidermoid
  Adenoid cystic carcinoma

Other: sarcoma, hemangioma, histiocytosis X, leukemia, lymphoma, epidermoids

Trauma

Temporal bone fracture

Facial trauma

Miscellaneous

Congenital facial paralysis

Guillain-Barré syndrome

Sarcoidosis

Metabolic
  Diabetes mellitus
  Uremia
  Hypothyroidism

Vasculitis
  Polyarteritis nodosa
  Wegener granulomatosis

Melkersson-Rosenthal syndrome

Mimics of facial nerve paralysis
  Myasthenia gravis
  Myotonic dystrophy

Although the etiology of Bell's palsy is unknown, it may be caused by auto-immune or viral-induced inflammatory or ischemic injury with swelling of the peripheral nerve. The external auditory canal and ear should be examined for vesicles caused by herpes zoster (Ramsay Hunt syndrome). The incidence of Bell's palsy is higher in patients with diabetes or a family history of Bell's palsy and in pregnant women. If the facial weakness progresses over a period of more than 3 weeks, a neoplastic etiology must be ruled out.

About 84% of patients with Bell's palsy experience a satisfactory spontaneous recovery, although subtle signs of aberrant regeneration are commonly found (see discussion on p 153). In these patients, recovery typically begins within 3 weeks and is complete by 2–3 months. In the remaining patients, recovery is incomplete, and aberrant regeneration is common. Complete facial palsy at the time of presentation, impairment of lacrimation, dysacusis, and advanced age are all poor prognostic signs. Electrical stimulation testing provides an assessment of the degree of nerve degeneration and has been reported to be helpful in predicting recovery.

Corticosteroids are commonly used to treat Bell's palsy, although little evidence supports their beneficial effect. Since it is postulated, however, that edema of the nerve within a tight fallopian canal contributes to nerve damage, a 7–10 day course of oral corticosteroids is not unreasonable for patients without specific systemic contraindications who are seen within the first 48 hours.

In cases of orbicularis oculi involvement, treatment of corneal exposure may be necessary. Artificial tear preparations and lubricants are sufficient in mild cases. Taping the eyelid shut with lubricating ointment in the eye for sleep may be necessary. Breakdown of corneal epithelium indicates the need for a tarsorrhaphy or other surgical procedure or the injection of botulinum toxin type A (Botox) to induce ptosis.

Adour KK. Current concepts in neurology: diagnosis and management of facial paralysis. *N Engl J Med.* 1982;307:348–351.

Katusic SK, Beard CM, Wiederholt WC, et al. Incidence, clinical features, and prognosis in Bell's palsy, Rochester, Minnesota, 1968–1982. *Ann Neurol.* 1986;20:622–627.

May M, Galetta S. The facial nerve. In: Tasman W, Jaeger EA, eds. *Duane's Clinical Ophthalmology.* Philadelphia: JB Lippincott Co; 1994; vol 2; chap 8:15–17.

Neoplasms may involve the seventh nerve in the cerebellopontine angle (acoustic neuroma, meningioma), within the fallopian canal, or in the parotid gland. Most of these lesions are histologically benign and slow growing. When small, they may be missed with CT; MRI with intravenous contrast is recommended. Such lesions can compress the seventh nerve, resulting in facial synkinesis.

Infections may spread to involve the seventh nerve from otitis media, or the nerve may be impaired from meningitis. *Lyme disease,* caused by infection with the tick-borne spirochete *Borrelia burgdorferi,* can cause unilateral or bilateral facial palsies. Classic manifestations include a characteristic rash (erythema chronicum migrans), arthritis, and meningopolyneuritis. The prognosis for seventh nerve recovery is excellent.

Clark JR, Carlson RD, Sasaki CT, et al. Facial paralysis in Lyme disease. *Laryngoscope.* 1985;95:1341–1345.

Herpes zoster involving the seventh nerve is called *Ramsay Hunt syndrome.* It is diagnosed by the identification of vesicles along the posterior aspect of the external auditory canal, over the tympanic membrane, or on the pinna. Pain is often severe, and postherpetic neuralgia may result. The prognosis for recovery is less promising than with Bell's palsy.

May M, Galetta S. The facial nerve. In: Tasman W, Jaeger EA, eds. *Duane's Clinical Ophthalmology.* Philadelphia: JB Lippincott Co; 1994; vol 2; chap 8:17–18.

An isolated seventh nerve palsy, as well as other isolated or multiple cranial nerve palsies, may be the first sign of human immunodeficiency virus (HIV) seroconversion.

Parry GJ. Peripheral neuropathies associated with human immunodeficiency virus infection. *Ann Neurol.* 1988;23(suppl):S49–S53.

The seventh nerve is the cranial nerve most commonly involved in *sarcoidosis.* The site of involvement is usually the parotid gland, which becomes infiltrated with noncaseating granulomatous material. Seventh nerve involvement is frequently bilateral yet asymmetric.

Facial diplegia may occur in *Guillain-Barré syndrome,* especially in the Fisher variant when ophthalmoplegia and ataxia are also present. Cerebrospinal fluid analysis reveals elevated protein with a normal cell count, and deep tendon reflexes should be absent. Recovery is generally complete.

A seventh nerve palsy may occur with head trauma. Battle's sign (ecchymosis over the mastoid) may be present, and fractures of the temporal bone should be suspected. A congenital facial palsy is frequently related to birth trauma from forceps and tends to resolve.

In *Melkersson-Rosenthal syndrome* recurrent facial paralysis, unilateral or bilateral, is accompanied by chronic facial swelling and lingua plicata (furrowing of the tongue). The etiology of this disorder, which usually begins in childhood or adolescence, is unknown. The facial swelling is frequently marked, and it may be bilateral even when facial paresis is only unilateral.

May M, Galetta S. The facial nerve. In: Tasman W, Jaeger EA, eds. *Duane's Clinical Ophthalmology.* Philadelphia: JB Lippincott Co; 1994; vol 2; chap 8:18, 20–22, 23, 25–26.

Disorders of Overactivity of the Seventh Nerve

Disorders of the seventh nerve, its nucleus, or the pyramidal or extrapyramidal pathways may produce hyperexcitable states. Essential blepharospasm, hemifacial spasm, and facial myokymia are the three most important disorders of overactivity (Table VII-2).

Essential blepharospasm This condition is bilateral. Onset consists of episodic contraction of the orbicularis oculi, usually occurring between ages 40 and 60. Initially, the spasms are mild and infrequent, but they may progress to the point that the patient's daily activities are severely disrupted. In advanced cases the patient's eyelids cannot be pried open during an episode of spasm. Facial grimacing and other movements may be associated with blepharospasm (Meige syndrome), and cogwheeling in the neck and extremities or other extrapyramidal signs may be

TABLE VII-2

COMPARISON OF THE MAJOR CAUSES OF SEVENTH NERVE OVERACTIVITY

	LATERALITY	SITE OF DYSFUNCTION*	ETIOLOGY	TREATMENT
Essential blepharospasm	Bilateral	Basal ganglia	Unknown	Medical: haloperidol, clonazepam, other drugs
				Surgical: botulinum toxin, extirpation of eyelid protractors, selective seventh nerve section
Hemifacial spasm	Unilateral	Facial root in cerebellopontine angle	Unknown or nerve compression by blood vessels or tumors	Medical: carbamazepine, baclofen
				Surgical: botulinum toxin, decompression of facial root
Facial myokymia	Unilateral	Facial nucleus or fascicle in pons	Glioma, multiple sclerosis	Medical: carbamazepine, phenytoin sodium
Eyelid myokymia	Unilateral	Unknown	Unknown	None

*Presumed

noted. Tardive dystonia secondary to neuroleptic and antipsychotic drugs can produce a condition similar to Meige syndrome. Extrapyramidal disorders such as parkinsonism, Huntington disease, and basal ganglia infarction may be accompanied by some degree of blepharospasm.

The exact cause of benign essential blepharospasm is unknown, but it is believed to be related to basal ganglia dysfunction. The clinician evaluating a patient with blepharospasm should rule out causes of reflex blepharospasm, in particular severely dry eyes, intraocular inflammation, and meningeal irritation. Stress may exacerbate the condition. Neuroradiologic studies are generally unrevealing.

Medical therapy for blepharospasm can be attempted, although it is rarely successful. Haloperidol, clonazepam, bromocriptine, baclofen, and other drugs have demonstrated limited usefulness. Currently, the treatment of choice for essential blepharospasm is injection of botulinum toxin type A into the orbicularis oculi muscle. The duration of the effect of the toxin is temporary, lasting only a few months, so that repeated injections are necessary. The effectiveness of the drug relates to its ability to cause muscle weakness. Complications such as ptosis, exposure of the cornea, diplopia, and local ecchymosis are usually mild and transient.

Occasionally, when medical treatment fails, surgical therapy—the meticulous extirpation of the eyelid protractors—may be indicated. Selective ablation of the seventh nerve is an alternative procedure that carries greater complications and a lower success rate.

Gillum WN, Anderson RL. Blepharospasm surgery. An anatomical approach. *Arch Ophthalmol.* 1981;99:1056–1062.

Grandas F, Elston J, Quinn N, et al. Blepharospasm: a review of 264 patients. *J Neurol Neurosurg Psychiatry.* 1988;51:767–772.

Jordan DR, Anderson RL. Essential blepharospasm. In: *Focal Points: Clinical Modules for Ophthalmologists.* San Francisco: American Academy of Ophthalmology; 1988;6:6.

Jordan DR, Patrinely JR, Anderson RL, et al. Essential blepharospasm and related dystonias. *Surv Ophthalmol.* 1989;34:123–132.

McCord CD Jr, Coles WH, Shore JW, et al. Treatment of essential blepharospasm. I. Comparison of facial nerve avulsion and eyebrow-eyelid muscle stripping procedure. *Arch Ophthalmol.* 1984;102:266–268.

Osako M, Keltner JL. Botulinum A toxin (Oculinum®) in ophthalmology. *Surv Ophthalmol.* 1991;36:28–46.

Hemifacial spasm   This condition is characterized by unilateral episodic spasm involving the facial musculature that typically lasts from seconds to minutes. The disorder frequently begins as intermittent twitching of the orbicularis oculi muscle and spreads over several years to involve all of the facial muscles. Episodes may increase in frequency for weeks to months and then abate for months at a time. Seventh nerve function is usually intact.

The pathogenesis of some cases of hemifacial spasm may relate to abnormalities of the seventh nerve at the root entry zone. Abnormal firing in the motor nucleus or ephaptic transmission of nerve impulses causes innervation directed toward one muscle group to excite adjacent nerve fibers directed to another muscle group. Compression of the seventh nerve by anomalous vessels in the cerebellopontine angle, tumors in the angle (in 1% of cases), or previous seventh nerve injury may result in hemifacial spasm. But in most cases a specific etiology is not identified.

Carbamazepine, clonazepam, or baclofen may provide improvement in some patients. Facial myectomy and neurectomy have been shown to give patients with hemifacial spasm limited relief. Suboccipital craniotomy with placement of a sponge between the seventh nerve and the offending blood vessel (Jannetta procedure) may be considered in advanced cases. Botulinum toxin type A injection into the facial muscles has proved very effective. Reinjection is required at intervals of several months. Hemifacial spasm responds to lower doses of botulinum toxin than does blepharospasm. Side effects are similar to those seen in patients with blepharospasm treated with botulinum toxin.

Barker FG 2nd, Jannetta PJ, Bissonette DJ, et al. Microvascular decompression for hemifacial spasm. *J Neurosurg.* 1995;82:201–210.

Digre K, Corbett JJ. Hemifacial spasm: differential diagnosis, mechanism, and treatment. *Adv Neurol.* 1988;49:151–176.

Mauriello JA Jr, Coniaris H, Haupt EJ. Use of botulinum toxin in the treatment of one hundred patients with facial dyskinesias. *Ophthalmology.* 1987;94:976–979.

Sprik C, Wirtschafter JD. Hemifacial spasm due to intracranial tumor. An international survey of botulinum investigators. *Ophthalmology.* 1988;95:1042–1045.

Facial myokymia   This disorder is characterized by continuous unilateral fibrillary or undulating contraction of facial muscle bundles. These rippling movements usually begin within a portion of the orbicularis oculi and may spread to involve most of the facial muscles.

Facial myokymia typically signifies intramedullary disease of the pons involving the seventh nerve nucleus or fascicle. It is usually the result of a pontine glioma in children and multiple sclerosis in adults. The myokymia may be relieved with carbamazepine or phenytoin sodium (Dilantin).

Occasionally, the myokymia progresses over weeks to months to place all facial muscles in spasm with concomitant weakness of volitional facial movement. This condition, spastic paretic facial contracture, is generally indicative of a pontine glioma. Rarely, myokymia occurs in Guillain-Barré syndrome.

Intermittent fluttering of one eyelid, *orbicularis oculi myokymia,* is relatively common. The phenomenon usually lasts days or weeks. It is benign.

Andermann F, Cosgrove JBR, Lloyd-Smith DL, et al. Facial myokymia in multiple sclerosis. *Brain.* 1961;84:31–44.

Tenser RB, Corbett JJ. Myokymia and facial contracture in brain stem glioma. An electromyographic study. *Arch Neurol.* 1974;30:425–427.

Van Zandycke M, Martin JJ, Vande Gaer L, et al. Facial myokymia in the Guillain-Barré syndrome: a clinicopathologic study. *Neurology.* 1982;32:744–748.

Other conditions   Rarely, focal cortical seizures are manifested by gross clonic movements involving one side of the face only. The eyes may deviate to the involved side during the episode, and the patient's ipsilateral hand may also have clonic movements. Frequently, a transient supranuclear facial paresis, *Todd's paralysis,* follows the seizure. The electroencephalogram should be abnormal during the clonic episodes.

Habit spasm such as facial tic or nervous twitch is relatively common, particularly in childhood, and is characterized by stereotyped, repetitive, reproducible facial movements that can be promptly inhibited on command. These movements tend to disappear in time without treatment. Only very rarely does Tourette syndrome present with facial twitching alone.

Reflex blepharospasm results from fifth nerve irritation, usually from a severely dry eye, intraocular inflammation, or meningeal irritation. Treatment of the underlying cause alleviates the symptom. Oral facial dyskinesias seen after long-term use of major tranquilizers may persist even after the drugs are stopped. This condition is called *tardive dyskinesia.*

CHAPTER VIII

Selected Systemic Conditions With Neuro-Ophthalmic Signs

Certain neurologic and medical disorders are seen commonly enough and affect vision with such regularity that they deserve separate emphasis. While the discussion that follows is not comprehensive, it is intended to cover many aspects of diseases with which ophthalmologists should be familiar.

Immunologic Disorders

Multiple Sclerosis

Patients with multiple sclerosis (MS) frequently have visual complaints, and often the ophthalmologist is the first physician consulted. Familiarity with both the ocular and neurologic consequences of MS is important to guide the ophthalmologist to the appropriate diagnosis.

Epidemiology and genetics The incidence of MS varies considerably in different geographic areas, increasing with latitude north and south of the equator. Prevalence in the United States ranges from 6 to 80 per 100,000. MS is relatively rare throughout Asia and Africa. MS affects women more often than men (2:1 in some series). The disease is relatively uncommon in children under 10 years of age, and the incidence is highest among young adults (25–40 years of age). However, examples of onset even after the age of 50 are not rare.

Although the cause of MS remains unknown, multiple factors appear contributory. Epidemiological studies suggest that both genetic and environmental factors play a role. The risk of developing MS is approximately 20 times greater in first-degree relatives of patients with the disease. Furthermore, identical twins show a tenfold greater concordance of the disease than do fraternal twins. Population-based concordance studies suggest that two or more genes are operative for MS susceptibility, and there is a strong association with HLA-DR2 antigen.

Supporting the theory of an environmental causative agent are migration studies that show that individuals moving after the age of 15 carry the same risk of developing MS as those in their native location, while those migrating before age 15 acquire the risk level of their new locale. No specific viral etiology has been identified, but an acquired agent, such as a virus, may precipitate an autoimmune process that attacks myelin.

Haegert DG, Marrosu MG. Genetic susceptibility to multiple sclerosis. *Ann Neurol.* 1994;36(Suppl2):S204–S210.

Matthews WB, Compston A, Allen IV, et al. *McAlpine's Multiple Sclerosis.* 2nd ed. New York: Churchill Livingstone; 1991.

Poser CM. The epidemiology of multiple sclerosis: a general overview. *Ann Neurol.* 1994;36(Suppl2):S180–S193.

Course and prognosis   Multiple sclerosis is usually a chronic, relapsing disease, but the course of the disease is variable. Spontaneous remissions occur, and 90% of patients have a relapsing course in the early stages. An interval of months or years may precede a relapse. A slow, apparently continuous deterioration of the neurologic status may be observed late in the course of the disease. In 10%–20% of patients the disease progresses inexorably from onset. Progressive MS is more common when onset occurs in older patients, whose overall disability tends to be greater. Near total disability and, rarely, death within 1–2 years of onset may result. In contrast, numerous patients have a somewhat mild illness with intervals of several years between relapses. Approximately one third of patients experience a relatively benign course without serious disability or reduction of life span.

The prognosis of MS is difficult to predict, since most of the studies are retrospective. In a series of 241 patients studied and followed for a minimum of 10 years, approximately one third had died, one third were disabled, and one third had no physical restrictions or disabilities interfering with work or home life. Indicators of a favorable prognosis include the following:

▫ Early age at onset

▫ Female gender

▫ Relapsing-remitting course

▫ Optic neuritis or sensory symptoms at onset

▫ Few attacks or minimal disability in the first 2–3 years

As a rule, the longer the interval between the initial attack and first relapse, the better the prognosis.

Weinshenker BG. Natural history of multiple sclerosis. *Ann Neurol.* 1994;36(Suppl): S6–S11.

Pathology   Pathologic examination reveals discrete foci of inflammatory demyelination in the central nervous system. The myelin forming the sheath for the axonal processes of neurons undergoes patchy destruction in the brain, spinal cord, and optic nerves. Initially, the axons generally remain intact but no longer conduct nerve impulses efficiently. Eventually, the axons themselves may suffer irreparable damage.

MS is a disease of white matter; demyelination is the primary pathologic event. Myelin destruction is seen in association with local perivascular mononuclear cell infiltration and is followed by myelin removal by macrophages. The next stage is characterized by astrocytic proliferation with production of glial fibrils. The term *multiple sclerosis* stems from the presence of these numerous gliotic (sclerotic) lesions, which take on spherical, ovoid, or other three-dimensional configurations but appear as "plaques" on the surface of brain sections. The axons or nerve cell bodies are more or less uninvolved, but destruction of axons is noted in some of the oldest lesions. Plaques are frequently situated in the white matter at the ventricular margins, the optic nerves and chiasm, the corpus collosum, the spinal cord, and throughout the brain stem and cerebellar peduncles. Peripheral nerves are not involved, and all other organs are normal in uncomplicated cases.

Ebers GC. Immunogenetics and CSF studies in multiple sclerosis. In: Vandenbark AA, Raus JCM, eds. *Immunoregulatory Processes in Experimental Allergic Encephalomyelitis and Multiple Sclerosis.* New York: Elsevier Science Publishing Co; 1984.

Clinical presentation The diagnosis of MS is made by identifying neurologic symptoms that occur over time and affect different areas of the central nervous system. Ocular symptomatology is commonly part of the clinical picture of multiple sclerosis, and various ocular complications are discussed below. Other signs and symptoms attributable to MS may precede, follow, or coincide with the ocular signs. Many symptoms of MS are so transient or benign that the patient may fail to remember previous episodes. Typically, significant episodes last for weeks or months. The physician must ask specifically about transient diplopia, ataxia, vertigo, patchy paresthesias, bladder or bowel dysfunction, and extremity weakness. Fatigue and depression are common and may precede the onset of focal neurologic deficits. Because the symptoms of MS are often so evanescent and unaccompanied by objective neurologic findings, patients are sometimes considered hysterical.

The cerebellum, brain stem, and spinal cord may be involved singly or simultaneously, thus producing mono- or polysymptomatic complaints. Some of the more common nonocular symptoms include the following:

- *Cerebellar dysfunction*: Ataxia, dysarthria, intention tremor, truncal or head titubation, dysmetria (sometimes described by the patient as poor depth perception)

- *Motor symptoms*: Extremity weakness, facial weakness (Bell's palsy), hemiparesis, or paraplegia

- *Sensory symptoms*: Paresthesias of face or body (especially in a bandlike distribution around the trunk), Lhermitte's sign (an electric shock–like sensation in the limbs and trunk produced by neck flexion), pain (occasionally trigeminal neuralgia)

- *Mental changes*: Emotional instability, depression, irritability, fatigue; later in the course, euphoria in the face of severe neurologic symptoms; dementia with severe, widespread demyelination

- *Sphincter disturbances*: Frequency, urgency, hesitancy, incontinence; urinary retention leading to urinary tract infection

It has been suggested that infection, trauma, abnormal reaction to certain foreign substances such as drugs, vaccinations, stress, exertion and fatigue, and increased body temperature may induce attacks of MS. No adequately controlled studies examine these issues. MS is typically quiescent during pregnancy and may flare up after delivery.

Matthews WB, Compston A, Allen IV, et al. *McAlpine's Multiple Sclerosis.* 2nd ed. New York: Churchill Livingstone; 1991.

Sadovnick AD, Eisen K, Hashimoto SA, et al. Pregnancy and multiple sclerosis. A prospective study. *Arch Neurol.* 1994;51:1120–1124.

Optic neuritis The clinical signs and symptoms of optic neuritis are discussed on pp 81–83. Even after recovery of the visual loss of demyelinating optic neuritis, transient deterioration of vision may be brought on by exercise and by even small elevations of body temperature (Uhthoff's symptom). Some patients with optic neuritis note phosphenes with movement of the affected eye or with sudden loud noises (sound-induced photisms). This symptom is thought to arise from ephaptic transmission between the medial and lateral geniculate bodies.

Optic neuritis is recognized clinically during the patient's course of MS in up to 75% of cases. It is one of the presenting features of MS in approximately 25% of patients. Evidence of optic nerve involvement appears in over 90% of cases, regardless of symptoms, according to visually evoked cortical potential response data. Furthermore, autopsy studies show anterior visual pathway demyelination in virtually all patients with clinical multiple sclerosis.

Visual recovery to a level of 20/40 or better occurs in 95% of untreated patients with optic neuritis. Recovery is unrelated to the presence of pain, the occurrence of optic disc swelling, or the severity of visual loss. Overall, after 5 years of follow-up in the Optic Neuritis Treatment Trial (ONTT), visual acuity was 20/25 or better in 87% of cases, 20/25 to 20/40 in 7%, 20/50 to 20/190 in 3%, and 20/200 or worse in 3%. Recurrent optic neuritis occurred in 28%. Most eyes with a recurrence retained normal or almost normal vision. Despite the seemingly excellent prognosis of optic neuritis, patients usually remain aware of visual deficits in the affected eye after recovery. Studies using measures of visual function other than Snellen acuity (such as contrast sensitivity function, light brightness sense, stereopsis, visual fields, and color vision) have shown residual abnormalities in up to 90% of patients with at least 20/30 vision.

What is the risk of developing clinical multiple sclerosis after an initial isolated attack of optic neuritis? The presence or absence of abnormalities on MRI of the brain obtained at study entry during an episode of optic neuritis was the strongest predictive factor in determining the likelihood of developing MS in the ONTT. Clinically definite MS developed in 27% of patients and probable MS in 9%. The probability of developing clinically definite MS by MRI appearance was the following: 16% no lesions, 44% with one lesion, 24% with two lesions, and 51% with three or more lesions. Patients with a prior history of optic neuritis and nonspecific neurologic symptoms were at higher risk of developing MS.

Beck RW. The Optic Neuritis Treatment Trial. Three-year follow-up results. Optic Neuritis Study Group. *Arch Ophthalmol.* 1995;113:136–137.

Fleishman JA, Beck RW, Linares DA, et al. Deficits in visual function after resolution of optic neuritis. *Ophthalmology.* 1987;94:1029–1035.

Jacobs L, Karpik A, Bozian D, et al. Auditory-visual synesthesia: sound-induced photisms. *Arch Neurol.* 1981;38:211–216.

Optic Neuritis Study Group. The 5-year risk of MS after optic neuritis. Experience of the Optic Neuritis Treatment Trial. *Neurology.* 1997;49:1404–1418.

Optic Neuritis Study Group. Visual function 5 years after optic neuritis. Experience of the Optic Neuritis Treatment Trial. *Arch Ophthalmol.* 1997;15:1545–1552.

Rizzo JF 3rd, Lessell S. Risk of developing multiple sclerosis after uncomplicated optic neuritis: A long-term prospective study. *Neurology.* 1988;38:185–190.

Slamovits TL, Rosen CE, Cheng KP, et al. Visual recovery in patients with optic neuritis and visual loss to no light perception. *Am J Ophthalmol.* 1991;111:209–214.

Treatment of optic neuritis. The ONTT clarified the role of corticosteroid therapy in the management of patients with optic neuritis. The 457 patients between the ages of 18 and 45 with acute unilateral optic neuritis were randomized to one of three treatment regimens:

□ Oral prednisone (1 mg/kg/day for 14 days)

□ IV methylprednisolone (250 mg every 6 hours for 3 days) followed by oral prednisone (1 mg/kg/day for 11 days)

□ Oral placebo (14 days)

Patients treated with oral prednisone alone showed no faster recovery and had no better vision at the end of 6 months of follow-up than did patients treated with placebo. Most important, patients treated with oral prednisone had a higher rate of development of new attacks of optic neuritis in either eye. *Therefore, oral prednisone alone is contraindicated for acute optic neuritis.*

Patients treated with IV methylprednisolone recovered vision faster than did patients treated with placebo, but only within the first 2 weeks. At 6 months' follow-up, there was no statistically significant difference in visual acuity between the IV-treated and placebo-treated patients. Patients with demyelinating lesions on MRI who were treated with IV corticosteroids had a reduced incidence in subsequent signs and symptoms of MS within the first 2 years. This benefit was observed within the first 2 years, however, and not at 3 years.

The ONTT Study Group recommended obtaining an MRI in all patients with optic neuritis and treating those with severe loss of vision or those with other evidence of MS using IV methylprednisolone for 3 days followed by oral prednisone as indicated above. Various strategies for implementing the ONTT results may be acceptable, and the options should be discussed with the individual patient to determine the most appropriate course of action. Other considerations, such as employment or financial and personal issues, often influence the decision to proceed with an MRI or IV methylprednisolone.

Beck RW, Cleary PA, Anderson MM Jr, et al. A randomized, controlled trial of corticosteroids in the treatment of acute optic neuritis. The Optic Neuritis Study Group. *N Engl J Med.* 1992;326:581–588.

Beck RW, Cleary PA, Trobe JD, et al. The effect of corticosteroids for acute optic neuritis on the subsequent development of multiple sclerosis. *N Engl J Med.* 1993;329: 1764–1769.

Optic Neuritis Study Group. The clinical profile of optic neuritis. Experience of the Optic Neuritis Treatment Trial. *Arch Ophthalmol.* 1991;109:1673–1678.

Chiasmal and retrochiasmal abnormalities Although the white matter within the optic chiasm, optic tracts, and visual radiations is frequently involved pathologically with MS lesions, chiasmal and retrochiasmal visual field defects are only infrequently reported. This discrepancy appears to have two causes: concurrent optic nerve disease masks the findings and perimetry is inadequate. Nevertheless, bitemporal and homonymous visual field defects may occur with MS and then generally follow a course of recovery similar to that seen with optic neuritis.

Hawkins K, Behrens MM. Homonymous hemianopia in multiple sclerosis. With report of bilateral case. *Br J Ophthalmol.* 1975;59:334.

Newman NJ, Lessell S, Winterkorn JM. Optic chiasmal neuritis. *Neurology.* 1991;41: 1203–1210.

Ocular motility disturbances Diplopia is a frequent symptom of MS. Several attacks of transient diplopia may occur before an observable ocular motor defect
becomes clinically apparent. Since MS is a disease of central nervous system white
matter, motility abnormalities are typically localized to the supranuclear, nuclear,
and fascicular portions of the ocular motor system. Internuclear ophthalmoplegia,
especially when bilateral, is highly suggestive of MS in someone under age 50 years.
Other signs include complete or partial paralysis of horizontal or vertical gaze or a
vertical misalignment (skew deviation) not attributable to single nerve or muscle
dysfunction. Although uncommon, MS must be considered in a young adult with an
isolated ocular motor palsy and no history of trauma. Since they likely reflect
fascicular involvement, ocular motor palsies are frequently accompanied by other
brain stem findings. The sixth nerve is the most commonly reported ocular motor
nerve involved, but partial third nerve paresis has been described.

Nystagmus is frequently seen in MS. It may be horizontal, rotary, or vertical.
Both pendular and jerk types of nystagmus may occur. Various types of cerebellar eye findings are common, including rebound nystagmus, fixation instability
(macrosaccadic oscillations), saccadic dysmetria, and abnormal pursuit movements.
Concomitant vertical and horizontal nystagmus occurring out of phase produce
circular or elliptical eye movements that are highly suggestive of MS. Occasionally,
MS lesions produce Parinaud (dorsal midbrain) syndrome. Patients with eye movement abnormalities typically complain of diplopia, blurred vision, or oscillopsia.
Chapter VI discusses ocular motility disorders in detail.

Funduscopic abnormalities in multiple sclerosis Nerve fiber layer defects have
been discussed in chapter III (see pp 52–53). Perivenous sheathing and fluorescein
leakage occur along peripheral veins in approximately 10% of patients with MS.
Autopsy studies of 47 MS patients confirmed retinitis and periphlebitis in 5%–10%.
Posterior or anterior uveitis occurs in 2.5% of MS patients, an incidence approximately 10 times higher than in the general population. Pars planitis associated with
HLA-DR2 infrequently occurs in MS.

Arnold AC, Pepose JS, Hepler RS, et al. Retinal periphlebitis and retinitis in multiple
sclerosis. I. Pathologic characteristics. *Ophthalmology.* 1984;91:255–262.

Graham EM, Francis DA, Sanders MD, et al. Ocular inflammatory changes in established multiple sclerosis. *J Neurol Neurosurg Psychiatry.* 1989;52:1360–1363.

Lightman S, McDonald WI, Bird AC, et al. Retinal venous sheathing in optic neuritis. Its
significance for the pathogenesis of multiple sclerosis. *Brain.* 1987;110:405–414.

Laboratory evaluation No test unequivocally establishes the presence of MS,
which remains a *clinical* diagnosis. Laboratory tests such as MRI, CT, or VECP (also
known as VEP or VER) may help to support the diagnosis. The Poser criteria specifically define the requirements for clinical and laboratory-supported diagnoses of definite and probable MS (Table VIII-1). Visually evoked cortical potential responses are
discussed in chapter I. The cerebrospinal fluid (CSF) in patients with clinically definite MS is abnormal in more than 90% of cases. The most common abnormalities
are the elevation of immunoglobulin G (IgG), the elevation of the IgG/albumin
index, and the presence of oligoclonal IgG bands. None of these findings, however,
is specific for demyelinating disease.

Hershey LA, Trotter JL. The use and abuse of the cerebrospinal fluid IgG profile in the
adult: a practical evaluation. *Ann Neurol.* 1980;8:426–434.

Table VIII-1

Poser Criteria for Diagnosis of MS

CATEGORY	ATTACK*	CLINICAL EVIDENCE	PARACLINICAL EVIDENCE†	CSF OB IgG‡
Clinically definite				
CDMS A1	2	2		
CDMS A2	2	1	and 1	
Laboratory-supported definite				
LSDMS B1	2	1	or 1	+
LSDMS B2	1	2		+
LSDMS B3	1	1	and 1	+
Clinically probable				
CPMS C1	2	1		
CPMS C2	1	2		
CPMS C3	1	1	and 1	
Laboratory-supported probable				
LSPMS D1	2			+

* Attacks must be >24 hr long, be separated by at least 1 month, and be in separate parts of the CNS

† Paraclinical evidence: demonstration of a lesion that has *not* produced signs but which may have caused symptoms in the past (MRI CT, evoked potentials, urologic testing)

‡ CSF OB/IgG = CSF Oligoclonal bands IgG (2 more in CSF than serum required)

Poser CM, Paty DW, Scheinberg L, et al. New diagnostic criteria for multiple sclerosis: guidelines for research protocols. *Ann Neurol.* 1983;13:227–231.

CT scan with double-dose infusion of IV contrast material may reveal white-matter demyelinating lesions; however, MRI is the neuroimaging study of choice for MS. MRI is particularly sensitive for identification of white-matter plaques in the central nervous system, and it is far superior to CT for visualizing the posterior fossa and spinal cord (Fig VIII-1) (see p 46). MRI shows multiple lesions in 85%–95% of patients with clinically definite MS and in 66%–76% of patients with suspected MS. Although the MRI abnormalities are not specific for MS, multifocal (four or more) lesions that are periventricular and ovoid are most consistent with the condition. The lesions seen with MRI fluctuate over time. Active lesions will enhance with gadolinium-DPTA administration. Lesions in the optic nerves of patients with symptomatic optic neuritis have been visualized on MRI enhanced by special fat-suppression techniques.

Jacobs L, Munschauer FE, Kaba SE. Clinical and magnetic resonance imaging in optic neuritis. *Neurology.* 1991;41:15–19.

Miller DH, Newton MR, van der Poel JC, et al. Magnetic resonance imaging of the optic nerve in optic neuritis. *Neurology.* 1988;38:175–179.

Paty DW. Magnetic resonance in multiple sclerosis. *Curr Opin Neurol Neurosurg.* 1993; 6:202–208.

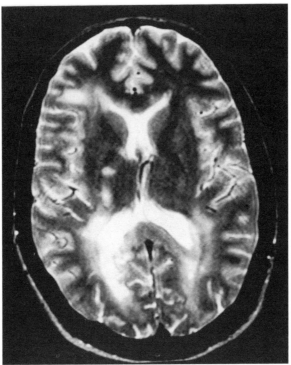

FIG VIII-1—T2-weighted MRI of the brain in a patient with multiple sclerosis demonstrates typical periventricular white-matter lesion.

Paty DW, Oger JJ, Kastrukoff LF, et al. MRI in the diagnosis of MS: a prospective study with comparison of clinical evaluation, evoked potentials, oligoclonal banding and CT. *Neurology.* 1988;38:180–185.

Treatment of multiple sclerosis There is no proven treatment for MS. As in the management of optic neuritis, corticosteroids are often used to treat acute exacerbations of MS, but no evidence shows lasting improvement or alteration of prognosis with corticosteroid administration. Immunosuppressant and immunomodulating agents may be useful for long-term treatment. Interferon ß1b (Betaseron) reduces the number of MS exacerbations by approximately one third in patients with relapsing-remitting disease. Copolymer-1 has a similar efficacy with fewer side effects. Interferon ß1a (AVONEX) reduces MS attacks by 30% and lessens disease activity as measured by gadolinium-enhanced MRI. Other agents being tested in clinical trials include oral myelin; retinoic acid; linomide; and cladribine (Leustatin), a T-cell-specific agent. Low-dose oral methotrexate may be beneficial for patients with chronic, progressive MS. Other immunosuppressant agents have not proven helpful.

The IFNB Multiple Sclerosis Study Group. Interferon beta-1b is effective in relapsing-remitting multiple sclerosis. I. Clinical results of a multicenter, randomized, double-blind, placebo-controlled trial. *Neurology.* 1993;43:655–661.

Myasthenia Gravis

Myasthenia gravis (MG) is an immunological disorder characterized by weakness. It improves with rest. Most patients with MG develop neuro-ophthalmic abnormalities during its course. Although the disease is usually a systemic disorder, half of the affected patients have ocular symptoms and signs at onset, so the ophthalmologist is frequently the first physician encountered. The muscles and nerves are intact in MG, but the acetylcholine receptor sites for neuromuscular transmission are blocked by immune complexes. MG may be caused, unmasked, or worsened by drugs such as procainamide, quinidine, polymixin and aminoglycoside antibiotics, monobasic amino acid antibiotics, corticosteroids, beta blockers, chloroquine, lithium, phenytoin, cisplatin, and magnesium.

Drachman DB. Myasthenia gravis. *N Engl J Med.* 1978;298:136–142, 186–193.

Katz B. Myasthenia gravis. In: *Focal Points: Clinical Modules for Ophthalmologists.* San Francisco: American Academy of Ophthalmology; 1989;7:7.

Clinical presentation   The most common sign of MG is ptosis, which may be unilateral or bilateral. It tends to vary, with the eyelid being more ptotic in the evening, after exertion, or after prolonged upward gaze. Cogan's lid twitch, elicited following downgaze, is a brief overelevation of the upper eyelid with an upward saccade. In keeping with Hering's law of innervation, when the more ptotic eyelid is manually elevated, the less ptotic eyelid inevitably falls.

MG frequently causes diplopia. The diplopia, like the ptosis, is variable, both during the day and from one day to another. The diplopia pattern may simulate any cranial nerve paresis (usually sixth or partial third nerve palsy), a supranuclear motility disturbance (e.g., internuclear ophthalmoplegia, gaze palsies), an isolated muscle "palsy" (e.g., isolated inferior rectus), or total ophthalmoplegia.

The hallmarks of MG are fluctuation and fatigue. Clinical signs and symptoms usually worsen in the evening and with usage and improve with rest. Any changing pattern of diplopia, with or without ptosis, should suggest myasthenia gravis. Orbicularis oculi weakness is nearly always present in patients with ocular myasthenia gravis. The eyelids or globes may fatigue with prolonged upgaze. Pupillary abnormalities and sensory disturbances are not encountered with myasthenia gravis, however, and their presence should provoke a search for another diagnosis.

Systemic symptoms and signs include weakness of the jaw, neck extensors, trunk, and limbs; dysphagia; hoarseness; dysarthria; and dyspnea. Dysphagia and dyspnea can be life threatening, and they require prompt treatment. Graves disease occurs in about 5% of myasthenia gravis patients. Its appearance can occasionally complicate the clinical findings.

Diagnosis   The diagnosis of myasthenia gravis is made clinically by identifying typical signs and symptoms, pharmacologically by overcoming the receptor block through the administration of acetylcholinergic agents, and serologically by demonstrating elevated anti–acetylcholine receptor antibody titers. A diagnosis of myasthenia gravis does not necessarily rule out other pathology.

If a demonstrable, measurable abnormality is present on the examination, an *edrophonium chloride (Tensilon) test,* a *sleep test,* or an *ice-pack test* can confirm the diagnosis of MG. Before performing the Tensilon test, the clinician should warn the patient of the short-lived but often discomforting potential side effects of

Tensilon, including diaphoresis, lacrimation, abdominal cramping, nausea, vomiting, and salivation. Atropine sulfate (0.4–0.6 mg) should be immediately available, and some physicians treat with atropine (0.6 mg IM) prior to administering the Tensilon test.

In most protocols, 2 mg (0.2 cc) of Tensilon are first injected intravenously through a butterfly needle as a test dose. The patient is observed for 60 seconds. If the symptoms disappear or decrease (e.g., eyelid elevates, motility improves), the test can be discontinued, for it is positive. If no response is elicited, the remaining 8 mg are administered. Alternatively, the physician can administer 4 mg of Tensilon, observe for improvement, and administer the final 4 mg. This divided dose seems to cause fewer adverse effects. However, many patients develop minor side effects (fasciculations, warmth, nausea) no matter how the medication is given. If the defect is marked (complete ptosis), the endpoint (eyelid elevation) is dramatic (Fig VIII-2). However, a subtle deficit such as minimal diplopia may require other means to better define the endpoint. Lancaster red-green or Maddox rod tests with prisms or diplopia fields can be given before and after Tensilon (see chapter I). False-positive and false-negative Tensilon tests may occur.

It is important to remember that although major side effects from Tensilon are rare, bradycardia, respiratory arrest, syncopal episodes, or cholinergic crisis may be precipitated by IV edrophonium administration. It is necessary to monitor the patient's pulse and blood pressure throughout the procedure. The procedure should be done in a chair that can be reclined, and resuscitation equipment should be on hand. The ophthalmologist must be prepared to deal with severe side effects by injecting atropine sulfate IV and maintaining vital signs.

An alternative to the Tensilon test is the *neostigmine methylsulfate (Prostigmin) test*. This test is particularly useful in children and in adults without ptosis who may require a longer observation period than that allowed by Tensilon. Adverse reactions are similar to those with Tensilon. The most frequent side effects are salivation, fasciculations, and gastrointestinal discomfort. Intramuscular neostigmine and atropine are injected concurrently. A positive test produces resolution of signs within 30–45 minutes. The dosage formula is:

$$\frac{\text{Weight (kg)} \times \text{adult dose*}}{70}$$

*Adult dose: 1.5 mg neostigmine with 0.4 mg atropine.

The *sleep test* is a safe, simple office test that eliminates the need for Tensilon testing in many patients. After having the baseline deficit (measurements of ptosis, motility) documented, the patient rests quietly with eyes closed for 30 minutes. The measurements are repeated immediately after the patient "wakes up" and opens his or her eyes. Improvement after rest is highly suggestive of MG.

Since neuromuscular transmission improves in the cold, the *ice-pack test* is often helpful to diagnose patients with ocular signs. An ice pack is placed over lightly closed eyes for 2 minutes or to the limit of the patient's tolerance. Improved ptosis occurs with MG.

Katz B. Myasthenia gravis. In: *Focal Points: Clinical Modules for Ophthalmologists.* San Francisco: American Academy of Ophthalmology, 1989;7:7.

Moorthy G, Behrens MM, Drachman DB, et al. Ocular pseudomyasthenia or ocular myasthenia "plus": a warning to clinicians. *Neurology.* 1989;39:1150–1154.

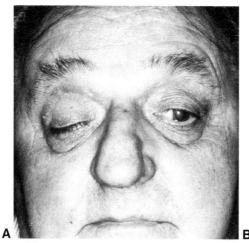

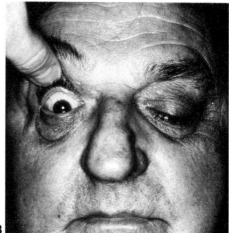

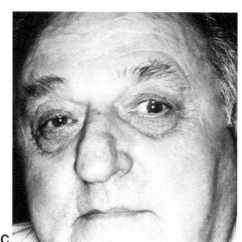

FIG VIII-2—*A,* Patient with complete right ptosis and partial left ptosis. Eyelid opening is achieved primarily by frontalis overaction. *B,* Manual opening of the right eyelid produces complete left ptosis. This sign, while usually present in myasthenia gravis, is not specific. It may be seen with other disorders producing asymmetrical ptosis and is a manifestation of Hering's law of equal innervation. *C,* A Tensilon test produces marked improvement in eyelid position bilaterally.

Odel JG, Winterkorn JM, Behrens MM. The sleep test for myasthenia gravis. A safe alternative to Tensilon. *J Clin Neuroophthalmol.* 1991;11:288–292.

Sethi KD, Rivner MH, Swift TR. Ice-pack test for myasthenia gravis. *Neurology.* 1987;37: 1383–1385.

Seybold ME. The office Tensilon test for ocular myasthenia gravis. *Arch Neurol.* 1986;43: 842–843.

Other diagnostic tests for myasthenia gravis include the serum assay for anti–acetylcholine receptor antibodies and electrophysiologic testing. There are three types of *acetylcholine receptor antibody tests* commercially available. *Binding* antibodies are usually requested, because they are detected in approximately 90% of patients with generalized MG and 70% of patients with ocular MG. *Blocking* antibodies are rarely present (1%) without binding antibodies. *Modulating* antibodies are present as frequently as binding antibodies. Blocking and modulating antibody testing is usually reserved for patients who are negative for the binding antibody and for whom evidence of autoimmune MG is necessary. *Electromyographic repetitive nerve stimulation* shows a characteristic decremental response in many patients with systemic myasthenia gravis. Single-fiber electromyograms also show findings that are fairly typical in patients with MG. All myasthenic patients must be investigated radiologically for thymomas, which are visible on CT scan in 10% of these patients. Since there is a high coexistence of myasthenia gravis with other autoimmune disorders, serologic screening tests for thyroid dysfunction and systemic lupus erythematosis are also warranted.

Treatment Medical treatment for myasthenia gravis uses acetylcholinesterase inhibitors, corticosteroids, and other immunosuppressant agents. Thymectomy is the treatment of choice in myasthenic patients who have thymic enlargement and is necessary for those with thymoma.

Myasthenia gravis is a systemic disease with disastrous potential. Although purely ocular myasthenia gravis does exist, more frequently the disease is a systemic one that presents initially with ophthalmologic findings alone. Given the possibility of having to deal with respiratory and other life-threatening manifestations of the disease, it is prudent to manage myasthenic patients in cooperation with a neurologist. If ocular signs remain truly isolated for more than 2 years, the disease is likely to remain purely ocular.

Table VIII-2 summarizes points of differentiation between myasthenia gravis, chronic progressive external ophthalmoplegia (CPEO), and thyroid ophthalmopathy, which is discussed in detail below.

Inherited Disorders

Myopathies

Oculopharyngeal dystrophy This hereditary condition is usually autosomal dominant with onset in the fifth and sixth decades of life. The typical presentation is progressive dysphagia followed by ptosis. Most patients develop chronic progressive external ophthalmoplegia. Pathological studies show a vacuolar myopathy. The disease is classically seen in patients of French-Canadian ancestry.

Myotonic dystrophy This dominantly inherited (chromosome 19), multisystem disorder also produces ophthalmoplegia that may mimic CPEO. Symptoms usually start in late childhood or early adulthood with myotonia that is worsened with excitement, cold, and fatigue. It is easily detected by asking the patient to shake hands; the patient will not be able to release his or her grasp. This myopathy is unusual, since it affects distal limb musculature first. Wasting of the temporalis and masseter produces the typical "hatchet face." The myopathic facies, frontal balding, and ptosis cause a distinct and remarkably similar appearance.

Ocular findings include ptosis, pigmentary retinopathy, ophthalmoparesis, and polychromatic lenticular deposits ("Christmas tree" cataracts). The pupils are miotic and respond sluggishly to light. Other features include low intelligence, insulin resistance, hearing loss, cardiomyopathy, cardiac conduction abnormalities, testicular atrophy, and uterine atony. Electromyography provides the definite diagnosis by demonstrating the typical myotonic discharges.

TABLE VIII-2

DIFFERENTIATION OF CONDITIONS PRODUCING PTOSIS
AND EXTRAOCULAR MUSCULAR INVOLVEMENT

	MYASTHENIA GRAVIS	THYROID OPHTHALMOPATHY	CHRONIC PROGRESSIVE EXTERNAL OPHTHALMOPLEGIA (CPEO)
Age	Any age	Any age	Any age
Muscle preferentially involved	Levator Extraocular muscles	Inferior rectus Medial rectus muscles	Levator Extraocular
Fatiguability	Yes	No, unless coexistent myasthenia gravis	No
Response to Tensilon	Yes	No, unless coexistent myasthenia gravis	No
Other eye signs	No	External eye signs	Pigmentary retinopathy Optic neuropathy
Forced ductions	Normal	Restriction	Restriction if long-standing
Clinical course	Fluctuation May have generalized weakness	May resolve or progress	Slowly progressive
Eyelids	Ptosis	Retraction	Ptosis
Diplopia	Yes	Yes	No
Other signs and symptoms	Dysphagia, jaw weakness, limb weakness, dyspnea	Tachycardia, arrhythmia, tremor, weight loss, diarrhea, heat intolerance	Heart block Manifestation of Kearns-Sayre syndrome

Neurocutaneous Syndromes

(See BCSC Section 6, *Pediatric Ophthalmology and Strabismus,* for additional discussion of these disorders.)

The *phakomatoses* are disorders characterized by the presence of hamartias and hamartomas involving different organ systems such as skin, eyes, central nervous system, and viscera. Six entities are classically grouped under this category: neurofibromatosis, tuberous sclerosis, cerebrofacial angiomatosis (Sturge-Weber syndrome), retinal angiomatosis, ataxia-telangiectasia, and Wyburn-Mason syndrome. Klippel-Trénaunay-Weber syndrome has been included by some authors. A syndrome of cavernous hemangioma of the retina associated with central nervous system angiomas (von Hippel–Lindau) is yet another variant of the phakomatoses.

These disorders are characterized by tumors formed from normal tissue elements: hamartomas and choristomas. A *hamartoma* is composed of elements normally found at the involved site. The glial retinal tumors of tuberous sclerosis are a type of hamartoma. *Choristas* and *choristomas* are anomalies containing tissues

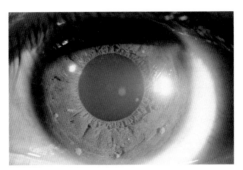

FIG VIII-3—Lisch nodules of iris, left eye, in child with type 1 neurofibromatosis. (Photograph courtesy of Mark J. Greenwald, MD.)

not normally present at the involved site. A limbal dermoid is a commonly encountered example of choristoma. Hamartomas and choristomas differ from true neoplasms in that they seem to be anomalies of tissue formation rather than cellular proliferations arising in previously normal tissue. They lack the capacity for limitless proliferation exhibited by true neoplasms. Except for the vascular hamartia of ataxia-telangiectasia, all phakomatosis lesions are hamartomas.

Neurofibromatosis The two most common forms of neurofibromatosis are *von Recklinghausen neurofibromatosis (NF-1)* and *bilateral acoustic neurofibromatosis (NF-2)*. NF-1 is the more common form of the disease. It is inherited in an autosomal dominant manner and has been linked to chromosome 17. General features include multiple neurofibromas, pigmented skin lesions, osseous malformations, and associated tumors. The disease is defined by the presence of multiple cutaneous pigmented macules (café-au-lait spots), neurofibromas, and iris (Lisch) nodules (Fig VIII-3). Mild cases may show only iris nodules associated with café-au-lait spots.

Neurofibromas are histologically benign and may take the form of either fibroma molluscum or plexiform neurofibromas. They may involve the eyelid and face, occasionally causing marked deformities (Fig VIII-4). Lisch nodules are pigmented iris hamartomas present in 94%–97% of patients with type 1 neurofibromatosis who are age 6 years or older. These nodules do not become symptomatic but may prove helpful in establishing the diagnosis, especially when discovered in asymptomatic relatives.

Other ocular involvement in neurofibromatosis includes congenital glaucoma and retinal astrocytomas. Osseous defects may involve the orbit, commonly the greater wing of the sphenoid, with associated orbital encephalocele. Vertebral and long-bone defects are seen as well. Multiple tumors of the brain, spinal cord, and meninges as well as of cranial, peripheral, and sympathetic nerves may be encountered in these patients. Optic nerve or chiasmal gliomas in children are frequently associated with neurofibromatosis (Fig VIII-5). These lesions cause proptosis and visual loss but are rarely life threatening. Treatment of these lesions is controversial. Additional neoplastic associations include pheochromocytoma and meningioma.

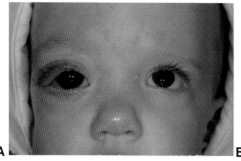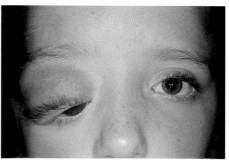

A   B

FIG VIII-4—Plexiform neurofibroma involving the right upper eyelid, associated with ipsilateral buphthalmos, in girl with NF-1. *A,* Age 8 months. *B,* Age 8 years. (Photographs courtesy of Mark J. Greenwald, MD.)

Huson S, Jones D, Beck L. Ophthalmic manifestations of neurofibromatosis. *Br J Ophthalmol.* 1987;71:235–238.

Lubs ML, Bauer MS, Formas ME, et al. Lisch nodules in neurofibromatosis type I. *N Engl J Med.* 1991;324:1264–1266.

Riccardi VM. Von Recklinghausen neurofibromatosis. *N Engl J Med.* 1981;305:1617–1627.

Bilateral acoustic neurofibromatosis (NF-2) is less common than NF-1. Also transmitted as an autosomal dominant trait, it is linked to chromosome 22. Only about 60% of these patients have café-au-lait spots or peripheral neurofibromas, and Lisch nodules are not a feature of this disease. Bilateral acoustic neuromas usually present symptomatically in young adulthood. Other central nervous system tumors may occur but not as frequently as in NF-1.

Mulvihill JJ, Parry DM, Sherman JL, et al. NIH conference. Neurofibromatosis 1 (Recklinghausen disease) and neurofibromatosis 2 (bilateral acoustic neurofibromatosis). An update. *Ann Intern Med.* 1990;113:39–52.

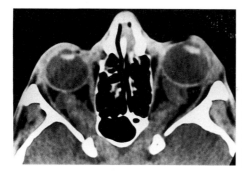

FIG VIII-5—Axial CT image showing bilateral optic glioma with chiasmal involvement associated with severe bilateral visual loss in an adolescent boy with NF-1. Note relatively low density of tissue surrounding the central core of the enlarged optic nerve. (Photograph courtesy of Mark J. Greenwald, MD.)

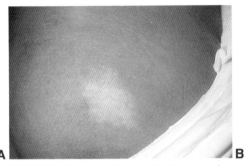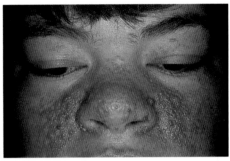

FIG VIII-6—Cutaneous lesions of tuberous sclerosis. *A,* Hypopigmented macule ("ash-leaf spot"). *B,* Adenoma sebaceum of the face. (Photographs courtesy of Mark J. Greenwald, MD.)

Tuberous sclerosis Also known as Bourneville syndrome, tuberous sclerosis is transmitted as an autosomal dominant trait linked to chromosome 9. It has classically been characterized by the triad of adenoma sebaceum, mental deficiency, and epilepsy, although presentation shows great variability. The majority of patients have seizures, but many patients have normal mentation. The so-called sebaceous adenomas are actually hamartomatous angiofibromas that commonly appear in a butterfly distribution over the nose and cheeks (Fig VIII-6). Other skin lesions include periungual fibromas, café-au-lait spots, and shagreen patches (large, leatherlike, hyperpigmented, raised patches that are typically located on the trunk). The "ash-leaf spot," a leaf-shaped area of skin depigmentation that fluoresces under a Woods lamp, is considered pathognomonic for tuberous sclerosis.

Calcified astrocytic hamartomas are frequently evident on plain skull x-ray ("brain stones") and CT scan (Fig VIII-7). Other visceral involvement that has been described includes cardiac rhabdomyomata, renal cysts, and angiomyolipomata. The characteristic ocular finding is an astrocytic hamartoma of the retina or optic disc (Fig VIII-8).

Cerebrofacial (encephalotrigeminal) angiomatosis (Sturge-Weber syndrome) The characteristic skin lesion in Sturge-Weber syndrome is nevus flammeus, an angioma involving skin and subcutaneous tissues in the distribution of the fifth nerve (Fig VIII-9). This lesion is present from birth, is usually unilateral, and is commonly associated with a parietal-occipital leptomeningeal hemangioma ipsilateral to the facial vascular hamartoma (Fig VIII-10). Calcification of the cortex underlying the hemangioma can be seen radiographically. CT is the imaging method of choice. Convulsions are a major problem in these patients.

Unilateral congenital open-angle glaucoma is seen in approximately 25% of patients with Sturge-Weber syndrome and is usually associated with an angioma of the upper eyelid. Onset of glaucoma may occur at any time; tonometry should be performed early and repeated periodically. Heterochromia iridis has been described. The characteristic fundus lesion is a choroidal hemangioma, a solitary, yellow-

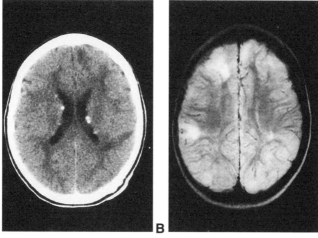

FIG VIII-7—Brain lesions of tuberous sclerosis. *A,* Axial CT image showing small periventricular calcifications in the basal ganglia bilaterally. *B,* Axial T2-weighted MRI showing two tuberous malformations of the right hemisphere cortex. (Photographs courtesy of Mark J. Greenwald, MD.)

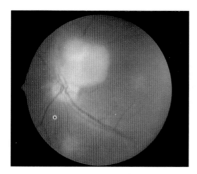

FIG VIII-8—Fundus lesions of tuberous sclerosis, left eye. In addition to the large phakoma partially overlying the optic disc, note a small hypopigmented lesion in the temporal macula and partial obscuration of a retinal blood vessel near the edge of the photograph directly below the disc by a barely visible second phakoma. (Photograph courtesy of Mark J. Greenwald, MD.)

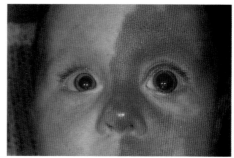

FIG VIII-9—Facial port-wine nevus involving the left eyelids, associated with ipsilateral buphthalmos in an infant girl with Sturge-Weber syndrome. (Photograph courtesy of Mark J. Greenwald, MD.)

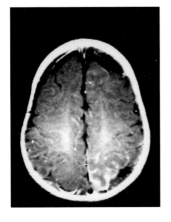

FIG VIII-10—Axial T1-weighted MRI, after gadolinium infusion, showing vascular malformation with underlying cortical atrophy in the left occipital lobe of a 4-month-old girl with Sturge-Weber syndrome. (Photograph courtesy of Mark J. Greenwald, MD.)

orange, moderately elevated mass seen in the posterior pole of up to 50% of these patients. More diffuse uveal involvement can give the fundus a confluent "tomato catsup" appearance (Fig VIII-11). Exudative retinal detachments may occur in association with these lesions.

Klippel-Trénaunay-Weber syndrome may be a variant of cerebrofacial angiomatosis. Nonocular findings include cutaneous nevus flammeus and hemangiomas, varicosities, associated hemihypertrophy of the limbs, and intracranial angiomas. The cutaneous lesions and vascular anomalies are sometimes amenable to laser treatment. Ocular involvement, usually congenital glaucoma and conjunctival telangiectasia, is uncommon.

Retinal angiomatosis   Also known as *von Hippel disease,* retinal angiomatosis is transmitted by autosomal dominant inheritance. The disease may also occur sporadically. The characteristic ocular lesion is a retinal capillary angioma: a globular, smooth-surfaced, pink retinal tumor fed by a single, dilated, tortuous retinal artery

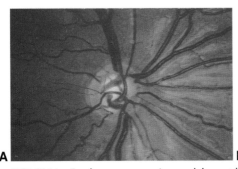
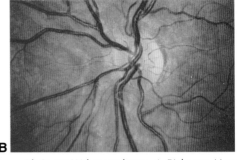

A   **B**

FIG VIII-11—Fundus appearance in an adolescent boy with Sturge-Weber syndrome. *A,* Right eye. Note glaucomatous disc cupping and deeper red color of surrounding choroid, compared with normal fellow eye. *B,* Left eye. (Photographs courtesy of Mark J. Greenwald, MD.)

and drained by a similar-appearing vein. These lesions are often multiple and are bilateral in 50% of cases. Serous exudation can cause retinal detachment.

Cerebellar hemangioblastomas are seen in approximately 25% of patients with retinal angiomatosis, and this association is known as *von Hippel–Lindau disease* (Fig VIII-12). Hemangioblastomas may also occur in the brain stem or spinal cord and may be associated with syrinxes in these regions.

Patients with cerebellar angiomas may also have renal, pancreatic, hepatic, or epididymal cysts and pheochromocytomas or renal cell carcinoma. Several of these multisystem manifestations are potentially lethal. Early detection of the retinal abnormality by the ophthalmologist should prompt referral of the patient for a thorough systemic investigation.

Ataxia-telangiectasia   Ataxia-telangiectasia, or Louis-Bar syndrome, is considered the most common cause of progressive ataxia in early childhood. It is characterized by progressive cerebellar ataxia and oculocutaneous telangiectasia. Thymic hypo-plasia, with defective T-cell function and immunoglobulin deficiency, predisposes patients to recurrent sinopulmonary infections. The genetic abnormality is localized to chromosome 11, and the inheritance pattern is generally autosomal recessive. Conjunctival telangiectasia is almost always seen, especially as the child grows older (Fig VIII-13).

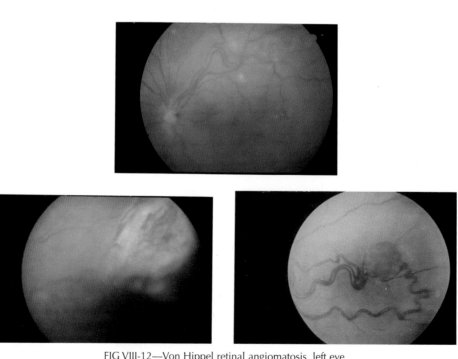

FIG VIII-12—Von Hippel retinal angiomatosis, left eye.

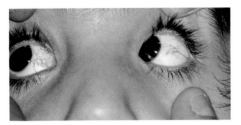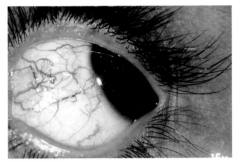

FIG VIII-13—Abnormally dilated and tortuous conjunctival vessles, left eye, in a child who has ataxia-telangiectasia.

Ocular motility deficits are the classic eye findings, specifically horizontal and vertical supranuclear gaze palsies. Initially, the patient shows an inability to initiate saccades, which may be associated with head thrusting and abnormalities of the fast phase of optokinetic nystagmus. Pursuit becomes impaired, and eventually the disease leads to total ophthalmoplegia. However, oculocephalic responses remain intact. There is a high incidence of malignant lymphoma and leukemia in those patients who do not succumb to recurrent infections.

Wyburn-Mason syndrome Wyburn-Mason syndrome refers to an association of an intracranial arteriovenous malformation (AVM) with an arteriovenous malformation of the ipsilateral retina (racemose angioma) (Fig VIII-14). The lesions consist of direct communications between the arteries and the veins without an intervening capillary bed. The vessels are usually fully developed and may involve any part of the posterior pole. They are usually increased in number, size, and tortuosity. Spontaneous hemorrhage from these lesions may cause decreased vision. Because of the association between retinal and intracranial AVMs, an MRI of the brain should be obtained in patients with a retinal AVM.

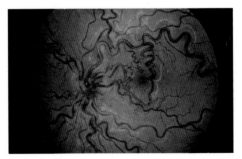

FIG VIII-14—Racemose angioma of the retina, left eye.

Associated AVMs may be seen in the midbrain, basofrontal region, or posterior fossa, and they may be associated with spontaneous intracranial hemorrhage or convulsions. AVMs can also involve the maxilla, pterygoid fossa, or mandible. Orbital AVMs may be associated with mild proptosis, conjunctival vascular dilation, or a bruit.

Endocrinologic Disorders

Thyroid Ophthalmopathy (Graves Disease)

Graves disease is generally believed to be an autoimmune disorder characterized by one or more of the following three clinical entities:

□ Hyperthyroidism associated with diffuse hyperplasia of the thyroid gland

□ Infiltrative orbitopathy

□ Infiltrative dermopathy (localized pretibial myxedema)

Orbital involvement in Graves disease may appear prior to or concomitant with systemic signs of dysthyroidism (usually hyperthyroidism), or it may appear only when the thyrotoxic state is controlled.

Clinical presentation and diagnosis Symptoms and signs of *hyperthyroidism* include nervousness, emotional lability, inability to sleep, excessive sweating, tremors, heat intolerance, weight loss, weakness, frequent bowel movements, hyperreflexia, sinus tachycardia, atrial arrhythmias, and pretibial myxedema. Screening tests for hyperthyroidism should include measurements of total thyroxine (T_4), free T_4, and triiodothyronine (T_3). *Hypothyroidism* typically results in lethargy, decreased energy, constipation, cold intolerance, stiffness and cramping of muscles, weight gain, carpal tunnel syndrome, sleep apnea, hair loss, dry skin, periorbital edema, enlarged tongue, and "hung-up" tendon reflexes (reflexes with prolonged relaxation phase). An elevated level of thyroid-stimulating hormone (TSH) should create suspicion of hypothyroidism.

The diagnosis of thyroid ophthalmopathy is a clinical one. It is convenient to think of three components of the disorder:

□ External symptoms

□ Motility abnormalities

□ Optic neuropathy

The initial symptoms of Graves ophthalmolopathy are usually a result of external eye disease. Conjunctival injection is typically localized over the horizontal rectus muscles, with the muscles themselves often being easily visible through the conjunctiva (Fig VIII-15). The conjunctiva is often chemotic. Symptoms of dry eyes are common, as a result of lacrimal gland infiltration. Eyelid signs of dysthyroidism are important clinical diagnostic clues. The most specific eyelid sign is retraction (Figs VIII-16, VIII-17), which is often associated with lid lag and retraction on downward gaze (Fig VIII-18). Periorbital erythema and edema create a fullness to the eyelids. Concurrent myasthenia gravis should be suspected if ptosis is present.

As the extraocular muscles become infiltrated and enlarged, patients develop diplopia. The most frequently affected muscle in thyroid ophthalmopathy is the inferior rectus; therefore, inability to elevate the eye in either abduction or adduction is the earliest motility disturbance. Commonly known as *double elevator palsy,* this is now also termed *monocular elevation deficiency.* The medial rectus is the

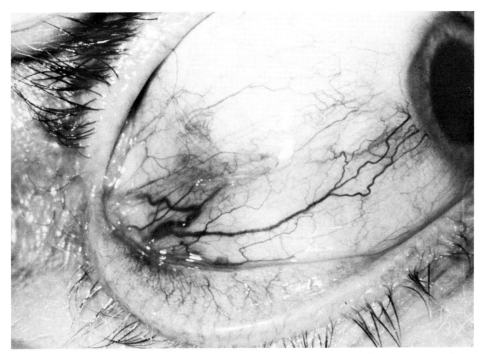

FIG VIII-15—Conjunctival injection, most marked over the lateral rectus. Note the engorgement of vessels over the muscle.

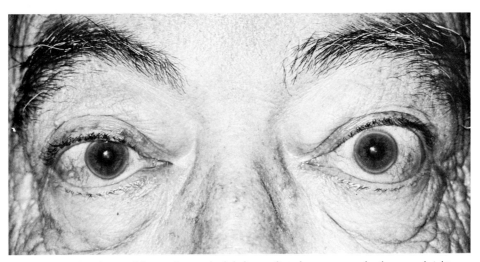

FIG VIII-16—Patient has eyelid retraction on the left that, at first glance, may make the normal right eyelid appear ptotic. Note also the bilateral conjunctival injection.

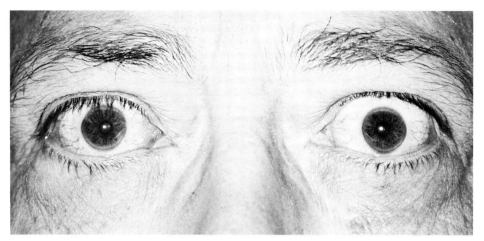

FIG VIII-17—Bilateral eyelid retraction with sclera easily visible above the superior limbus bilaterally. Note again the conjunctival injection.

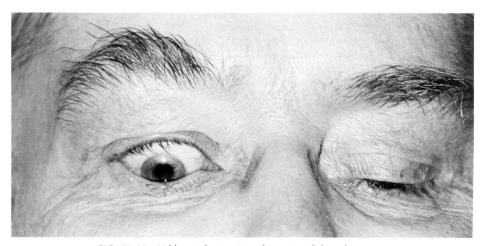

FIG VIII-18—Lid lag and retraction of upper eyelid on downgaze.

second most frequently affected muscle, resulting in an abduction defect that may simulate a sixth nerve palsy. Any muscle or group of muscles may be involved, resulting in bizarre motility patterns. The forced duction test is always positive when restrictive diplopia is present and can be very helpful in identifying the restrictive myopathy of dysthyroidism.

With increasing muscle enlargement and orbital congestion, exophthalmos occurs. Proptosis may be unilateral or bilateral. The most frequent cause of unilateral and bilateral proptosis is dysthyroidism. The orbits are "tight," with increased resistance of the globes to retropulsion. With worsening exophthalmos and eyelid retraction, the risk of corneal exposure increases. (Other frequent causes of proptosis in children and adults are described in BCSC Section 7, *Orbit, Eyelids, and Lacrimal System.*)

If the orbit is tight, intraocular pressure (IOP) may become elevated. With inferior rectus restriction, IOP increases on attempted upgaze. Applanation tonometry in primary position and upgaze can document this increase. Elevated IOP in eccentric gaze rarely affects the optic nerve and does not require treatment.

Optic neuropathy, leading to blindness, is an infrequent but dreaded complication of thyroid ophthalmopathy. Dysthyroid optic neuropathy must be considered in any patient with thyroid eye disease whose loss of vision cannot be accounted for by corneal changes or retinal folds. Optic nerve function in such cases is probably compromised by compression caused by crowding of the nerve by grossly enlarged extraocular muscles and orbital fat at the orbital apex. Extensive proptosis need not be present to provoke suspicion of optic neuropathy.

The diagnosis of thyroid ophthalmopathy remains a clinical one and may be made even in the absence of supporting endocrinologic abnormalities. Not infrequently, patients with typical thyroid ophthalmopathy have normal thyroid function studies (T_3, T_4). TSH is most often reduced, but referral to an endocrinologist for further testing may be necessary. Even if dysthyroidism is absent, regular follow-up of affected patients is important, since changes in their hormonal and metabolic status can occur over time. Graves ophthalmopathy may worsen during treatment with radioactive iodine. The worsening of ophthalmopathy during radioiodine therapy is often transient and can be prevented by the administration of prednisone (0.4–0.5 mg/kg for 1 month, starting 2–3 days after radioiodine therapy and tapered over the next 2 months).

Orbital ultrasonography may show thickening of extraocular muscles and can help in diagnosis. The abnormalities of thyroid ophthalmopathy on CT and MRI are characteristic. Proptosis can be measured and enlargement of one or more extraocular muscles can be seen. The inferior and medial rectus are the muscles most often involved, while the lateral rectus is sometimes spared. Muscle involvement is almost always bilateral. Coronal sections illustrate the enlarged muscles in relation to the optic nerve (Fig VIII-19). The sparing of the tendons is characteristic, unlike the typical CT or MRI appearance of orbital myositis.

If the clinical presentation is typical for thyroid ophthalmopathy and no evidence indicates optic nerve compromise, neuroimaging studies are not needed. If the diagnosis is doubtful, or if orbital decompression surgery is being considered to treat optic neuropathy, an unenhanced orbital CT scan is recommended.

Bartalena L, Marcocci C, Bogazzi F, et al. Relation between therapy for hyperthyroidism and the course of Graves' ophthalmopathy. *N Engl J Med.* 1998;338:73–78.

Dresner SC, Kennerdell JS. Dysthyroid orbitopathy. *Neurology.* 1985;35:1628–1634.

Frueh BR. Graves' eye disease: orbital compliance and other physical measurements. *Trans Am Ophthalmol Soc.* 1984;82:492–598.

Treatment   The primary treatment of Graves disease is control of the dysthyroid state, which may have no effect on the eye signs. Initial ocular treatment serves to protect against corneal exposure with use of artificial tears, ointment before bedtime, taping the eyelids closed at night, plastic shields as moisture chambers, or tarsorrhaphy. Rare cases that present with rapidly progressing orbitopathy with optic neuropathy require orbital decompression as initial treatment.

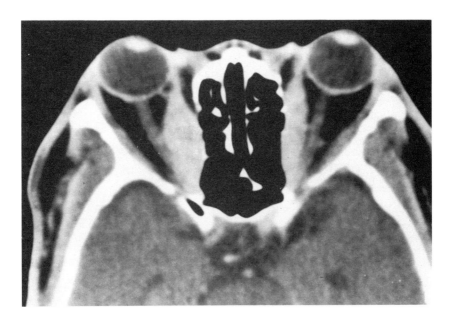

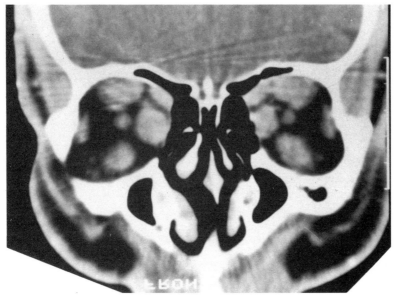

FIG VIII-19—CT scan with contrast. Axial *(top)* and coronal *(bottom)* views of the orbits demonstrate bilateral extraocular muscle enlargement with sparing of the tendinous insertions. The lateral recti are relatively spared in comparison to the other extraocular muscles.

Treatment of the ocular myopathy varies, depending on the acuteness or chronicity of the condition. Most patients with chronic or subacute disease can be observed. Systemic corticosteroids may be effective during the acute congestive phase, but they are of no use during the fibrotic period. Dosage may begin with the equivalent of 80 mg/day of prednisone, tapered according to clinical response. If no response is seen within 3 weeks, tapering should begin and another mode of treatment instituted. Long-term corticosteroid treatment without significant clinical improvement is not appropriate, and intraorbital corticosteroids are of no benefit. Other immunosuppressive agents, such as cyclosporine, have also been used with limited success.

Utiger RD. Treatment of Graves' ophthalmopathy. *N Engl J Med.* 1989;321:1403–1405.

Extraocular muscle surgery should be considered only when repeated measurement has shown the ocular misalignment to be stable for at least 6 months, and when no indication of active orbital inflammation is present.

Dysthyroid optic neuropathy must be treated aggressively and promptly. High-dose oral or IV corticosteroids may be used. If no improvement occurs within 1 week, the corticosteroids should either be discontinued or maintained for a short period in conjunction with alternative therapy such as radiation or decompression.

Orbital radiation, 1500–2000 cGy over a period of 10 days, is administered to retrobulbar tissue, sparing the lens. During these 10 days, the congestive orbitopathy may worsen transiently. Systemic corticosteroids are useful during this period.

Hurbli T, Char DH, Harris J. Radiation therapy for thyroid eye diseases. *Am J Ophthalmol.* 1985;99:633–637.

Kazim M, Trokel S, Moore S. Treatment of acute Graves orbitopathy. *Ophthalmology.* 1991;98:1443–1448.

Orbital decompression through a transantral or transeyelid approach allows the orbital contents to expand into the maxillary or ethmoid sinus spaces. Another approach is lateral wall decompression with fracture of the orbital floor, which provides less potential for decompression of the optic nerve than the transantral approach. Orbital decompression frequently has an adverse effect on ocular motility. If a multistaged procedure is required, the decompression should be followed by strabismus surgery, then eyelid surgery.

Kennerdell JS, Maroon JC, Buerger GF. Comprehensive surgical management of proptosis in dysthyroid orbitopathy. *Orbit.* 1987;6:153–179.

Lyons CJ, Rootman J. Orbital decompression for disfiguring exophthalmos in thyroid orbitopathy. *Ophthalmology.* 1004;101:223–230.

Warren SD, Spector SG, Burde RM. Long-term follow-up and recent observations on 305 cases of orbital decompression for dysthyroid orbitopathy. *Laryngoscope.* 1989; 99:35–40.

The exact cause of thyroid ophthalmopathy remains an enigma. No doubt it is in some way connected to thyroid dysfunction, but the mechanism is unknown. Current research has implicated an immunologic response as the underlying cause of the thyroid disease. It is likely that the orbital disease is caused by a similar mechanism with different target organs such as retrobulbar fat, extraocular muscles, and lacrimal glands. Whether this mechanism is humoral or cellular or a combination of the two is under continuing investigation.

Bahn RS, Heufelder AE. Pathogenesis of Graves' ophthalmopathy. *N Engl J Med.* 1993;329:1468–1475.

Weetman AP, Cohen S, Gatter KC, et al. Immunohistochemical analysis of the retro-bulbar tissues in Graves' ophthalmopathy. *Clin Exp Immunol.* 1989;75:222–227.

Neuro-Ophthalmic Disorders Associated with Pregnancy

Several ophthalmic and neuro-ophthalmic abnormalities occur with greater frequency during pregnancy or the postpartum period. These include the following:

☐ Central serous chorioretinopathy

☐ Hypertensive retinopathy

☐ Purtscher-like retinopathy

☐ Retinal detachment

☐ Thrombotic thrombocytopenic purpura

☐ Cerebral venous thrombosis

☐ Cerebral arterial occlusion

☐ Carotid cavernous fistula

Pregnancy can also aggravate the following preexisting conditions:

☐ Uveal melanoma

☐ Pituitary adenoma

☐ Meningioma

☐ Hemangioma

☐ Diabetes

☐ Graves disease

Royburt M, Seidman DS, Serr DM, et al. Neurologic involvement in hypertensive disease of pregnancy. *Obstet Gynecol Surv.* 1991;46:656–664.

Sunness JS. The pregnant woman's eye. *Surv Ophthalmol.* 1988;32:219–238.

Pathology can often be related to hypertension-induced damage and occurs most frequently in those patients with *eclampsia* and *preeclampsia* (toxemia of pregnancy). Transient visual disturbances, including scotomata, photopsias, dimming of vision, and diplopia, occur in up to 50% of patients with preeclampsia. Cerebral blindness may occur in up to 1%–5%. CT may show hypodensity, and MRI may reveal increased signal on T2 images; both are consistent with cerebral edema. Because of a posterior predilection for these changes, it is not surprising that the retrogeniculate visual system is frequently involved. The abnormalities seen on neuroimaging appear to be as potentially reversible as the patient's symptoms.

Raroque HG Jr, Orrison WW, Rosenberg GA. Neurologic involvement in toxemia of pregnancy: reversible MRI lesions. *Neurology.* 1990;40:167–169.

Ischemic cerebrovascular complications occur during pregnancy and the post-partum period approximately 13 times more frequently than the expected rate in age-matched controls. Predisposing conditions include cardiac emboli, cervical arterial disease, cranial arterial disease, intracranial aneurysm, and intracranial venous occlusion secondary to a relative hypercoagulable state. Abnormalities are of arterial etiology in 60%–90% of cases, typically occurring during the second and third trimesters and first week postpartum. Problems attributable to venous occlusive disease typically occur later, during the first 6 weeks postpartum. Venous sinus thrombosis classically presents with headaches and papilledema.

Digre KB, Varner MW. Diagnosis and treatment of cerebrovascular disorders in pregnancy. In: Adams HP Jr, ed. *Handbook of Cerebrovascular Diseases*. New York: Marcel Dekker; 1993:255–286.

Donaldson JO, Lee NS. Arterial and venous stroke associated with pregnancy. *Neurol Clin*. 1994;12:583–599.

In *Sheehan syndrome* pituitary infarction occurs in the postpartum period, resulting in hypopituitarism. Secondary hemorrhage may cause cranial nerve palsies (II, III, IV, V, VI) and loss of consciousness from subarachnoid blood. Preexisting pituitary macroadenomas may enlarge during pregnancy, and monthly visual field examinations are warranted in such cases. Orbital and choroidal hemangiomas can undergo rapid expansion during pregnancy. Other preexisting conditions, such as many of the autoimmune disorders, may actually improve during pregnancy, only to flare up in the postpartum period. Multiple sclerosis, optic neuritis, sarcoidosis, and possibly lupus are among these disorders. Migraine without aura frequently remits during pregnancy, but other women experience migraine attacks (including acephalgic migraine) only when they are pregnant. Occurrence or recurrence of pseudotumor cerebri is *not* more frequent during pregnancy. Management of this condition is the same during pregnancy as in patients who are not pregnant, in cooperation with the patient's obstetrician.

Digre KB, Varner MW, Corbett JJ. Pseudotumor cerebri and pregnancy. *Neurology*. 1984;34:721–729.

Disorders of the Cerebral Circulation

Approach to the Patient with Transient Visual Loss

Transient visual loss is an important sign of cerebrovascular disease, but the large differential diagnosis and overlapping clinical profiles make the approach to these patients confusing at times. Disorders such as migraine rarely cause permanent visual loss, but other vascular conditions can lead to blindness or stroke. Therefore, a systematic approach to patients with transient visual loss is imperative. The fundus examination may provide additional clues to the underlying etiology. Several factors in the history can guide the ophthalmolgist to the appropriate testing and management in these patients.

Is the visual loss monocular or binocular?   Monocular transient visual loss suggests a problem with the ipsilateral carotid or retinal circulation, or the optic nerve. Binocular, simultaneous visual loss indicates posterior circulation dysfunction affecting the occipital lobes.

What is the duration of visual loss?   Monocular or binocular visual loss lasting seconds may be a result of optic disc drusen or papilledema (transient obscurations of vision). With papilledema the visual loss is often precipitated by a change in posture or eye movement. Cerebrovascular disease typically causes transient visual loss lasting less than 15 minutes. Visual loss from vasospasm or migraine may last from seconds to an hour and may be accompanied by positive visual phenomena such as flashes, sparkles, or heat waves. The typical scintillating scotoma of migraine is binocular and lasts 20–30 minutes. Transient monocular visual loss caused by impending central retinal artery occlusion is usually brief, lasting minutes.

What was the pattern of visual loss and recovery?   Classic amaurosis fugax from carotid artery disease is described as a shade coming down over the vision and eventually lifting. However, others describe a closing in of vision or sudden loss of vision in the affected eye. With vasospasm or migraine, the description may resemble that of carotid disease, and the attacks are sometimes precipitated by exercise. Uhthoff's symptom of transient visual blurring with physical activity or elevation in body temperature occurs after optic neuritis. Transient visual loss resulting from posterior circulation ischemia is typically an abrupt change in vision, causing a homonymous hemianopia or complete, bilateral visual loss. If the visual loss is preceded by fortification spectra, it is a result of migraine. A hexagonal "chicken wire" pattern in the vision or a whiteout of vision suggests occipital ischemia. Gradual peripheral constriction ("closing in") of vision without positive visual phenomena occurs with cerebrovascular disease or migraine affecting the occipital lobes.

How old is the patient?   In a patient under age 45, migraine is the most likely cause of transient visual loss. One important exception in pregnant women is eclampsia that usually causes transient visual loss within days of delivery. Older patients, especially those with known risk factors for cerebrovascular disease, should be investigated for treatable causes of transient ischemic attacks. Giant cell arteritis is a consideration in patients over age 65.

Does the patient show other associated symptoms or signs?   Typical symptoms associated with cerebrovascular ischemia and migraine are described below. Headache following transient visual loss suggests migraine, although headache need not be present. Apparent monocular positive visual phenomena also suggest migraine. Persistent headaches and intracranial noises are typical for pseudotumor cerebri. In an elderly patient transient visual loss associated with headaches, weight loss, fever, malaise, and scalp tenderness may indicate giant cell arteritis. Other neurologic symptoms and signs can help localize the vascular territory involved.

Cerebrovascular Disease

Decreased cerebral perfusion in both the anterior (*carotid*) and posterior (*vertebrobasilar*) circulation systems can be the source of visual problems. The ophthalmologist may be challenged by a variety of symptoms resulting from brain ischemia including transient monocular or binocular visual loss, positive visual phenomena, visual field defects, diplopia, and vertigo. Ischemic neurologic deficits of duration shorter than 24 hours are termed *transient ischemic attacks (TIA).* They often presage a subsequent stroke. Patients with TIAs require a diligent evaluation for underlying risk factors predisposing them to stroke. A systematic approach to the patient that determines the vascular territory involved and potential etiology is essential to guide the clinician in choosing the proper laboratory investigations and treatment.

Carotid system disease The ophthalmologist is most likely to encounter carotid system disease producing ipsilateral transient or permanent monocular visual loss without other neurologic symptoms.

Transient monocular visual loss. An attack of transient monocular blindness, or *amaurosis fugax,* associated with carotid disease is typically described as a curtain or shade coming from above or below. Others describe the appearance of a black spot in the center of the visual field extending out to the periphery, or constriction of the visual field like a camera shutter. Visual loss is usually complete within 30 seconds, and most attacks are over within 15 minutes. Attacks of up to 1–2 hours are less commonly reported.

Emboli in the retinal arteries may be seen following an attack. Bright plaques (cholesterol emboli, or Hollenhorst plaques) rarely occlude retinal arteries and may or may not produce visual symptoms (Fig VIII-20). Platelet thrombi (fibrin-platelet emboli) often occlude the retinal arterioles and produce transient monocular blindness. Either cholesterol or fibrin-platelet emboli are strongly indicative of atheromatous disease of the carotid arteries or aortic arch. They are independently associated with a high incidence of ischemic heart disease, peripheral ischemic disease, and aortic abdominal aneurysms, and they correlate with an adverse survival rate. These emboli demand investigation of not only the carotid vascular system but the entire cardiovascular system. Calcific plaques suggest a cardiac source.

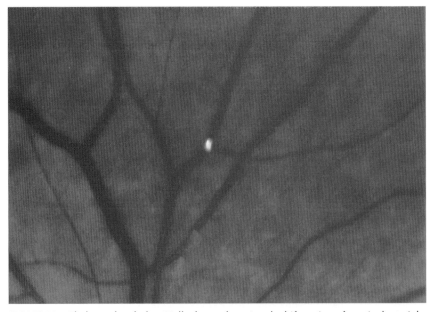

FIG VIII-20—Cholesterol embolus (Hollenhorst plaque) at the bifurcation of a retinal arteriole.

Fisher CM. "Transient monocular blindness" versus "amaurosis fugax." *Neurology.* 1989;39:1622–1624.

Fisher CM. Observations of the fundus oculi and transient monocular blindness. *Neurology.* 1959;9:333–347.

Howard RS, Russell RW. Prognosis of patients with retinal embolism. *J Neurol Neurosurg Psychiatry.* 1987;50:1142–1147.

Central retinal artery occlusion. Carotid artery disease can produce central retinal artery occlusion (CRAO), usually as the result of an embolus. After the embolus lodges, blindness occurs immediately. The retinal vessels may narrow with box-carring or sludging of the blood in the arteries and veins. The retina becomes pale, and a cherry-red spot develops in the macula. Approximately 2–3 weeks later the vessels remain narrow but are blood filled. Occasionally, the size of the vessels returns to normal. When emboli are present, they are most often found in the distribution of the superior temporal retinal arteries.

The prognosis for recovery of vision from CRAO is generally poor. In some cases of cilioretinal artery sparing, useful acuity is preserved. No established treatment regimen has been shown to be effective in producing visual recovery. Acute lowering of IOP by anterior chamber paracentesis, ocular massage, and administration of IV acetazolamide, topical beta blockers, or oral nitrates has been tried. Rhesus monkey studies demonstrate that recovery of the visual acuity, ERG, and visual fields occurs after up to 60–100 minutes of ischemia, but after 100 minutes of complete CRAO, the retina sustains irreversible ischemic damage. Efforts to reverse the ischemia should be pursued within the first day of presentation after CRAO.

Rossmann H. Treatment of retinal arterial occlusion. *Ophthalmologica.* 1980;180: 68–74.

Stone R, Zink H, Klingele T, et al. Visual recovery after central retinal artery occlusion: two cases. *Ann Ophthalmol.* 1977;9:445–450.

Most important, CRAO is an indication to search for evidence of the underlying systemic disease (Table VIII-3). The major cause of death in these patients is generalized cardiovascular disease and not stroke. It is clear that a systemic vasculopathy should be considered before all diagnostic and therapeutic efforts are directed exclusively at the carotid circulation. Giant cell arteritis is an important cause of CRAO that should be suspected in elderly patients.

Augsburger JJ, Magargal LE. Visual prognosis following treatment of acute central retinal artery obstruction. *Br J Ophthalmol.* 1980;64:913–917.

Hankey GJ, Slattery JM, Warlow CP. Prognosis and prognostic factors of retinal infarction: a prospective cohort study. *Br Med J.* 1991;302:499–504.

Savino PJ, Glaser JS. Retinal stroke. Is the patient at risk? *Arch Ophthalmol.* 1977;95: 1185–1189.

TABLE VIII-3

CAUSES OF CRAO

Thromboembolic disease
    Atherosclerotic carotid disease
    Cholesterol emboli
    Thrombus formation
    Cardiogenic emboli
        Valvular heart disease
        Mural thrombus
        Atrial fibrillation

Vasculitis
    Giant cell arteritis
    Systemic lupus erythematosis
    Sjögren syndrome

Hypercoagulability
    Hyperviscosity states
    Protein C, protein S deficiency
    Antiphospholipid antibody syndrome

Vasospasm
    Migraine

Carotid artery dissection

Branch retinal artery occlusion (BRAO) can also herald a serious systemic disorder. One large study found a high correlation between BRAO and hypertension. Embolic disease is frequently associated with BRAO. As with CRAO, a diligent search for an underlying vasculopathy is warranted.

Ros MA, Magargal LF, Uram M. Branch retinal artery obstruction: a review of 201 eyes. *Ann Ophthalmol.* 1989;21:103–107.

Ocular ischemic syndrome. Carotid artery disease may produce ocular ischemic syndrome or *venous stasis retinopathy (VSR)* secondary to chronic hypoperfusion of the eye. VSR is also called *carotid occlusive disease.* The etiology of VSR may be secondary to reduction in perfusion pressure from carotid stenosis with resultant ischemia and hypoxia in the retinal microcirculation. VSR can be caused from vascular occlusion anywhere between the heart and the optic disc. One study determined a 20% incidence of VSR in patients with carotid disease. If ocular perfusion can be restored, VSR usually resolves. Early detection is critical, since neovascularization and progressive ocular ischemia occur with prolonged hypoperfusion.

It is convenient to consider the ocular ischemic syndrome by stages of presentation. In the early stages, the patient may have transient or persistent blurred vision, or exposure to bright light may bring about transient visual loss. Dot-and-blot retinal hemorrhages characterize early ocular ischemia. With severe ischemia, anterior segment changes occur that may be confused with intraocular inflammation. The patient may have a red, painful eye with episcleral vascular injection and decreased visual acuity. *Ischemic uveitis* may be secondary to diffuse vascular occlusive disease of the aortic arch or carotid artery occlusion (usually bilateral) with poor cross or collateral circulation. Signs include aqueous flare, dilated and tortuous retinal veins, narrowed retinal arteries with microaneurysm formation, midperipheral dot-and-blot hemorrhages, and macular edema. Intraocular pressure may be low, normal, or high, and anterior chamber angle neovascularization may occur. Recurrent orbital or facial pain that improves when the patient lies down is highly suggestive of carotid occlusive disease.

Chronic hypoperfusion prompts the development of corneal edema, iris atrophy, iridoplegia, iris neovascularization, and cataract. Neovascularization of the iris and anterior chamber angle can produce a hyphema. Late complications include vitreous hemorrhage, progressive visual loss, and neovascular glaucoma (in some cases IOP may be unexpectedly low because decreased aqueous production results from decreased perfusion of the ciliary body).

Treatment of ocular ischemic syndrome involves carotid endarterectomy, IOP-lowering agents, corticosteroids for pain, and panretinal photocoagulation. If the preoperative IOP is low, restoration of blood flow by carotid endarterectomy may precipitate dangerously high intraocular pressures. Unfortunately, once the patient develops signs of chronic hypoperfusion, improvement is unlikely. In others carotid occulsion may be too advanced to be surgically correctable.

Brown GC, Magargal LE. The ocular ischemic syndrome. Clinical, fluorescein angiographic and carotid angiographic features. *Int Ophthalmol.* 1988;11:239–251.

Furlan AJ, Whisnant JP, Kearns TP. Unilateral visual loss in bright light. An unusual symptom of carotid artery occlusive disease. *Arch Neurol.* 1979;36:675–676.

Although VSR may resemble diabetic retinopathy, there are several distinctions between the two conditions (Table VIII-4).

TABLE VIII-4

DIFFERENTIATION OF DIABETES AND VSR

DIABETIC RETINOPATHY	VENOUS STASIS RETINOPATHY
Bilateral	Usually unilateral
Macula and posterior pole	Change first in midperiphery
IOP normal	IOP low, normal, or high (seen most often with carotid occlusion)

Anterior ischemic optic neuropathy (AION) from embolic carotid disease is probably rare but has been described. Most frequently, AION is a result of small-vessel occlusive disease, and carotid studies are not warranted (see pp 76–80).

Neurologic symptoms and signs. Carotid TIAs may produce other neurologic signs such as contralateral monoparesis, hemiparesis or clumsiness, contralateral numbness or paresthesia, and aphasia. Associated homonymous hemianopia may occur with infarction of the retrochiasmal visual pathways. A horizontal gaze preference toward the side of the cerebral lesion may follow middle cerebral artery infarction. Abnormal optokinetic nystagmus, reflecting ipsilateral parietal lobe dysfunction, may occur.

Etiologies of anterior circulation ischemia. Atherosclerosis is the most common cause of TIAs and stroke. In about 90% of patients with internal carotid occlusion, the initial site of obstruction is the carotid sinus. Atheroma formation is most common at the bifurcation of the common carotid artery into the internal and external carotid arteries and in the carotid siphon (Fig VIII-21). Atheromas can remain stationary, fibrose, regress, ulcerate, narrow and occlude the lumen, or release emboli. It is believed that the normal internal carotid lumen must be reduced by 50%–90% before distal flow is affected. Carotid dissection is an infrequent cause of stroke, but it should be considered in patients with ipsilateral monocular visual loss, Horner syndrome, pain in the face or neck, and contralateral neurologic signs.

Cardiac disease commonly causes TIA or stroke. Valvular heart disease, including mitral valve prolapse and emboli-producing atrial myxoma, is implicated in the production of both carotid and vertebrobasilar system TIAs. Cardiac emboli arise from many etiologies including ventricular aneurysms, hypokinetic wall segments, and endocarditis. Other cardiac causes include cardiac arrhythmia, particularly atrial fibrillation and other paroxysmal arrythmias, and unsuspected patent foramen ovale with right-to-left cardiac shunt.

Other possible causes of transient monocular blindness and carotid territory ischemia are ophthalmic artery disease, giant cell arteritis, Raynaud disease, vasculitis, hyperviscosity syndromes, antiphospholipid antibody syndrome, and migraine (vasospasm). Hypertension, diabetes, hypercholesterolemia, and smoking are treatable risk factors.

Trimble M, Bell DA, Brien W, et al. The antiphospholipid syndrome: prevalence among patients with stroke and transient ischemic attacks. *Am J Med.* 1990;88:593–597.

Clinical and laboratory evaluation. Evaluation of a patient with presumed carotid territory ischemia includes measurement of blood pressure, cardiac auscultation, and auscultation for carotid bruits, best heard at the angle of the jaw where the bifurcation is located. Unfortunately, the presence or absence of a bruit is not a reliable indicator of carotid disease. The presence of a bruit indicates turbulent flow within the vessel, and it may be heard with narrowing of the external or internal carotid artery. However, a bruit will be absent both if flow is undisturbed and if carotid occlusion is severe or complete.

Angiography remains the standard for assessment of carotid stenosis. The test is invasive, requiring the intra-arterial injection of iodinated contrast dye. Computerized techniques have lessened the amount of dye required. This technique offers the advantage of allowing visualization of the cerebral circulation, which can

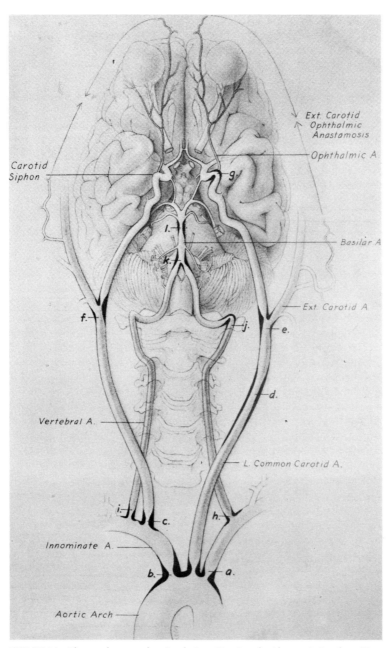

Carotid
Siphon

Ext. Carotid
Ophthalmic
Anastamosis

Ophthalmic A

g.

l.

k.

Basilar A

f.

j.

e.

Ext. Carotid A

d.

Vertebral A.

L. Common Carotid A.

i.

c.

h.

Innominate A

b.

a.

Aortic Arch

FIG VIII-21—The cerebrovascular circulation. (Reprinted with permission from Hoyt WF. Some neuro-ophthalmologic considerations in cerebral vascular insufficiency: Carotid and vertebral artery insufficiency. *Arch Ophthalmol.* 1959;62:264.)

help the clinician to formulate a treatment plan. In centers where angiography is performed regularly, the risk of serious complication such as stroke or death is 0.5%.

Carotid ultrasonagraphy (duplex scanning) is a noninvasive method used to assess the carotid arterial wall and estimate the degree of stenosis present. It is generally a good screening test, although the reliability varies and quality control (correlation of duplex scanning to angiography) is not rigid in many laboratories. Ultrasound is very sensitive for detection of ulcerated plaques.

Magnetic resonance angiography employs the same general technique as magnetic resonance imaging, using computer software to reconstruct the vascular system. No contrast agents are needed. MRA along with MRI is extremely useful for detecting carotid artery dissection. Currently, it does not assess the degree of carotid stenosis accurately, but it may become the test of choice for noninvasive carotid imaging in the near future.

Ross JS, Masaryk TJ, Modic MT, et al. Magnetic resonance angiography of the extra-cranial carotid arteries and intracranial vessels: A review. *Neurology.* 1989;39: 1369–1376.

Echocardiography is useful for detecting valvular and cardiac wall defects, intracardiac tumors, and large thrombi. Transesophageal echocardiography is more sensitive for these processes than conventional transmural echocardiography. A normal echocardiogram does not exclude the possibility of emboli, since very small particles will not be visualized. With carotid artery disease a routine echocardio-gram is mandatory. Coincident myocardial and cerebral ischemia should always be considered. Prolonged inpatient cardiac monitoring or ambulatory Holter monitor-ing may document previously undetected cardiac arrhythmias. In patients with suspected endocarditis, blood cultures should be obtained.

If a cardiac or carotid source is not found, other systemic processes may be contributing to stroke. Major risk factors include age, hypertension, hypotension and syncope (possibly iatrogenic from overly vigorous treatment of hypertension or from other medications), ischemic heart disease, diabetes, hypercholesterolemia, smok-ing, and sleep apnea. Most of these conditions are treatable. Laboratory studies should be obtained to look for these conditions and any others under clinical suspicion such as thyroid disease, hypercoagulable states, collagen-vascular dis-eases, vasculitis, or syphilis.

Prognosis. Symptoms produced by carotid stenosis and those produced by carotid occlusion may be clinically indistinguishable. More than 40% of patients with carotid artery disease have TIA symptoms before a permanent deficit develops. With cerebral hemisphere TIAs 20% of subsequent strokes occur within 1 month of the TIA, and 50% within 1 year. The stroke rate drops to 5%–8% per year thereafter. It is impossible to predict which patients with TIAs will have major strokes, although severe ipsilateral carotid stenosis is associated with higher risk. The major cause of death following TIA or stroke is myocardial infarction.

The risk of stroke following transient monocular blindness is lower than that following cerebral TIAs. The average annual incidence is approximately 2%. Carotid stenosis or occlusion may be demonstrated in about 60% of patients with transient monocular blindness.

Hollenhorst RW. Vascular status of patients who have cholesterol emboli in the retina. *Am J Ophthalmol.* 1966;61:1159–1165.

Hurwitz BJ, Heyman A, Wilkinson WE, et al. Comparison of amaurosis fugax and transient cerebral ischemia: a prospective clinical and arteriographic study. *Ann Neurol.* 1985;18:698–704.

Savino PJ, Glaser JS. Retinal stroke. Is the patient at risk? *Arch·Ophthalmol.* 1977;95: 1185–1189.

Treatment. The North American Symptomatic Carotid Endarterectomy Trial (NASCET) prospectively evaluated the effectiveness of carotid endarterectomy compared to medical management in patients with symptomatic carotid artery stenosis. Patients with amaurosis fugax, carotid transient ischemic attacks, or mild strokes were randomized to one of two treatment groups:

□ Best medical management, including daily aspirin

□ Carotid endarterectomy, followed by best medical management

A significant reduction in subsequent stroke was found in patients with 70%–99% carotid stenosis who underwent surgery. Therefore, carotid endarterectomy was recommended for patients with severe (>70%) symptomatic carotid stenosis, providing that the morbidity and mortality rates for angiography and surgery at the treating facility were acceptable. Surgery was not beneficial in patients with moderate (50%–69%) carotid stenosis compared to medical therapy. The Asymptomatic Carotid Atherosclerosis Study and Veterans Affairs Cooperative Study Group found that carotid endarterectomy significantly reduced stroke rate in asymptomatic patients with >60% stenosis.

The patient's general health and other factors also influence the decision of whether to operate. When angiography and surgery are being contemplated, referral to a medical center with a thoroughly experienced team of neurologist, cardiologist, neuroradiologist, and vascular surgeon is essential.

Barnett HJM, Taylor W, Eliasziw M, et al. Benefit of carotid endarterectomy in patients with symptomatic moderate or severe stenosis. *N Engl J Med.* 1998;339:1415–1425.

Kistler JP, Buonanno FS, Gress DR. Carotid endarterectomy—specific therapy based on pathophysiology. *N Engl J Med.* 1991;325:505–507.

When medical treatment is desirable for patients with carotid artery stenosis, antiplatelet treatment is initiated. Daily aspirin remains the most common therapy. For stroke prevention, doses of 650–1300 mg/day may be used. The addition of dipyridamole is not beneficial. Ticlopidine and clopidogrel are useful in patients who are intolerant of or allergic to aspirin. Anticoagulation is sometimes necessary if antiplatelet agents are ineffective, in the presence of an embolic source, or with intermittent atrial fibrillation.

Retinal artery vasospasm has been seen in a small subgroup of patients with transient monocular visual loss, who have no other demonstrable etiology for their symptoms. In these patients daily aspirin or calcium channel blockers are usually effective in preventing further episodes of visual loss.

Winterkorn JM, Kupersmith MJ, Wirtschafter JD, et al. Brief report: treatment of vasospastic amaurosis fugax with calcium-channel blockers. *N Engl J Med.* 1993;329: 396–398.

Vertebrobasilar system disease   The vertebrobasilar arterial system is composed of the vertebral, basilar, and posterior cerebral arteries (Fig VIII-21, p 203). The blood vessels supply the occipital cortex and many areas concerned with ocular motility in the brain stem and cerebellum.

Clinical features. Patients with vertebrobasilar insufficiency often present to the ophthalmologist first, because ocular motor and visual symptoms are prominent. Nonophthalmic symptoms of transient ischemic attacks in the vertebrobasilar system include the following:

- Ataxia, imbalance, or staggering
- Vertigo alone or in combination with other brain stem symptoms such as tinnitus, deafness, or vomiting (central vertigo may be described as light-headedness, spinning dizziness, or a sensation of environmental tilt)
- Transient dysarthria and dysphagia
- Hemiparesis, hemiplegia, and hemisensory disturbances
- Drop attacks (patient suddenly falls to the ground with no warning and no loss of consciousness)

Bilateral blurring or dimming of vision occurs almost as frequently as vertigo. The patient may complain of sudden bilateral graying or a whiteout of vision. The attacks of dimming last seconds to minutes and may be accompanied by flickering or flashing stars. Photopsias may occur that closely mimic the scintillating scotomata of migraine. (The visual aura of migraine is likely caused by electrical or hemodynamic changes in the parieto-occipital cortex.) These attacks are frequently repetitive and may occur alone or in combination with the other transient symptoms of vertebrobasilar insufficiency mentioned above. Migraine can produce similar symptoms, with or without an associated headache.

Homonymous visual field changes without other neurologic symptoms suggest involvement of the posterior circulation. Highly congruous homonymous visual field defects are typical of occipital lobe infarcts. Patients complaining of reading difficulties without obvious cause should have a careful visual field and Amsler grid examination in search of small congruous homonymous visual field defects. These defects are occasionally found on routine visual field examination and might be confused with macular disease because of their central location, especially if they are printed out asymmetrically on a computerized perimeter.

> Trobe JD, Lorber ML, Schlezinger NS. Isolated homonymous hemianopia. A review of 104 cases. *Arch Ophthalmol.* 1973;89:377–381.

Cerebral blindness, or cortical blindness, caused by bilateral occipital lobe lesions is characterized by amaurosis and normally reactive pupils. Frequently, patients with cerebral blindness will deny their blindness (Anton syndrome).

Ocular motor disturbances are common with vertebrobasilar insufficiency, and diplopia is a frequent complaint. Examination may reveal horizontal or vertical gaze palsies, internuclear ophthalmoplegia, skew deviation, ocular motor nerve palsies, or nystagmus. A central Horner syndrome may be present with pontine or medullary infarcts.

Etiologies of posterior circulation ischemia. The most frequent causes of vertebrobasilar TIAs and stroke are atheromatous occlusion, hypertensive vascular disease, microembolization (either from the vertebrobasilar arteries or from the heart), fluctuations in cardiac output, and arterial dissection. Infarction in the distribution of the posterior cerebral arteries is most commonly caused by embolism.

The following have all been associated with symptoms and signs of vertebrobasilar ischemia: polycythemia, hypercoagulable states, congenital aplasia or hypoplasia of a vertebral or posterior communicating artery, anemia, and vasospasm. Mechanical factors secondary to cervical spondylosis and chiropractic manipulation of the cervical spine have also been implicated in vertebrobasilar occlusions resulting in severe neurologic deficits. A less common cause of vertebrobasilar dysfunction is a reversal of blood flow in the vertebral artery (subclavian steal), caused by a proximal occlusion of the subclavian artery that produces an unusual alteration in the direction of flow in the ipsilateral vertebral artery. Lowered pressure in the distal segment of the subclavian artery can siphon, or steal, blood from the vertebral artery and produce fluctuating symptoms of vertebrobasilar artery insufficiency.

Clinical and laboratory evaluation. The evaluation of posterior circulation ischemia is similar to the medical work-up for carotid system disease. Neuroimaging should be performed on all patients with homonymous visual field defects and other signs of brain stem or cerebellar dysfunction. MRI is preferred, since CT shows considerable bony artifact in the posterior fossa. Sometimes angiography is necessary to visualize the aortic arch, the configuration of the vertebrobasilar vessels, and the extent of filling from the anterior circulation through the circle of Willis.

The examiner is much less likely to find a treatable structural vascular abnormality with posterior circulation ischemia than with carotid system disease. The evaluation of these patients generally emphasizes a search for underlying cardiac or systemic and blood pressure disorders, including postural hypotension.

Treatment. The majority of patients with vertebrobasilar TIAs are treated medically with antiplatelet therapy (aspirin or ticlopidine) or anticoagulants.

Conclusion   Transient neurologic or ophthalmic symptoms in middle-aged or elderly patients suggest a vascular origin. Localization of the symptoms and signs determines whether they result from ischemia in the vertebrobasilar or the carotid artery territory. Although recurrent cerebrovascular ischemia is a concern, the major cause of death in these patients is coronary artery disease. Thus, efforts to control cardiovascular disease, hypertension, diabetes mellitus, and hyperlipidemias, accompanied by cessation of smoking, should be considered before diagnostic and therapeutic efforts are directed exclusively at the cerebrovascular circulation.

Cerebral Aneurysms

Cerebral aneurysms are localized dilations of the vessel wall. Table VIII-5 classifies these aneurysms by shape and etiology. They are present in approximately 5% of the population but rarely become symptomatic before age 20. They may be an isolated finding and are commonly associated with hypertension. Less common predisposing conditions include arteriovenous malformations, coarctation of the aorta, polycystic kidney disease, and connective tissue diseases (e.g., fibromuscular dysplasia, Marfan syndrome, Ehlers-Danlos syndrome). A familial occurrence is possible.

Table VIII-6 breaks down the locations of cerebral aneurysms with their frequencies of occurrence. The most common type of intracranial aneurysm is the saccular, or "berry," aneurysm that arises at arterial bifurcations. Of these aneurysms 90% are supratentorial and 10% are infratentorial. Aneurysms arising from the internal carotid artery and basilar artery produce neuro-ophthalmic manifestations. In general, those >10 mm in size are most likely to rupture. Since high morbidity and mortality result from aneurysm rupture, early detection and surgical intervention can be lifesaving.

TABLE VIII-5

CLASSIFICATION OF ANEURYSMS

Shape
    Saccular
    Fusiform

Cause
    Development defect in vessel wall
    Acquired degenerative change
    Atherosclerosis
    Infection and inflammation
    Neoplasm
    Trauma

Clinical presentation   Unruptured aneurysms cause progressive neurologic dysfunction because of their mass effect. Transient ischemic attacks, cerebral infarction, and seizures may occur. An ophthalmic artery aneurysm causes a progressive unilateral optic neuropathy. Usually, the patient has developed optic atrophy before any symptoms are noticed. Ipsilateral periocular pain often occurs. Anterior communicating artery aneurysms produce visual loss by compressing the optic chiasm or optic tract. Aneurysms at the junction of the internal carotid and posterior communicating arteries produce an ipsilateral third nerve palsy. Typically, pain occurs around the ipsilateral eye or the forehead. *The combination of headache and a partial or complete third nerve palsy should raise suspicion of an aneurysm, particularly in persons under age 50.* Pain may be present or absent with unruptured aneurysms.

    Intracavernous carotid aneurysms typically produce a cavernous sinus syndrome. Cranial nerves III, IV, and VI and the ophthalmic branch of cranial nerve V are involved, singly or in combination. Since they are confined by the walls of the

TABLE VIII-6

LIKELIHOOD OF ANEURYSM BY LOCATION

LOCATION	FREQUENCY OF OCCURRENCE
Internal carotid artery and branches	85%
Main trunk	25%–40%
Posterior communicating artery	
Ophthalmic artery	
Cavernous sinus	
Anterior communicating artery	25%–30%
Middle cerebral artery trifurcation	13%–30%
Anterior cerebral artery	5%
Basilar artery	3%–9%
Vertebral artery	5%

cavernous sinus, these aneurysms typically do not rupture but cause progressive neurologic dysfunction.

A ruptured aneurysm is a neurosurgical emergency. Patients develop symptoms and signs of subarachnoid, intraparenchymal, or subdural hemorrhage. The headache of a ruptured aneurysm is often described as "the worst of my life" and may be localized or generalized. Nausea, vomiting, and neck stiffness signify meningeal irritation from subarachnoid blood. Focal neurologic deficits including third nerve palsy, aphasia, and hemiparesis occur, depending on the location of the aneurysm and hemorrhage. Rarely, fever may be present. Elevated intracranial pressure may produce papilledema and sixth nerve palsies. Patients may be disoriented, lethargic, or comatose. Alterated mental status is a poor prognostic sign.

Ocular hemorrhage frequently accompanies subarachnoid hemorrhage. Intraretinal, preretinal, subhyaloid, vitreous, subconjunctival, orbital, or optic nerve sheath hemorrhage may be present. The ocular hemorrhages are likely produced when intracranial pressure in the optic nerve sheath exceeds ocular venous pressure, reducing ophthalmic venous drainage and causing venous rupture. The combination of vitreous and subarachnoid hemorrhage is called *Terson syndrome*.

Many patients recall symptoms of a "sentinel bleed" before major rupture has occurred. Transient or mild neurologic symptoms with headache are most commonly described.

Laboratory investigation   The definitive diagnostic test for suspected aneurysm is a cerebral arteriogram. A four-vessel study of both carotid and vertebral arteries is imperative, since 10% of patients have multiple aneurysms. If the aneurysm has ruptured, vasospasm may prevent visualization of the aneurysm acutely. Likewise, a thrombosed aneurysm may not be seen on arteriography, because the lumen will not fill.

MRI demonstrates most aneurysms >5 mm in size. High-quality MRA can detect aneurysms as small as 3 mm. MRA is useful as a screening test for unruptured aneurysms; it is less expensive than angiography and has no associated morbidity (Fig VIII-22).

CT scanning is useful acutely after aneurysm rupture to detect the presence of intraparenchymal and subarachnoid blood. With a severe hemorrhage blood may appear in the basal cisterns, Sylvian fissure, or interhemispheric fissue or over the convexity. A study obtained for suspected aneurysm rupture should never be enhanced unless unenhanced scans are also performed, since areas of enhancement cannot be distinguished from blood. Focal hemorrhage and edema will often identify the location of the aneurysm. The CT scan is abnormal in 85%–90% of cases of aneurysmal rupture. An enhanced CT can demonstrate large aneurysms, but CT is not an acceptable screening test for unruptured aneurysms.

If subarachnoid hemorrhage is suspected and the CT scan is negative, lumbar puncture will confirm the presence of subarachnoid blood. However, a lumbar puncture should not be attempted in the face of midline shift or evidence of cerebral (uncal) herniation.

Prognosis   The risk that an aneurysm will rupture is approximately 1% per year. Once an aneurysm has ruptured, the morbidity and mortality rate is significant. The proportion of patients who die at the time of rupture is 30%. If untreated, another 33% die within 6 months of rupture and 15% die within 10 years. Many of those who survive suffer severe neurologic deficits.

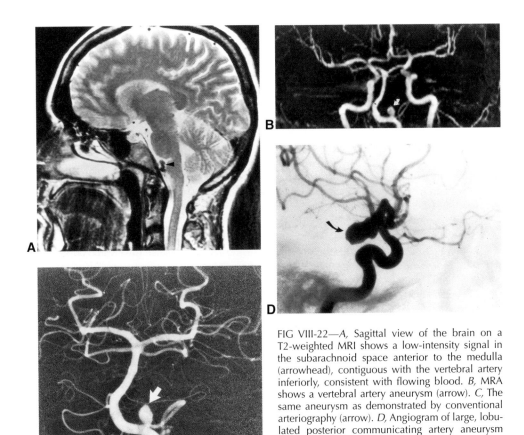

FIG VIII-22—*A*, Sagittal view of the brain on a T2-weighted MRI shows a low-intensity signal in the subarachnoid space anterior to the medulla (arrowhead), contiguous with the vertebral artery inferiorly, consistent with flowing blood. *B*, MRA shows a vertebral artery aneurysm (arrow). *C*, The same aneurysm as demonstrated by conventional arteriography (arrow). *D*, Angiogram of large, lobulated posterior communicating artery aneurysm (arrow). (Photographs courtesy of Leo Hochhauser, MD.)

Rebleeding is a serious consequence of aneurysm rupture, and risk is highest in the first 24 hours. In untreated patients the cumulative risk of rebleeding in the first 2 weeks is 25%. Delayed neurologic deficits occur from rebleeding, vasospasm, and hydrocephalus.

Vasospasm is a major cause of delayed morbidity and death. It occurs in 30% of patients within the first 2 weeks with a peak incidence in 4–10 days. Infarction may result. Surgical intervention is timed to avoid the period of vasospasm.

Following subarachnoid hemorrhage, patients who are awake or have only mild mental status impairment with minimal neurologic deficits on presentation have the best prognosis for successful aneurysm surgery. The outcome for patients who present in coma with massive neurologic impairment is poor.

Treatment Treatment of symptomatic aneurysms prior to rupture is ideal. Supportive treatment to stabilize the patient includes efforts to lower intracranial pressure with hyperventilation or mannitol, treatment of cerebral vasospasm with calcium channel blockers and blood volume expansion, and control of blood pressure.

The definitive treatment is surgical clipping of the aneurysm. Large aneurysms can be treated using interventional radiologic techniques, such as balloon occlusion. When aneurysm clipping is technically impossible, ligation of the feeding artery or carotid artery is sometimes necessary.

Arteriovenous Malformations

Like aneurysms, arteriovenous malformations (AVMs) are usually congenital and may be familial. Symptoms typically develop before age 30 with a slight male preponderance, and 6% of patients also have an intracranial aneurysm. Intracranial hemorrhage with or without subarachnoid hemorrhage is the initial presentation in half of the cases. In contrast to patients with saccular aneurysms, those with AVMs are much more likely to become symptomatic before a hemorrhage occurs. Seizures are the first manifestation in 30% of affected patients, while 20% have headaches or other focal neurologic deficits initially. The neurologic symptoms may be progressive or transient.

Of the 90% of AVMs that are supratentorial, about 70% are cortical and 20% are deep. The remaining 10% are located in the posterior fossa or dura mater. Early mortality occurs in up to 20% of cases when bleeding takes place, and the rebleeding rate is 2.5% each year. Most AVMs bleed into the brain, producing headaches and focal neurologic deficits.

The neuro-ophthalmic manifestations of an AVM depend on its location. Cortical AVMs in the occipital lobe may produce visual symptoms and headaches that resemble migraine. The visual phenomena are usually brief and unformed, but typical migrainous scintillating scotomata do rarely occur. Hemispheric AVMs may produce homonymous visual field defects (Fig VIII-23). Signs and symptoms of brain stem AVMs are not specific and may include diplopia, nystagmus, dizziness, ocular motor nerve palsy, gaze palsy, anisocoria, or pupillary light–near dissociation. Reports of transient monocular visual loss caused by a steal phenomenon from an intracranial AVM are rare.

Some patients with AVMs report a subjective intracranial bruit, and occasionally the examiner will detect a bruit with auscultation of the skull over the AVM.

Diagnosis If bleeding is suspected, an unenhanced CT will show the hemorrhage. Although unruptured AVMs are typically seen on an enhanced CT scan, MRI is more sensitive for visualization of small AVMs. MRI nicely demonstrates the heterogeneous signals representing the various elements of the lesion: blood vessels, brain, flowing and clotted blood, calcium, hemorrhage, or edema (Fig VIII-24). AVMs that calcify are sometimes identifiable on plain radiographs or CT. Cerebral angiography is required to clearly show the anatomy and to define the feeding and draining vessels of the AVM (Fig VIII-25).

Treatment The location of the AVM, the anatomy of feeding and draining vessels, and the size of the lesion all affect choice of treatment. Surgical resection, ligation of feeding vessels, embolization, and stereotactic radiosurgery can be used alone or in combination. Seizures usually improve with anticonvulsant therapy.

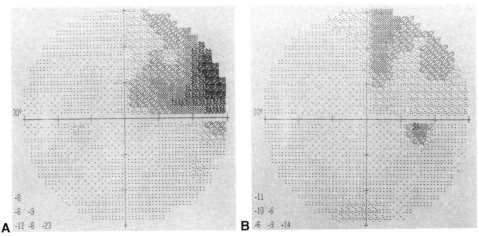

FIG VIII-23—Automated perimetry shows a noncongruous homonymous right superior quandrantanopia in a 32-year-old man with partial complex seizures and headaches. *A,* Left eye. *B,* Right eye.

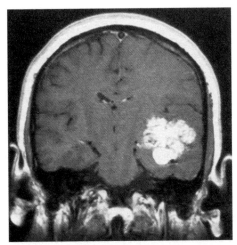

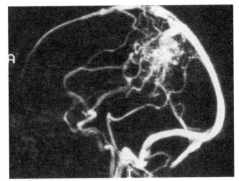

FIG VIII-24—Coronal view of the brain on a T1-weighted, contrast-enhanced MRI demonstrates a large left temporal lobe AVM. The irregular contour and heterogeneous enhancement pattern are typical for this type of vascular lesion. The mass effect (note that the left temporal lobe is larger than the right) without surrounding edema suggests that this is a long-standing, benign process.

FIG VIII-25—Arteriogram shows a tangle of blood vessels and multiple draining veins. (Photograph courtesy of Leo Hochhauser, MD.)

Kupersmith MJ, Vargas ME, Yashar A, et al. Occipital arteriovenous malformations: Visual disturbances and presentation. *Neurology.* 1996;46:953–957.

Dissecting Aneurysms

Dissecting aneurysms may develop in the internal carotid artery or in any of its branches, and they may arise either extracranially or intracranially. Extracranial carotid artery dissection can be traumatic or spontaneous (Table VIII-7).

Clinical presentation   The clinical features of a dissecting aneurysm are variable. Severe cases may present with cerebral ischemia and coma. Sometimes symptoms are delayed for weeks or months following trauma. The most common presentation of *traumatic dissection* is headache with ipsilateral ophthalmic signs and contra-lateral neurologic deficits. The headache is usually located on the ipsilateral fore-head, around the orbit, or in the neck. A bruit may be present.

Spontaneous dissection of the carotid artery produces either transient or per-manent neurologic symptoms and signs. These include amaurosis fugax, acute stroke, monocular blindness, and ipsilateral Horner syndrome. If the dissection extends to the intracranial carotid segment, cranial neuropathies can occur, produc-ing diplopia, dysgeusia, tongue paralysis, or facial numbness.

Visual loss associated with carotid dissection may be a result of embolic occlusion of the ophthalmic artery, central retinal artery, short posterior ciliary arteries, or retinal branch arteries. Alternatively, ophthalmic artery occlusion may be caused by the dissection itself. Reduced blood flow from carotid dissection is a rare cause of ocular ischemic syndrome.

Forty percent of dissecting aneurysms affect the vertebral and basilar arteries. General features of these dissections are headache, neck pain, and signs of brain

TABLE VIII-7

CAUSES OF DISSECTING ANEURYSMS

Traumatic
    Blunt head or neck injury
    Motor vehicle accidents
    Blows to the head or neck
    Carotid artery compression
    Hanging by the neck
    Manipulative neck therapy
    Surgery
    Rapid neck rotation, flexion, or hyperextension
    Carotid artery cannulation during angiography

Spontaneous
    Fibromuscular dysplasia
    Moyamoya disease
    Marfan syndrome
    Ehlers-Danlos syndrome
    Polycystic kidney disease
    Syphilis
    Atherosclerosis
    Migraine
    Idiopathic

stem and cerebellum dysfunction. *Basilar artery dissection* is more common than vertebral artery dissection; it causes headache followed by brain stem and cerebellar signs. Ocular motor nerve palsies are commonly seen, and many patients progress to tetraplegia, coma, and death. *Vertebral artery dissection* produces four syndromes:

□ Fatal brain stem infarction, usually affecting young adults

□ Subarachnoid hemorrhage

□ Aneurysmal dilation causing brain stem and lower cranial nerve signs from mass effect

□ Chronic dissection causing extensive bilateral aneurysm formation and repeated TIAs, strokes, and subarachnoid hemorrhage

Diagnosis　MRI is the diagnostic test of choice for extracranial carotid artery dissection. Routine MRI (not MR angiography) demonstrates a false lumen or area of clot in the cervical portion of the carotid artery and may identify areas of brain infarction. Selective arteriography is useful to define extracranial and intracranial dissection and visualize the vertebrobasilar system (Fig VIII-26).

Treatment　The treatment of arterial dissection is controversial, depending on the extent and location of the dissection and the patient's overall condition. Extracranial carotid dissections involving the proximal portion of the internal carotid artery may be treated surgically. Anticoagulation is often used, although recanalization of the artery can occur with or without its use. Vertebrobasilar dissections cannot be approached surgically, but bypass procedures are sometimes employed.

Caplan LR, Baquis GD, Pessin MS, et al. Dissection of the intracranial vertebral artery. *Neurology.* 1988;38:868–877.

Newman NJ, Kline LB, Leifer D, et al. Ocular stroke and carotid artery dissection. *Neurology.* 1989;39:1462–1464.

Cerebral Venous and Dural Sinus Thrombosis

Occlusion of the cortical and subcortical veins produces focal neurologic symptoms and signs, including neuro-ophthalmic findings. The lateral sinus, cavernous sinus, and superior sagittal sinus are most commonly affected. Each produces a distinct clinical syndrome. Table VIII-8 lists various causes of different types of occlusion.

Cavernous sinus thrombosis　*Septic cavernous sinus thrombosis (CST)* is a result of infection of the face, sphenoid or ethmoid sinuses, or oral cavity. Rarely, otitis media or orbital cellulitis is the cause. Patients develop headache, nausea, vomiting, and somnolence. There may be fever, chills, tachycardia, evidence of meningitis, or generalized sepsis. Ocular signs from anterior infection (facial, dental, orbital) are initially unilateral but frequently become bilateral. They include orbital congestion, lacrimation, conjunctival edema, eyelid swelling, ptosis, proptosis, and ophthalmo-plegia. A sixth nerve palsy is the most consistent early neurologic sign. Corneal anesthesia, facial numbness, Horner syndrome, and venous stasis retinopathy can occur. Treatment can include administration of antibiotics, anticoagulants, or corti-costeroids and surgery.

　　The signs and symptoms of *aseptic CST* resemble those of septic CST, but clinical or laboratory examination shows no evidence of infection. Pain around the

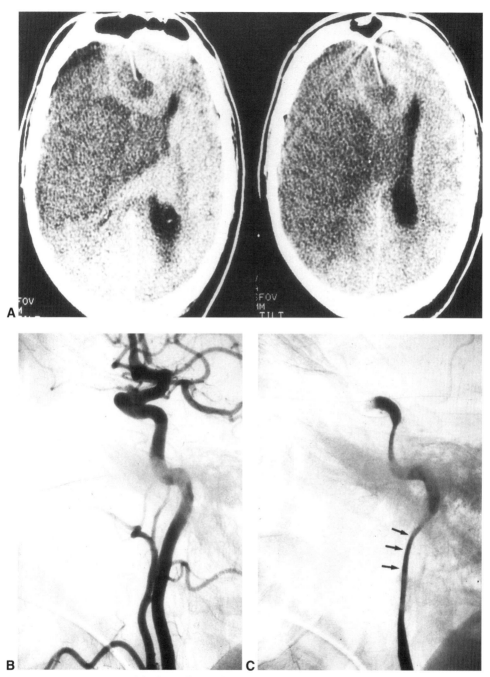

FIG VIII-26—*A,* CT scan of the brain shows a large area of hypodensity corresponding to a right internal carotid artery infarction. There is mass effect with shift of the midline structures to the left. *B,* Arteriogram demonstrates the normal left carotid circulation. *C,* Injection of the right carotid artery shows a dissection with narrowing of the vessel in the neck (arrows) and an abrupt cessation of flow in the carotid siphon. (Photographs courtesy of Leo Hochhauser, MD.)

TABLE VIII-8

CAUSES OF VENOUS AND DURAL SINUS THROMBOSIS

Inflammation
  Behçet disease
  Systemic lupus erythematosis

Septic occlusion
  Pyogenic sinus infection
  Osteomyelitis

Aseptic occlusion
  Hypercoagulability
  Oral contraceptives
  Pregnancy
  Antithrombin III deficiency
  Protein C, protein S deficiency
  Thrombocytosis
  Antiphospholipid antibody syndrome
  Sickle cell disease
  Pelvic or deep vein thrombosis

Trauma
  Skull fracture
  Epidural hematoma

Surgical ligation

Invasion of vessel wall by tumors
  Leukemia
  Lymphoma
  Meningioma
  Sarcoidosis
  Granulomatous disorders

Changes in blood flow
  Hypoperfusion
  Hematologic disorders
  Myeloproliferative disorders
  Venous emboli
  Arterial occlusive disease

eye is common, but orbital congestion is typically less severe than with septic CST. Anticoagulation or antiplatelet therapy is frequently used.

Lateral (transverse) sinus thrombosis Lateral sinus thrombosis is usually septic. Because of widespread antibiotic usage, infection is rarely a result of acute otitis media, and chronic otitis media is the common cause. Because most of the venous drainage from the brain is through the right lateral sinus, the right side is more frequently affected.

Patients develop features of systemic infection as well as neck pain, tenderness of the ipsilateral jugular vein, and retroauricular edema. There may be facial weakness. The most common ophthalmic sign is a sixth nerve palsy. If the sixth cranial nerve is compressed against the petroclinoid ligament, severe facial pain also occurs (*Gradenigo syndrome*). Papilledema will be present if intracranial pressure is increased.

The pseudotumor cerebri syndrome caused by lateral sinus thrombosis was originally called *otitic hydrocephalus.* Complications include meningitis and extension of the thrombosis. It is treated with antibiotics, mastoidectomy with incision and drainage of the lateral sinus, and intracranial pressure–lowering agents. Prompt treatment yields an excellent prognosis.

Superior sagittal sinus thrombosis   Aseptic thrombosis is more common than septic thromobis in the superior sagittal sinus (SSS). Septic thrombosis is most commonly a result of meningitis. Other causes of septic SSS thrombosis include paranasal sinus infection, pulmonary infections, tonsillitis, dental infections, pelvic inflammatory disease, and otitis media. SSS thrombosis can occur during pregnancy, immediately postpartum, or with oral contraceptive use. Vasculitis and systemic inflammatory disorders predispose to this condition.

The symptoms and signs depend on the extent and location of the occlusion within the SSS. With thrombosis of the anterior third of the sinus, symptoms are mild or absent. Posterior SSS thrombosis is a cause of pseudotumor cerebri, producing headaches and papilledema. (It is a diagnosis to consider in "atypical" pseudotumor cerebi patients, such as slim women and men.) If impairment of cerebral venous drainage is marked, altered mental status, seizures, and focal neurologic signs may develop. Cerebral blindness is a rare complication. With increasing intracranial pressure the condition can be fatal, as a result of intracerebral hemorrhage and brain herniation. Treatment is directed toward the underlying condition. Anticoagulation, fibrinolytic agents, and intracranial pressure–lowering treatments are used.

Diagnosis   Abnormalities can be seen on unenhanced and enhanced CT and MRI, although neither test is sensitive enough to be used alone. Standard MRI is useful to determine whether a brain abscess, infarction, hemorrhage, or edema is present. MRA, with images of the venous phase, is a sensitive and noninvasive method used to visualize the thrombosed vessels directly. Cerebral angiography demonstrates vascular occlusion and is particularly useful for visualizing the internal carotid and ophthalmic arteries.

Headache and Facial Pain

Headache is a common complaint presented to the ophthalmologist. When pain extends to the orbits, the patient and referring physician may assume that the eyes are in some way responsible for the discomfort. Often the patient may have fears, perhaps unspoken, of a brain tumor.

The history is the most important part of a headache evaluation, since the ocular examination is normal in the vast majority of patients with headache. Specific historical questions include the following:

□ Nature of the headache (sharp or dull, throbbing or constant, "squeezing")

□ Daily pattern of headache (worse in the morning or later in the day, waking the patient from sleep)

□ Location of the headache (unilateral or bilateral, localized or diffuse)

□ Associated phenomena (scintillating scotomata, flashing lights, nausea or vomiting, vertigo, ptosis, tearing)

□ Precipitating or alleviating factors (bending over, coughing, foods)

□ Overall pattern (when headaches began, chronicity, recent change in pattern)

□ Family history of headaches

In addition to a complete ophthalmologic examination, the patient complaining of headache should be screened systemically by measurement of blood pressure and pulse and examined neurologically for meningeal signs (neck stiffness), point tenderness, and symmetry of cranial nerve and motor functions. Any complaint of visual phenomena should prompt careful visual field testing. Any permanent homonymous deficit requires neuroimaging.

Headaches truly secondary to ocular causes are rare. Local eye diseases such as iritis, scleritis, acute glaucoma, subacute angle-closure glaucoma, and orbital disease should be discernible on examination. Headaches related to refractive error or strabismus should be relieved by appropriate correction.

Any patient over age 60 who presents with headache is a suspect for giant cell arteritis. Other symptoms of this condition include jaw claudication, fever, weight loss, scalp tenderness, polymyalgia, fatigue, and visual complaints. An erythrocyte sedimentation rate (Westergren method) helps screen such a patient, but a normal ESR does not exclude the diagnosis.

Headache caused by elevated intracranial pressure, as with intracranial mass lesions or pseudotumor cerebri, is typically global, constant, and worse in the morning. It is frequently worsened by bending over, head movement, or Valsalva maneuvers such as coughing and straining. Vomiting may occur, even without nausea. Other focal neurologic signs, nonlocalizing signs such as sixth nerve palsy, or papilledema may be present.

A sudden severe headache with stiff neck, changes in mentation, or focal neurologic signs suggests intracranial hemorrhage. Neuroimaging is urgently required in these cases. Headache caused by meningitis may be chronic and not associated with focal neurologic deficits. Neck stiffness and pain on flexion, back pain, pain on eye movement, and photophobia may reflect meningeal inflammation.

Mills RP. Headache. In: *Focal Points: Clinical Modules for Ophthalmologists.* San Francisco: American Academy of Ophthalmology; 1988;6:8.

Raskin NH. *Headache.* 2nd ed. New York: Churchill Livingstone; 1988.

Migraine and Tension-Type Headache

Migraine is a condition consisting of repetitive bouts of headache, more common in women than men. Familial tendency is strong, and the patient may report motion sickness as a child. Onset typically occurs at puberty or young adulthood, and the headaches may decrease after menopause. There may be hormonal variation.

Spector RH. Migraine. *Surv Ophthalmol.* 1984;29:193–207.

Migraine with aura (previously termed *classic migraine*) is heralded by neurologic symptoms that are usually visual. Imagery builds up over minutes with positive phenomena that typically have movement. The classic fortification spectrum begins with a small scotoma near fixation that gradually expands. The scotoma is bounded by a zig-zag, shimmering, colorful or silver visual image that moves temporally into the periphery and then breaks up. Loss of vision may occur, most commonly hemianopic but frequently perceived by the patient as monocular (in the eye ipsilateral to the hemianopia). The aura usually lasts less than 45 minutes and is typically followed by a throbbing headache on the contralateral side of the head. Most patients experience associated nausea, photophobia, and phonophobia.

The typical headache lasts several hours. In complicated migraine a focal neurologic deficit may be part of the aura, or it may occur with the headache and then persist. This deficit is usually transient, but permanent deficits related to intracranial infarction do occur.

Hupp SL, Kline LB, Corbett JJ. Visual disturbances of migraine. *Surv Ophthalmol.* 1989;33:221–236.

Migraine without aura (previously called *common migraine*) has no preceding neurologic symptoms. The headache may be global, not strictly unilateral, and it can last hours to days. The other features of sick headache are present. Distinguishing between this type of headache and the very common tension-type headache is frequently quite difficult. *Tension-type headaches* are chronic, described as aching or vicelike, typically worse at the end of the day, and often precipitated by stress. They may be associated with depression.

Some patients, especially the elderly, may report only the visual symptomatology of classic migraine without any associated headache. These *acephalgic migraines,* or migraine equivalents, must be differentiated from TIAs. Visual migraine equivalents include scintillating scotomata, transient homonymous hemianopia without positive visual phenomena, peripheral visual field constriction progressing to tunnel vision or complete visual loss, transient monocular visual loss, and episodic diplopia (usually vertical and accompanied by other neurologic symptoms). Symptoms typically last less than 60 minutes and tend to progressively develop and remit during that time. A positive patient history or family history of classic migraine is helpful, as is a description of the deficit. The classic scintillating scotoma with fortification spectrum is essentially pathognomonic of migraine. If the visual disturbances do not completely resolve, visual field testing is appropriate. Residual visual field defects may indicate another underlying process, such as cerebrovascular disease or a vascular malformation.

Evaluation of patients with migraine If the patient has a typical history for migraine and a normal neurologic and ophthalmologic examination, neuroimaging studies are unlikely to show an intracranial abnormality. A history of alternating hemicranial headaches suggests a benign etiology, but most patients with headaches that always occur on the same side of the head are also likely to have migraine. Occasionally, a mass lesion or a large vascular malformation is heralded by typical migraine headaches. Referral of patients with suspicious headaches to a neurologist is prudent.

Frishberg BM. The utility of neuroimaging in the evaluation of headache in patients with normal neurologic examinations. *Neurology.* 1994;44:1191–1197.

Treatment of migraine and tension-type headache Treatment of headache should be guided by the specific type of headache and the needs of the patient. Some patients, for example, only need reassurance that they do not have serious intracranial disease. Precipitating or contributing factors should be eliminated as much as possible. Certain foods provoke headaches in some people, and patients should consider avoiding chocolate, nitrates, monosodium glutamate, aged cheese, caffeine, wine and other alcohol, aspartame (NutraSweet), nuts, and shellfish. The role of estrogens and oral contraceptives is uncertain, but a temporal relationship between initiation of hormone therapy and the development of migraine symptoms indicates that the hormones should be discontinued.

Other environmental migraine triggers include stress or relief from stress (e.g., after a final exam or presentation, first day of vacation, weekends), change in sleep patterns, fumes or strong scents such as perfumes and cigarette smoke, and exercise.

Migraine therapy can be divided into acute and prophylactic management. Acutely, analgesics can be used. These include ergotamines, serotonergic agents, nonsteroidal anti-inflammatory drugs (NSAIDs), and other combined preparations that include caffeine, although *chronic* caffeine intake worsens headaches. An antiemetic agent may also be necessary. The "triptans," including sumatriptan, naratriptan, rizatriptan, and zolmitriptan are available in different formulations (oral, injection, nasal spray). They are useful for symptomatic relief of migraine but are contraindicated in patients with basilar artery migraine. These drugs can, rarely, produce myocardial infarction and should not be used in patients with suspected or known coronary artery disease.

Symptomatic treatment has its limitations, since use of pain medications more than a few times weekly can lead to *analgesic rebound headache*. Patients with migraine may overuse analgesics and develop a constant headache that is only relieved with the continuous use of pain medications. Therefore, it is important to take a thorough medication history from headache patients, who may be taking over-the-counter analgesics frequently. Analgesic rebound headaches require the withdrawal of analgesics, and hospitalization may be needed.

Prophylactic treatment is warranted if headaches disrupt the functions of daily life beyond what the patient is willing to tolerate. Beta blockers, calcium channel blockers, tricyclic antidepressants, selective serotonin reuptake inhibitors (SSRI), sodium valproate, and NSAIDs may be used with caution, keeping analgesic rebound headaches in mind.

Tension-type headaches are more likely to respond to treatment with tricyclic antidepressants and nonsteroidal anti-inflammatory medications, although the overall success rate is not as high as with migraine. Various forms of biofeedback may be helpful.

Icepick Pains and Idiopathic Stabbing Headache

Episodic, brief, sharp, jabbing pains occur more commonly in migraineurs than in people with other types of headaches. Cluster headache sufferers also have a high incidence of idiopathic stabbing headache, typically located in the same area as the cluster pain. The distribution of the ophthalmic division of the fifth nerve—the parietal area, orbit, and temple—is the most common location. The pain lasts less than a second or may occur as a series of stabs. A variant of this entity, the *jabs and jolts syndrome*, consists of knifelike pain lasting less than a minute. Idiopathic stabbing headache often responds to indomethacin, and many patients improve with standard headache prophylactic agents.

Cluster Headache

Cluster headache is a type of headache that occurs most frequently in men in their 30s and 40s, usually cigarette smokers. It is characterized by excruciating bouts of pain localized behind one eye, in the distribution of the ophthalmic division of cranial nerve V. Associated symptoms include ipsilateral tearing, conjunctival injection, rhinorrhea, and postganglionic Horner syndrome. The pain may wake patients from sleep and cause them to pace, rather than sleep it off. It typically lasts less than 2 hours. Headaches occur in clusters of episodes over days or weeks, then remit for months or years.

Treatment of cluster headache   Cluster headaches can be difficult to treat. The headache may respond acutely to methysergide (Sansert), subcutaneous sumatriptan, or dihydroergotamine. A 10–14 day tapering dose of prednisone is often successful in aborting the cluster cycle. Verapamil is useful for prophylaxis.

Facial Pain

Patients may relate localized facial pain to the eye. Common sources of facial pain include dental disorders and sinus disease. Other facial pain syndromes include trigeminal neuralgia, glossopharyngeal neuralgia, carotidynia, temporomandibular joint syndrome (TMJ), and herpes zoster neuralgia. The onset of facial pain in an elderly patient raises the possibility of giant cell arteritis. Facial pain is occasionally a sign of metastatic carcinoma.

Raskin NH. *Headache.* 2nd ed. New York: Churchill Livingstone; 1988:333–373.

Trigeminal neuralgia, also known as *tic douloureux,* typically occurs during middle age or later. It may be related to vascular compression of the fifth nerve, although in a few cases it represents demyelinating disease or a posterior fossa mass lesion. The pain is almost always unilateral (95%) and usually involves the maxillary or mandibular distribution of the fifth cranial nerve, only rarely (<5%) involving the ophthalmic division alone. Paroxysmal burning or electric shock–like jabs, lasting seconds to minutes, may be precipitated by chewing, tooth brushing, or a cold wind. There may be periods of remission. Sensory function in the face should be normal on testing. Any abnormality increases likelihood of a neoplasm. All patients should have neuroimaging of the posterior fossa, preferably with MRI. Treatment options include gabapentin, carbamazepine, phenytoin, baclofen, clonazepam, valproic acid, selective destruction of trigeminal fibers percutaneously, or surgical decompression of the fifth nerve in the posterior fossa.

In *glossopharyngeal neuralgia* paroxysmal pain occurs unilaterally in the region of the larynx, tongue, tonsil, and ear. Hoarseness and coughing may be present. Pain can be triggered by swallowing and pungent tastes. It is treated with the same medications used for trigeminal neuralgia. *Carotidynia* refers to pain arising from the cervical carotid artery and is typically neck pain that radiates to the ipsilateral face and ear. Carotid dissection must be ruled out. *Temporomandibular joint syndrome* is characterized by unilateral ear or preauricular pain that radiates to the temple, jaw, or neck and is worse with chewing. Limitation of normal jaw movement and clicking of the jaw on opening are usually present.

When *herpes zoster* involves the trigeminal dermatomes, pain may arise in the affected region days before a vesicular eruption is seen. Occasionally, no vesicles are apparent (zoster sine herpete). The pain may persist long after resolution of the acute infection (postherpetic neuralgia), and it can be extremely discomforting and difficult to treat.

Neuro-Ophthalmic Manifestations of Infectious Diseases

Acquired Immunodeficiency Syndrome (AIDS)

Ophthalmologists are often the first physicians that the patient with AIDS encounters, and they must be aware of the various presentations of AIDS. Although considered separately in the text, several factors may be involved in a single patient. Neuro-ophthalmic disorders may result from infection by the human immunodeficiency virus (HIV-1) or from secondary opportunistic infections and malignancy. The eye, afferent visual pathways, or ocular motor system can all be affected. BCSC Section 9, *Intraocular Inflammation and Uveitis,* discusses the following conditions in detail in the chapter "Ocular Involvement in AIDS."

Central nervous system lymphoma   High-grade, B-cell non-Hodgkin's lymphoma is the second most common malignancy in AIDS and the most common neoplasm to affect the central nervous system (CNS). CNS lymphoma can cause diplopia from third, fourth, or sixth nerve involvement. Lymphomatous infiltration of the orbit and optic nerve may lead to disc swelling and visual loss. The diagnosis is made by confirming the presence of lymphomatous cells in the spinal fluid or by performing stereotactic brain or meningeal biopsy. Changes shown on MRI may resemble those of toxoplasmosis, but they are typically periventricular with subependymal spread. Treatment consists of a combination of radiotherapy, surgery, and chemotherapy. However, most patients succumb within 3 months.

Cytomegalovirus (CMV)   CMV is most commonly encountered by the ophthalmologist when the patient develops retinal lesions. Often CMV retinitis is the presenting manifestation of AIDS. It is a common opportunistic infection in AIDS patients and a major cause of visual loss. The early lesions are dry, white, granular retinal opacifications that may look like cotton-wool spots or crumbled cheese, located at the posterior pole or peripheral retina. Subsequent findings include retinal exudates, vascular sheathing, retinal hemorrhages, choroidal inflammation, and exudative retinal detachment. Untreated CMV retinitis is a potentially blinding condition.

Within the central nervous system CMV causes optic neuritis and brain stem encephalitis. Anterior optic nerve infection produces acute visual loss with optic disc swelling. This condition usually occurs in patients with severe CMV retinitis. Others develop anterior optic neuropathy with minimal retinitis. Posterior optic neuropathy, which is rare, is characterized by slowly progressive visual loss without disc edema. Brain stem involvement may produce ptosis, internuclear ophthalmoplegia, sixth nerve palsy, horizontal and vertical gaze paresis, and nystagmus. Guillain-Barré syndrome associated with CMV infection follows the typical course seen in people not infected with HIV.

The diagnosis of CMV infection is made clinically, based on the characteristic ocular findings. Serologic tests and cultures may be inconclusive. CNS disease is often difficult to confirm, and the diagnosis is often made presumptively in the presence of elevated CMV titers in the blood and cerebrospinal fluid. Treatment with ganciclovir (Cytovene) and other acyclic nucleoside antiviral agents is useful for the retinitis and occasionally improves optic nerve disease.

Herpesvirus   Herpes simplex and herpes zoster can cause infection in patients with AIDS. Acute outer retinal necrosis produces photophobia, ocular pain, floaters, and decreased visual acuity. Ophthalmic findings include panuveitis, vitritis, and a

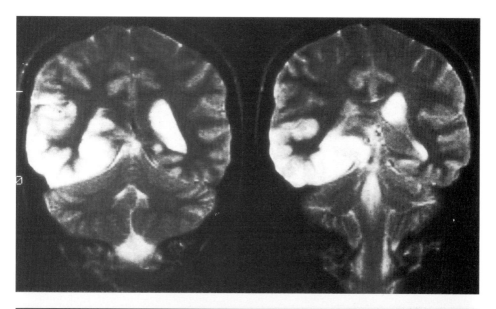

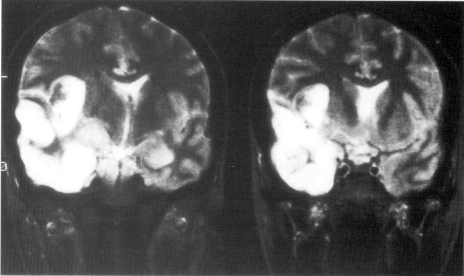

FIG VIII-27—Coronal T2-weighted MRIs reveal an area of high-signal intensity in the right temporal lobe, typical of herpes encephalitis. (Photographs courtesy of Leo Hochhauser, MD.)

necrotizing retinitis that initially spares the posterior pole. Disc edema and retinal arteritis may be found.

Central nervous system encephalitis is the most common manifestation of herpes infection (Fig VIII-27). Radiculitis may occur, producing herpes zoster ophthalmicus and Ramsay Hunt syndrome. In general, neuro-ophthalmic findings are uncommon with herpesvirus infection.

Human immunodeficiency virus HIV-1 infection causes acute and chronic CNS manifestations. Acute aseptic meningitis and meningoencephalitis affect 5%–10% of patients just after HIV-1 infection. Headache, fever, and meningeal signs may accompany a mononucleosis-like syndrome. Occasionally, altered mental status, seizures, and cranial neuropathies occur, most commonly seventh nerve paresis.

HIV encephalopathy, or the *AIDS dementia complex,* begins with impaired memory and concentration, behavior changes, and mental slowness. Abnormal pursuit and saccadic eye movements and saccadic intrusions (square-wave jerks) may be present. Late manifestations include profound dementia, behavior changes, psychosis, psychomotor impairment, weakness, visual neglect, visual hallucinations, seizures, and tremor. An optic neuropathy may develop. Ocular signs of HIV infection include cotton-wool spots, perivasculitis, and retinal hemorrhages.

MRI demonstrates cerebral atrophy and areas of white matter hyperintensity on T2-weighted images that correspond to areas of demyelination that are produced by the virus.

Mycobacterium *M tuberculosis* and *M avium-intracellulare* can infect the brain and eye. Neuro-ophthalmic manifestations of tuberculous meningitis include photophobia, third and sixth nerve paresis, papilledema, retrobulbar optic neuritis, anisocoria, and a poor pupillary light reaction. Cerebral infarction can result from obliterative endarteritis. Neuroimaging studies may show hydrocephalus, abscess formation, granulomas, and enhancement of the basal meninges with contrast administration.

Syphilis Syphilis frequently accompanies HIV infection, probably as a result of the shared risk of sexual transmission. Ophthalmic presentations include papillitis, retinal hemorrhages, arterial and venous occlusions, vasculitis, chorioretinitis, necrotizing vasculitis, optic neuritis, and uveitis. Meningovascular syphilis produces visual field defects and ocular motility disorders in some patients.

The diagnosis of syphilis may be difficult to make in an immunocompromised host. Most HIV-positive patients have abnormal serologic tests for syphilis (VDRL, RPR, FTA-ABS). The cerebrospinal fluid may show one or more of the following changes: positive syphilis serology, elevated protein, or pleocytosis. The cerebrospinal fluid VDRL alone cannot be relied upon to confirm CNS infection. A course of aqueous penicillin G (12–24 million U/day IV for 10–14 days) is recommended, with reexamination of the cerebrospinal fluid to determine the effectiveness of treatment.

Pneumocystis carinii Ocular infection with *P carinii* is uncommon. Reports have described yellow-white, slightly elevated lesions representing cysts containing the organism in the deep layers of the posterior pole.

Progressive multifocal leukoencephalopathy (PML) Originally described in patients with lymphoproliferative disorders and impaired cell-mediated immunity, PML occurs in 1%–4% of patients with AIDS. The disease is caused by a papovavirus that destroys oligodendrocytes. Gray matter is relatively spared. The central visual pathways and ocular motor fibers can be affected. Neuro-ophthalmic manifestations include homonymous hemianopia, blurred vision, cerebral blindness, prosopagnosia, and diplopia. Other neurologic findings are altered mental status, ataxia, dementia, hemiparesis, and focal deficits.

MRI shows areas of demyelination, most frequently in the parieto-occipital region. PML typically involves the subcortical white matter with focal or confluent lesions, and there may be faint contrast enhancement (Fig VIII-28). No effective treatment is known, and most patients die within 6 months of diagnosis.

Toxoplasmosis   Ocular toxoplasmosis is not a common complication of AIDS, but CNS toxoplasmosis affects approximately one third of patients with AIDS. Retinal lesions are usually found adjacent to blood vessels. Toxoplasmic optic neuritis is rare, characterized by subacute visual loss and optic nerve swelling. CNS toxoplasmosis produces multifocal lesions with a predilection for the basal ganglia, frontal, parietal, and occipital lobes (Fig VIII-29). Patients develop headaches, focal neurologic deficits, seizures, mental status changes, and fever. Neuro-ophthalmic findings include homonymous hemianopia and quadrantanopia, ocular motor palsies, and gaze palsies. Lifelong antitoxoplasmosis treatment is necessary in order to prevent recurrences.

MRI typically shows multiple lesions that are isointense with the brain on T1-weighted images and isointense or hyperintense on T2-weighted images. Gadolinium administration reveals enhancement.

Friedman DI. AIDS: neuro-ophthalmic considerations. *Ophthalmol Clin North Am.* 1991;4:449–462.

Friedman DI, Wasenko JJ. Magnetic resonance imaging findings in AIDS and other infectious diseases of the central nervous system. *Ophthalmol Clin North Am.* 1994;7: 301–331.

Hamed LM, Schatz NJ, Galetta SL. Brainstem ocular motility defects and AIDS. *Am J Ophthalmol.* 1988;106:437–442.

Jabs DA, Green WR, Fox R, et al. Ocular manifestations of acquired immune deficiency syndrome. *Ophthalmology.* 1989;96:1092–1099.

Lyme Disease

Lyme borreliosis is caused by infection with *Borrelia burgdorferi,* a spirochete transmitted by deer ticks. The disease typically occurs in three stages and can produce ocular and neuro-ophthalmic manifestations.

In *stage 1* 60%–80% of patients develop a localized infection characterized by a skin rash (*erythema chronicum migrans*) that is sometimes associated with fever, regional lymphadenopathy, and minor constitutional symptoms. This stage typically occurs within days or weeks of infection. The ocular findings include conjunctivitis, photophobia, periorbital edema, diffuse choroiditis, exudative retinal detachment, and iridocyclitis.

Stage 2 follows within days or weeks and represents disseminated infection via the blood or lymphatic system. Stage 2 is associated with symptoms in the skin, nervous system, or musculoskeletal sites. Annular or malar rash, arthralgia, pancarditis, lymphadenopathy, splenomegaly, arteriovenous block, hepatitis, hematuria, proteinura, malaise, and fatigue may be present. Neuro-ophthalmic findings at this stage consist of keratitis, panophthalmitis, papilledema (pseudotumor cerebri–like syndrome), granulomatous iritis, vitritis, pars planitis, and orbital myositis. Two thirds of patients have ocular findings at this stage. Cranial neuropathies can occur, most commonly Bell's palsy, optic neuritis, meningitis with headache and neck stiffness, and radiculopathies.

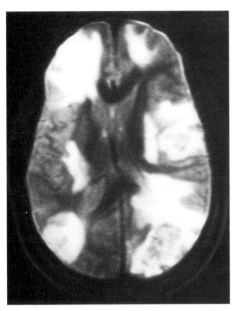

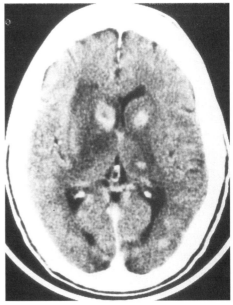

FIG VIII-28—Progressive multifocal leukoencephalopathy in a patient with AIDS. Multiple areas of high-signal intensity appear on this proton-density-weighted MRI. Note the fingerlike appearance in the left frontal lobe, conforming to the distribution of the white matter. (Photograph courtesy of Leo Hochhauser, MD.)

FIG VIII-29—CT scan of the brain with contrast shows multiple areas of enhancement in the caudate nuclei, basal ganglia, and occipital lobes in a patient with CNS toxoplasmosis. (Photograph courtesy of Leo Hochhauser, MD.)

Stage 3 represents persistent infection. Arthritis and scleroderma-like skin lesions are prominent. Keratitis and neurologic conditions predominate, including chronic encephalomyelitis, spastic paraparesis, ataxic gait, subtle mental disorders, and chronic radiculopathy. The neurologic picture may resemble multiple sclerosis, clinically and radiographically.

The diagnosis is made clinically, when the patient has been exposed to an endemic area (the patient may not recall a tick bite) and shows the typical rash of erythema chronicum migrans. The presence of an elevated Lyme antibody titer in the serum or cerebrospinal fluid is helpful. The ELISA is typically used for screening, but the Western blot technique confirms the diagnosis.

Stages 1 and 2 are treated with oral antibiotics such as tetracycline, erythromycin, doxycycline, or cefuroxime. Severe cases and stage 3 require IV penicillin G (20 million U/day for 14 days) or ceftriaxone.

Steere AC. Medical progress: Lyme disease. *N Engl J Med.* 1989;321:586–596.

Winterkorn JM. Lyme disease: Neurologic and ophthalmic manifestations. *Surv Ophthalmol.* 1990;35:191–204.

Fungal Infections

Fungal infections are cause by species that proliferate either with polymorpho-nuclear leukocyte deficiencies (aspergillosis, mucormycosis, blastomycosis, can-didiasis) or with opportunistic infections associated with defective T-cell function (cryptococcosis, histoplasmosis, coccidioidomycosis). The two main types of fungi are molds and yeasts, although some fungi can have characteristics of both.

Molds (filamentous fungi) are composed of hyphae, which extend and branch to form a mycelium, enabling the mold to grow. Molds reproduce when a portion of the hyphae breaks off. Aspergillosis and mucormycosis are CNS infections caused by molds.

Yeasts are round with outpouchings called buds or pseudohyphae. Yeasts are septated and reproduce by budding: the parent cell divides and one of the daughter nuclei migrates into a bud on the surface of a cell. Coccidioidomycosis, crypto-coccosus, and histoplasmosis are caused by yeasts. *Candida* can grow as a yeast or a mold.

> Miller NR, ed. *Walsh and Hoyt's Clinical Neuro-Ophthalmology.* 4th ed. Baltimore: Williams & Wilkins; 1995;5:3158–3317.

Aspergillosis The *Aspergillus* fungus grows in hay, grain, decaying vegetation, soil, and dung. It is contracted by inhaling or chewing grain, breathing in a hospital operating room or elsewhere in a hospital during renovation, or eating contaminated foods (pepper). The most frequent mode of transmission is inhalation of spores. Many species of *Aspergillus* infect humans. The three main types of infection are allergic aspergillosis, aspergillomas, and invasive aspergillosis.

Allergic aspergillosis affects the bronchopulmonary system and the paranasal sinuses. Neuro-ophthalmic findings are rare, and they occur secondarily with sphenoid sinus involvement. Signs and symptoms include optic neuropathy, prop-tosis, diplopia, and headache.

Aspergillomas, or *fungus balls,* may arise in the orbit, paranasal sinuses, or brain. They can occur in either immunocompromised or immunocompetent pa-tients. Orbital aspergillomas produce symptoms of orbital masses with proptosis, visual loss, diplopia, and pain. Orbital lesions also typically involve the sinuses or brain. Extension to the optic canal, cavernous sinus, optic nerves, and optic chiasm produces neuro-ophthalmic findings. Intracranial aspergillomas act like a mass lesion, causing progressive neurologic deficits.

Invasive aspergillosis typically occurs in immunocompromised patients. Most patients initially have pulmonary involvement, although the skin, orbit, or sinuses may be the nidus of infection. CNS infection occurs secondarily by either direct or hematogenous spread of organisms. Ophthalmic manifestations include acute retrobulbar optic neuropathy, endophthalmitis, orbital apex syndrome, and cavernous sinus syndrome. Vascular invasion produces cerebral infarction or hemorrhage. Meningitis, intracranial abscess, epidural and subdural hematoma, mycotic aneurysm formation, and encephalitis are serious sequelae of invasive aspergillosis.

Treatment includes systemic corticosteroids and antifungal agents, such as amphotericin B. Itraconazole and flucytosine are used to treat allergic aspergillosis. Surgical intervention is necessary to treat aspergillomas and invasive aspergillosis. The mortality for invasive aspergillosis is extremely high (>90%).

Denning DW, Stevens DA. Antifungal and surgical treatment of invasive aspergillosis: review of 2,121 published cases. *Rev Infect Dis.* 1990;12:1147–1201.

Levin LA, Avery R, Shore JW, et al. The spectrum of orbital aspergillosis: a clinico-pathological review. *Surv Ophthalmol.* 1996;41:142–154.

Mucormycosis   Mucormycosis is caused by several different mold fungi of the Zygomycetes class. These fungi, which inhabit decaying matter, are ubiquitous but of such low virulence that infection occurs only in debilitated hosts. The mold enters the body through the respiratory tract and proliferates, causing hyphal invasion of tissues. It grows rapidly, and produces a more acute infection than other fungi. These organisms have a predilection for blood vessels, and hemorrhage, thrombosis, and ischemic necrosis are hallmarks of mucormycosis. Aneurysm and pseudoaneurysm formation in the intracranial vasculature can produce devastating consequences when rupture occurs. The two types of mucormycosis producing ophthalmic involvement are rhinocerebral and CNS mucormycosis.

Rhinocerebral mucormycosis usually occurs in patients with diabetes, patients taking corticosteroids, or neutropenic patients who are receiving antibiotics. The initial infection spreads from the facial skin, nasal mucosa, paranasal sinuses, or the hard palate. The fungus spreads to the nearby blood vessels, affecting the orbital vessels, carotid arteries, cavernous sinuses, or jugular veins. Orbital and neurologic signs are produced by infarction, thrombosis, or hemorrhage. Untreated, rhinocerebral mucormycosis may bring about rapid deterioration leading to death within days. A few patients develop a chronic course.

Most patients have headache or facial pain. The other symptoms and signs depend on the location of the infection. Orbital involvement produces orbital swelling, pain on eye movement, conjunctival injection and chemosis, corneal ulceration, ophthalmoplegia, and visual loss. Retinal infarction, ophthalmic artery occlusion, and optic nerve infiltration are mechanisms of blindness. Other common presentations are painful diplopia and cranial neuropathy. An orbital apex, cavernous sinus, or chiasmal syndrome may be present. Neurologic signs include hemiparesis, aphasia, seizures, and altered mental status.

Central nervous system mucormycosis is very rare. The fungus usually gains access to the CNS from the nose or paranasal sinus, but there is no nasal sinus, ocular, or orbital disease when the neurologic manifestations appear. Infection of the orbit, palate, nose, and sinuses typically occurs secondarily. Meningitis, abscesses, cranial nerve involvement, and seizures are common.

The diagnosis of mucormycosis relies on a high index of suspicion, since many of the laboratory investigations are nonspecific. CT may demonstrate bone destruction, soft-tissue alteration in the paranasal sinuses and orbit, air-fluid levels in the sinuses and orbits, or brain abscess formation. MRI, MRA, and arteriography may be helpful to show vascular thrombosis. The definitive test is a biopsy that demonstrates vascular invasion, tissue necrosis, eschar formation, inflammatory cells, and nonseptate hyphae.

Mucormycosis has a mortality rate of about 50%. The underlying systemic disease should be treated and immunosuppressant agents eliminated, if possible. Surgical debridement of necrotic tissue and administration of amphotericin B are used, and hyperbaric oxygen may be helpful.

Blastomycosis   A yeast infection caused by *Blastomyces dermatitidis,* blastomycosis is endemic in the southeastern and south central United States, especially along the Mississippi and Ohio rivers. It is also found along the St. Lawrence River and the Great Lakes. The organism enters the body through the lung, typically following exposure to soil that has been contaminated with animal excrement. Most commonly, extrapulmonary involvement affects the skin, bone, and genitourinary tract. However, the eye, orbit, and brain may be involved even in the absence of pulmonary disease. The CNS is affected in 5% of cases.

Most CNS blastomycotic granuloma formation is intracranial, although the spine may also be infected. Meningitis occurs as a late finding. Blastomycosis produces eye disease in immunocompetent hosts with a predilection for the cornea and uveal tract. Corneal ulcer, hypopyon, uveitis, iridocyclitis, and endophthalmitis can occur. Orbital involvement is quite rare.

The diagnosis should be suspected in patients who develop chronic pulmonary disease and spend time outdoors in an endemic area. The organism is demonstrated in pus, sputum, cerebrospinal fluid, or other histopathologic sections. Cerebrospinal fluid sampling is notoriously unreliable for confirming the diagnosis, but presumptive treatment can be initiated if the organism is found in other body fluids. Treatment is with ketoconazole or amphotericin B. Intrathecal amphotericin B is given for CNS blastomycosis.

Candidiasis *Candida albicans* is a ubiquitous organism, and patients with diabetes mellitus, AIDS, malignancies, and other conditions in which the immune system is suppressed are highly susceptible. Candidiasis is the most common fungal infection in patients with cancer and accounts for a high percentage of fungal infections in patients who receive organ transplants. Infections usually affect mucocutaneous structures or deep organs. Neuro-ophthalmic and neurologic complications arise from deep organ or disseminated disease.

Ocular candidiasis can be either localized or diffuse, resulting from hematogenous spread or direct innoculation. Most cases arise following intraocular surgery, developing weeks to months after surgery and resembling an anaerobic infection. White, fluffy "cotton balls" may appear in the vitreous with areas of retinitis. Hypopyon, anterior chamber inflammation, retinal hemorrhages, Roth spots, and papillitis may be present. The diagnosis is made from the examination and culture of vitrectomy material.

Central nervous system candidiasis typically occurs in premature infants and patients with AIDS and other chronic, debilitating diseases. Occasionally, it occurs in otherwise healthy people. The infection may be part of disseminated candidiasis, or the organism can enter the CNS from septic embolization from the heart, lung, or other viscera. Early manifestations of *Candida* meningitis are headache, stiff neck, and irritability. Fever, altered mental status, and cranial nerve palsies are less common. Hydrocephalus occurs frequently in neonates. The cerebrospinal fluid shows a high protein in 60% of cases. The fungal organisms can be identified histologically in 40% of cases.

In the brain parenchyma, *Candida* causes abscess, vasculitis, aneurysm, or vascular thrombosis. Neuro-ophthalmic manifestations, including cerebral blindness, occur depending on the site of the lesion.

The heart, kidneys, eyes, and brain are preferentially involved in *disseminated candidiasis,* which can occur with cancer, AIDS, surgery, extensive burns, organ transplant, and central catheter placement. Pathologically, abcesses with suppurative and granulomatous reactions are found.

The treatment of candidiasis depends on the location and extent of infection. Amphotericin B and flucytosine are used for CNS and intraocular infections. Removal of organisms by vitrectomy often improves the visual outcome in ocular candidiasis.

Cryptococcosis *Cryptococcus neoformans,* the most common fungus causing cryptococcosis, is found in pigeon droppings and contaminated soil. Although it is ubiquitous, it rarely causes infection in otherwise healthy people. However, infection does occur in approximately 10% of patients with AIDS, and it is the most common life-threatening mycosis in these patients.

The most common neuro-ophthalmic abnormality is papilledema from crypto-coccal meningitis. The onset of symptoms is usually insidious with a waxing and waning course. Headache, nausea, vomiting, dizziness, and mental status changes are the most common complaints. Diplopia from unilateral or bilateral sixth nerve palsies may occur as a false-localizing sign of increased intracranial pressure. Inflammation at the base of the brain produces other cranial neuropathies. Photophobia, blurred vision, retrobulbar pain, homonymous visual field defects, or nystagmus may occur.

Optic nerve involvement manifests as a retrobulbar neuritis producing gradual visual loss over hours to days. It is postulated that adhesive arachnoiditis is one cause of visual loss with cryptococcal infections. Infiltration of organisms within the visual pathways and the perioptic meninges has been shown postmortem. Other ophthalmic complications include retinochoroiditis and cotton-wool spots.

The diagnosis is confirmed by demonstrating the *C neoformans* capsular antigen or isolating the yeast in the cerebrospinal fluid. Most patients with CNS crypto-coccosis have disseminated disease with evidence of infection in the blood, lungs, bone marrow, skin, kidneys, and other organs. Serum antigen titers are helpful for this reason.

Antifungal treatment consists of amphotericin B and flucytosine. Intrathecal amphotericin treatment may be necessary. Fluconazole or itraconazole are used for maintenance therapy. Visual loss caused by papilledema can be prevented with cerebrospinal fluid shunting or optic nerve sheath fenestration. The mortality rate of treated CNS cryptococcosis is 25%–30%. The prognosis is worse in patients with an underlying malignancy or AIDS.

Histoplasmosis *Histoplasma capsulatum* exists as a spore in the soil and in a yeast phase at body temperature. It is the only pathogenic fungus that grows intracellularly. Histoplasmosis is endemic in the eastern central United States, and infection occurs by inhalation of spores. Thus, pulmonary histoplasmosis is the most common manifestation. The size of the inoculum and the immune status of the patient determine whether or not systemic infection will result.

CNS involvement occurs with acute disseminated histoplasmosis, typically in the setting of an immunocompromised host. Meningitis in these patients is usually mild but is sometimes fatal. Encephalitis may affect the cerebral hemispheres, cerebellum, or brain stem, producing pyogranulomas or abscesses. Neurologic and neuro-ophthalmic manifestations are referable to the site of the infection. Ocular involvement is rare, but vitritis, retinitis, and uveitis have been described.

With chronic disseminated histoplasmosis, mild or severe meningitis occurs that is typically insidious in onset. Mild accompanying systemic manifestations often delay the diagnosis. Single or multiple intracranial lesions may be present. Rarely, patients develop isolated CNS histoplasmosis with meningitis or granuloma formation in the absence of other systemic involvement.

The diagnosis is made by detecting the antibody to *H capsulatum* by radioimmunoassay and ELISA. The DNA probe test and exoantigen test are more sensitive and specific. The skin test is not useful, since asymptomatic people living in an endemic area will test positive. Patients who are immunosuppressed or have CNS involvement are treated with amphotericin B.

Presumed ocular histoplasmosis syndrome (POHS) occurs in patients with serologic and radiographic evidence of prior histoplasmosis infection. (The word *presumed* in the name is now often dropped, as the causal relationship between fungus and disease has become clearer.) Chorioretinal scars, disciform macular lesions, and neovascularization without active inflammation characterize this condition. Choroidal neovascularization in the macula can cause permanent central visual loss. It is treated with photocoagulation. For further discussion of OHS, see BCSC Section 9, *Intraocular Inflammation and Uveitis;* and BCSC Section 12, *Retina and Vitreous.*

Cat-Scratch Disease

Bartonella henselae (formerly *Rochalimaea* sp) is a gram-negative rickettsia that causes cat-scratch disease. The condition is transmitted by cats or fleas from infected cats, usually by a scratch or a bite. It typically produces fever with painful lymphadenopathy. A variety of ophthalmic manifestations occur with cat-scratch disease. The most common is Parinaud oculoglandular syndrome (granulomatous conjunctivitis and preauricular adenopathy). Neuroretinitis is the most frequent neuro-ophthalmic finding. Visual loss with optic disc edema, uveitis, retinal edema with exudates, and white retinal inflammatory lesions are observed. The diagnosis is confirmed by detecting high titers of *B henselae* in the serum.

Cat-scratch disease is usually self-limited, and the neuroretinitis typically improves spontaneously. Various antibiotics have been used for treatment, including ciprofloxacin, trimethoprim-sulfamethoxazole, tetracycline, and clindamycin.

Golnick KC, Marotto ME, Fanous MM, et al. Ophthalmic manifestations of *Rochalimaea* species. *Am J Ophthalmol.* 1994;118:145–151.

CHAPTER IX

Functional Remediation and Management of Neuro-Ophthalmic Visual Dysfunction

Introduction

As with other therapeutic modalities, visual rehabilitation is a process that assesses the patient's residual abilities and attempts to match realistic visual goals with assistive devices, ocular motor and cognitive retraining, and environmental modifications. Some visual goals are simple and can be addressed during a general visual examination. More often, however, referral to specialists in optical/electronic assistive devices, mobility instruction, and home-based services is required.

With an increasing number of patients surviving traumatic brain injury and stroke and an aging population, the volume of patients with uncorrectable vision loss is rapidly expanding. The following is an overview of selected procedures useful to the clinician.

Further reading   BCSC Section 3, *Optics, Refraction, and Contact Lenses*, devotes a chapter to detailed discussion of magnifiers and telescopes as well as other devices such as prisms. Nonvisual assistance and daily living skills are also explored. The New York Association for the Blind, 111 East 59th St., New York, NY 10022, offers the *Lighthouse Catalogue of Optical Aids*, 3rd ed., free of charge.

Functional Assessment

History: A Questionnaire

Pretherapy structuring is useful to ready the patient to participate in the subsequent therapy session. Short, open-ended questions have been identified that address daily living tasks for near, intermediate, distance, and peripheral vision, as well as effects of lighting, distractibility, and general well-being. Sample questions are presented in Table IX-1.

TABLE IX-1

VISION ASSESSMENT SCREENING

1. Can you read well enough to sort your mail?
2. Can you distinguish foods on your plate?
3. Can you watch television at a comfortable distance (about what distance)?
4. Can you identify a person across the street?
5. Do you miss things to one side of you or the other?
6. How does lighting affect your vision (indoors and outdoors)?
7. When looking at one object, is it much harder for you to see when it is surrounded by other objects (i.e., do you get distracted)?
8. Do these problems vary from day to day? Does your vision fluctuate?
9. Are you generally a happy or sad person?
10. If there is one thing we can make an improvement upon today, what would that be?

Comments:

Functional Testing

The strategy used in rehabilitative evaluations is to find conditions that optimize visual performance.

Distance visual acuity   Measurements are made at variable distances, typically 10 feet or less, in good ambient illumination, using charts that have letters or numbers that are generally larger and more varied in size than the traditional Snellen chart. If useful, eccentric viewing, if not already present, is encouraged.

Near visual acuity   Measurements are made with reading cards containing simple text or isolated words or symbols, graded in size according to a point or metric scale. Samples of conventional newsprint, magazines, or phone books should also be used to demonstrate effects of print legibility. Effects of lighting type, intensity, and placement should be demonstrated at this point. Questions as to the availability of useful lighting in the home, at work, or in school are also valuable. Differences in near visual performance between single symbols, words, and continuous text give the examiner a general idea of the size of the useful field of view and the effects of any central field distortion and loss on reading.

Amsler grid   Plate #2 of the Amsler grid (with diagonal lines intersecting) allows the clinician to predict the ability of the patient to read normal newsprint and the potential for magnification to support reading. If the patient can easily find the central dot on the Amsler grid, he or she is using foveal or parafoveal fixation or has a low-density scotoma. In addition, if several squares around the fixation dot are also seen, the examiner can anticipate that the patient will be able to read normal print (with appropriate magnification, if necessary). To measure the diameter of a constricted central field, a white test object can be used to map out the central island of vision. Held at 33 cm, each square on the grid is equal to 1° of visual field.

An accurate manifest *refraction* is a basic starting point for all visual rehabilitation. However, when the patient is receiving multiple medical or surgical treatments or has active disease, ophthalmic specialists may not perform a refraction or may assume that a change of lens prescription would have little effect. A trial-frame refraction, using full-aperture lens, is recommended for each patient. The phoropter reduces eccentric viewing and creates a tunnel effect, reducing light reaching the eye. For patients who have significant central vision loss (≥20/200), larger dioptric changes should be demonstrated (±1.00 D sphere and cylinder, or greater) so that differences will be appreciated.

When fluctuating vision is reported or suspected, the refraction should be repeated on a different day to check reproducibility prior to dispensing a prescription. Checking monocular versus binocular visual performance will assess whether the use of a fogging lens, lens frosting, occlusion, or monocular bifocal segment should be employed. When high-plus reading prescriptions are to be used, base-in prisms (typically 2.00Δ more than the spherical power OU) should be ordered to ease the strain on convergence. (Example: +8.00 prismatic half-eyes incorporate 10.00Δ base-in prism OU.) Patients with nystagmus or other oscillatory eye movements may benefit from contact lenses, since the lens (and its optical center) moves with the eye, maximizing correction.

Magnification and Minification

Magnification

The retinal image of an object can be enlarged by several means:

☐ *Relative size*, or *linear, magnification* (making the object itself bigger). Some examples are large-print books and magazines, jumbo playing cards, or large-button phone pads.

☐ *Relative distance magnification* (moving closer to the object, increasing the size of the image on the retina). For example, the use of a reading add allows the viewer to move closer to the object and still maintain focus.

☐ *Angular magnification* (produced by a lens system that, independent of relative distance or size magnification, can increase the angular subtense of the image). Objects are made to appear closer and therefore larger. Telescopes and magnifiers are both examples.

The overwhelming variety of magnification devices can be broken down into three groups: convex lenses, telescopes, and electronic magnifiers.

Convex lenses *Spectacles.* The most functionally and cosmetically acceptable devices that allow for hands-free magnification are spectacles. However, as the lens power increases, the focal length decreases, and objects must be held closer with a loss of visual field and depth of field. When objects are held close to the eyes, the patient must learn new strategies to keep the object in focus (e.g., moving the text left to right without head movement), and illumination may require adjustment to avoid shadows from the head on the page. In general, however, the patient can often write by hand with prescriptions that are approximately half that used for reading.

Hand and stand magnifiers. Magnifiers typically allow for a greater viewing distance than spectacles and can have the advantage of an incorporated light source. The weight of these appliances can often create fatigue. Hand tremors are best handled with stand magnifiers that rest on the object's surface. Conventional reading adds (up to approximately +4.00 D) provide the converging power necessary for use of many stand magnifiers.

Telescopes   The only optical appliances that provide magnification for distance are telescopes. They can be used for independent travel (street and bus signs) and other distance viewing including television, movies, and plays. Telescopes can be hand-held or spectacle mounted; in each case, the patient must be trained to localize an object without use of a telescope and then focus rapidly through the telescopic sight. At higher powers of magnification, there is an increased perceived motion of objects (parallax), which may be difficult for patients to adapt to.

Telescopes magnify at the expense of visual field and illumination. Patients with restricted visual field are often poor candidates for telescopes. Using a telescope stops the dynamic scanning of the visual field that is an important adaptive response to field restriction. Additionally, the amount of magnification used may create an image that is too large for the available field of view. Patients with nystagmus may have difficulty maintaining alignment of their visual axis with the optics of a tele-scope. However, patients who are successful have reported a much-appreciated reduction in retinal image motion as well as improved acuity. The relative weight, cosmesis, cost, and required dexterity are all important issues for each patient attempting to use a focusing telescope.

Electronic magnifiers   Electronic magnification (e.g., closed-circuit television) has several advantages including

☐ Comfortable viewing distance

☐ Larger visual field (screen size)

☐ Adjustable contrast, brightness, and reversal of polarity (black letters on white background or white letters on black)

☐ High magnification (up to approximately 60×)

For patients with advanced central vision loss who have large central scotomata, electronic magnification may be the only way to see detail at near. Some models allow for an area underneath the camera sufficient to allow for writing and drawing and other tasks requiring hand-eye coordination.

Minification

Patients with highly restricted visual fields need to have the longest viewing distance possible to maximize the useful visual field. The two optical methods of reducing image size, condensing more information into the viewing field, are *minus lenses* and *reverse telescopes*. The obvious drawback of minification is the reduction in visual acuity. Patients with good central vision but restricted visual fields may benefit from this application. For example, a patient with 20/25 visual acuity and a visual field constricted to 5° around fixation (10° central field) may appreciate twofold expansion of the visual field to 20° by viewing through a 2× telescope in the reverse direction, despite the reduction in visual acuity to 20/50. Reverse telescopes may be handheld or mounted bioptically above the pupil in a spectacle form. Some practitioners also advocate the use of low-powered minus lenses carried in pocket form for a quick survey of the distance visual field as an aid to orientation and mobility.

Prisms: Partial and Full Diameter

For patients with uncorrectable vision loss ophthalmic prisms may provide correction of binocular vision anomalies, peripheral visual field enhancement, and image relocation. Prisms alter the perceived visual space, relocating part or all of the visual field. They may also cause distortion that reduces acuity and image contrast. The key to successful use of prisms is to find an acceptable balance between improved visual function and the degree of distortion inherent in their use. Prisms may help patients with hemianopic/sector visual field defects and those with visual fields with overall constriction.

Patients with hemifield peripheral visual loss sometimes learn adaptive head turns in the direction of the field loss, aiming the remaining visual field in the direction of the unseen one. Compensatory head posture can be an early indicator of field loss, whether lateral or altitudinal in nature, and should be noted during the examination.

Homonymous Hemianopia

Both partial and full-diameter yoked (oriented in the same direction) prisms can be used. However, the two formats use completely different strategies for helping patients compensate for visual field loss.

Partial prisms   Some patients with homonymous hemianopia benefit from a partial prism, typically a Fresnel press-on prism with the base in the direction of the field loss, covering a portion of the lens in the nonseeing field. Images of objects in the blind field are displaced closer to the seeing field, lessening the magnitude of eye scanning necessary to locate the object. The prism is used only for locating; a clear view of the object is provided by a head turn that allows for direct viewing through the unobstructed part of the spectacles. A 10.00–20.00Δ prism is placed with the apex as close to the visual axis in primary gaze as possible without interfering with central vision. Spontaneous eye movements will then allow for frequent eye excursions into the prism. The prism may have to be moved farther out to allow for more comfortable lateral scanning.

Weiss NJ, Brown WL. Uses of prism in low vision. In: Cotter SA, ed. *Clinical Uses of Prism: A Spectrum of Applications.* St Louis: Mosby–Year Book, 1995.

There are two drawbacks to the use of partial prisms:

□ Active participation by the patient is crucial. Patients with cognitive impairment may not be able to consistently initiate appropriate eye movements to use the prisms effectively.

□ A "jack-in-the-box" phenomenon can occur. As the eye enters the prism, a prismatic "jump" of the image may be observed, which is often startling and may be unacceptable to the patient.

Full-diameter prisms Full-diameter prisms (6–8Δ) placed in both spectacle lenses have been advocated for patients with visual neglect in one hemifield and in some patients who have difficulty with balance as a result of visual–spatial disorientation.

Cohen JM, Waiss B. Visual field remediation. In: Cole RG, Rosenthal BP, eds. *Remediation and Management of Low Vision.* St Louis: Mosby–Year Book; 1996.

Padula WV. *Neuro-Optometric Rehabilitation.* Santa Ana, CA: Optometric Extension Program; 1996.

Visual Field Constriction

Treatment of overall visual field loss incorporates methods for increasing the amount of information falling within the residual island of vision (minification) and expanding the dynamic visual field through rapid and systematic visual scanning. Efficient visual scanning relies on the ability of the patient to be cued to the area of field loss coupled with the use of prisms to reduce the eye excursions necessary to sample the visual field. The type and amount of illumination may also be modified to optimize visual acuity and image contrast.

Nystagmus

For some individuals involuntary ocular oscillations can be reduced or eliminated by an eccentric viewing position with the eyes in the position of least nystagmus, or null point. This positioning of the eyes may already be incorporated in a patient's head turn or can be identified on examination. Yoked prisms may be used to move the images (and therefore the eyes) to the null point, eliminating the need for exaggerated head turns. A gradual training period is used to allow for adaptation. Rotatable prisms mounted in light-weight frames that can be fitted over spectacles are valuable training tools to be used for office or home evaluation, prior to ordering the final prism power ground in to spectacles.

The Control of Illumination: Light Intensity and Spectrum

Both the quantity and quality of light reaching the eye are major considerations in the treatment of patients with vision loss, as are the associated problems of photophobia and glare control. Simple methods can be used to reduce light scatter and control lighting. Window blinds and drapes, rugs and floor mats on tile or shiny floor surfaces, and proper selection of lighting sources and fixtures can reduce glare and help customize illumination for patients with special lighting requirements.

For near tasks, including reading, the use of a typoscope (a piece of black, nonreflective material with a long rectangular window) can reduce reflected light scatter, allowing for illumination of isolated text lines. Colored acetate overlays may also be used to increase perceived contrast of text.

Numerous commercially available absorptive filters, some with photochromic properties, have been incorporated into spectacle prescriptions to reduce symptoms related to glare and light sensitivity. Attempts to correlate specific wavelength absorption and light intensity with categories of ocular disease have been made primarily by companies selling these products. The best approach for selection of these light-filtering lenses is by direct comparison of filters under those lighting conditions that are problematic to the patient. It is important to recognize that the selection of optimal filters is highly individualized and may vary for each patient as tasks change.

Photophobia

Although light sensitivity is anticipated in many patients with abnormal ocular structures, a nonocular or central photophobia can be found in patients as a result of traumatic brain injury or cerebrovascular accident. In one study patients reported a new, intense photophobia after trauma, immediately after and up to a decade after injury. Significant increases in contrast sensitivity and in visual performance (reading rate) were found when patients used absorptive filters that eliminated short-wavelength light transmission.

Jackowski MM, Stuff JF, Taub HA, et al. Photophobia in patients with traumatic brain injury: uses of light-filtering lenses to enhance contrast sensitivity and reading rate. *NeuroRehabilitation.* 1996;14:193–201.

High-Tech Low-Vision Appliances

Since the 1970s, technological and social changes have made access to information for the severely visually disabled a reality. Closed-circuit television is now a commonplace item in public libraries, schools, and work settings as well as in the home. Advances in speech and microprocessor technology have led to computer-based voice output, and text-enlargement programs. Viewing the computer screen may involve the use of conventional optical appliances, including high-plus reading spectacles and telemicroscopes. As a rule, however, patients with visual acuities of 20/200 or less will be served best by the added help of large-print software. Glare screens placed in front of monitors reduce visual fatigue for both normally sighted and visually impaired computer users.

The practical upper limit of text enlargement is often reached when the required magnification allows for only 5–6 characters to be displayed on the monitor at one time. At this level, reading performance is slow enough to require the use of non-visual process technologies. Stand-alone reading machines can allow access to most printed materials. Interactive systems include computers with optical character recognition devices (text scanners) and voice output terminals. Voice-activated computer systems with braille output displays aid patients with profound visual impairment.

Recent advances in microelectronics and microelectrode array fabrication have raised the possibility of providing a useful visual sense (pixelized vision) to patients with profound blindness by electrical stimulation of the visual pathways.

Reading

Hemianopic field losses without macular sparing present special problems for readers. Texts in English are scanned left to right. Patients with right homonymous hemianopia have trouble finishing a sentence, while those with left homonymous hemianopia have problems finding the beginning of a new line at the left margin. Many patients spontaneously demonstrate line tracing with their finger as a guide or use the left thumb as a margin marker. They should also be shown how to rotate the page away from the field loss, bringing more of the text into the useful field. If some magnification is necessary, the use of a bar magnifier (a planoconvex, or half, cylinder) that magnifies only in the vertical meridian is an inexpensive and helpful aid.

Driving

Central Vision Loss

Many states have some stipulation for limited or restricted driving when visual acuity falls below 20/40. In New York, for example, a restricted driver license can be obtained if best-corrected vision in the better seeing eye is not less than 20/70 *and* if the horizontal binocular visual field is at least 140°. Restrictions may include daylight-only driving, no limited-access roads, no adverse weather conditions, etc.

Homonymous Hemianopia

The question of driving with peripheral visual field loss is complicated. Although most states require and test for a best-corrected visual acuity of 20/40 in both eyes, fewer than half of the states routinely test for peripheral visual fields. Visual field testing may be poorly designed and administered and performed only along the horizontal meridian. Existing minimum standards for binocular visual fields range from 100° to 140° total horizontal visual field; monocular visual field limits are more variable, ranging from 140° to 20°. A study employing automated visual field screening of 10,000 volunteers reported that drivers with *binocular* visual field loss had accident and conviction rates twice as high as those with normal visual fields or with only monocular visual field loss.

> Johnson CA, Keltner JL. Incidence of visual field loss in 20,000 eyes and its relationship to driving performance. *Arch Ophthalmol.* 1983;101:371–375.

Visual field performance may spontaneously improve in the first 6–12 months after injury, requiring reevaluation of visual performance, including training and road testing by a rehabilitation-based agency. The use of wide-angle mirrors and compensatory driving strategies may, in some cases, be sufficient for selected individuals to return to restricted driving. However, the majority of eye care and medical professionals advise against driving for most patients with acquired visual field loss.

Approximately half of the states currently allow for driving with a telescopic aid. For example, the visual performance requirements for telescopic driving in New York are visual acuity of 20/100 through the spectacle carrier lens of the better seeing eye; visual acuity of 20/40 through the permanently mounted, bioptically placed telescope (in the patient's possession at least 60 days); and a horizontal binocular visual field of at least 140°. Static visual performance measurements do not ensure effective use of the telescope or safe driving. Training with the visual aid and road evaluation are both necessary to ready the patient for the challenges of using a telescopic device in a highly dynamic situation.

This chapter was prepared with the assistance of Mary M. Jackowski, PhD, OD.

CHAPTER X

Conclusion

As you complete your review of Section 5, *Neuro-Ophthalmology,* we hope that the experience has been useful. The field of neuro-ophthalmology is complex and bridges many specialties. Therefore, it often seems forbidding to the beginning resident. We hope that this trepidation has diminished as you have learned to think anatomically about optic neuropathy, visual field defects, pupillary abnormalities, ocular motor disorders, and the many other ocular signs and symptoms of neurologic disease.

Neuro-ophthalmic disease does not occur as commonly as many disorders that confront the ophthalmologist in daily practice. Yet the price paid by the patient who harbors a missed neuro-ophthalmic entity is often high. Neuro-ophthalmology thus assumes an importance beyond the frequency of occurrence of the disorders with which it deals. Ongoing changes in the delivery of health care in the United States indicate that the general ophthalmologist must develop cost-effective management strategies for all patients. We hope we have provided information that will obviate extensive work-up and allow for more appropriate and selective testing to confirm clinical diagnoses of neurologic and medical disorders that affect vision. If this manual succeeds in facilitating your understanding of neuro-ophthalmology, then its goal is accomplished.

BASIC TEXTS

Neuro-Ophthalmology

Brodsky MC, Baker RS, Hamed LM. *Pediatric Neuro-Ophthalmology.* New York: Springer-Verlag; 1996.
This book deals with special neuro-ophthalmic disorders of children and complements other pediatric texts.

Burde RM, Savino PJ, Trobe JD. *Clinical Decisions in Neuro-Ophthalmology.* 2nd ed. St Louis: Mosby; 1992.
This book is an excellent, up-to-date source for the clinician, emphasizing the diagnostic, how-to approach.

Daroff RB. *Eye Movement Disorders.* Dallas: Medical Information Alternatives.
This four-videotape set contains 39 case film segments, more than 170 diagrams, charts, graphs, and patient photographs that demonstrate all major eye movements and signs and how to recognize them.

Glaser JS. *Neuro-Ophthalmology.* 2nd ed. Philadelphia: Lippincott; 1990.
This source serves as the single basic text for the clinician. It is a valuable introduction to neuro-ophthalmology as well as a good review of the subject. A third edition is scheduled for release in December 1997.

Gold DH, Weingeist TA. *The Eye in Systemic Disease.* Philadelphia: Lippincott; 1990.
Three hundred twenty authors describe the essentials of as many diseases with ophthalmic manifestations. An excellent source for consultation.

Harrington DO, Drake MV. *The Visual Fields: Textbook and Atlas of Clinical Perimetry.* 6th ed. St Louis: Mosby; 1990.
This book is a clinical classic.

Leigh RJ, Zee DS. *The Neurology of Eye Movements.* 2nd ed. Philadephia: Davis; 1991.
Students of DG Cogan bring his classic work up to date; this book serves as the authority on eye movements.

Loewenfeld JE. *The Pupil. Anatomy, Physiology, and Clinical Applications.* Ames: Iowa State University Press; 1993.
This monumental work details centuries of information collected by the world's authority on the pupil and provides the final word on most problems affecting the iris and its innervation.

Miller NR, Newman NJ, eds. *Walsh and Hoyt's Clinical Neuro-Ophthalmology.* 5th ed. Baltimore: Williams & Wilkins; 1997.
This five-volume work is the ultimate encyclopedic reference in neuro-ophthalmology. It is so broad in scope and filled with so much information that it should be used as a reference source and digested in small and repeated bits. One should not contemplate reading it from beginning to end as a tour de force.

Miller NR, Fine SL. *Sights and Sounds in Ophthalmology.* Vol. 3, *The Ocular Fundus in Neuro-Ophthalmic Diagnosis.* St Louis: Mosby; 1977.

This book is a delightful and informative multimedia introductory study course and review of the various disorders of the optic nerve head. It is a must for the ophthalmology resident.

RELATED ACADEMY MATERIALS

Focal Points: Clinical Modules for Ophthalmologists

Beck RW. Anterior ischemic optic neuropathy (Module 3, 1986).

Borchert MS. Nystagmus in childhood (Module 8, 1991).

Brazis PW, Lee AG. Neuro-ophthalmic problems caused by medications (Module 11, 1998).

Chung SM. Update on NAION: the Ischemic Optic Neuropathy Decompression Trial (Module 6, 1998).

Corbett JJ. Diagnosis and management of idiopathic intracranial hypertension (pseudotumor cerebri) (Module 3, 1989).

Drake MV. A primer of automated perimetry (Module 8, 1993).

Ellis BD, Hogg JP. Neuroimaging for the general ophthalmologist (Module 8, 1998).

Goodwin JA. Temporal arteritis (Module 2, 1992).

Katz B. Myasthenia gravis (Module 7, 1989).

Kline LB. Computed tomography in ophthalmology (Module 9, 1985).

Mills RP. Headache (Module 8, 1988).

Newman SA. Automated Perimetry in Neuro-Ophthalmology (Module 6, 1995).

Newman SA. Diagnosis and treatment of chiasmal lesions (Module 1, 1987).

Purvin VA. Amaurosis fugax of carotid origin (Module 7, 1992).

Shults WT. Third, fourth, and sixth cranial nerve palsies (Module 7, 1983).

Siatkowski RM. Third, fourth, and sixth nerve palsies (Module 8, 1996).

Slavin ML. Functional visual loss (Module 2, 1991).

Tang RA, Pardo G. Ocular and periocular pain (Module 2, 1996).

Thompson HS, Kardon RH. Clinical importance of pupillary inequality (Module 10, 1992).

Tomsak RL. Magnetic resonance imaging in neuro-ophthalmology (Module 10, 1986).

Trobe JD. Managing optic neuritis: results of the optic neuritis treatment trial (Module 2, 1994).

Publications

Kline LB, ed. *Optic Nerve Disorders* (Ophthalmology Monograph 10, 1996).

Lane SS, Skuta GS, eds. *ProVision: Preferred Responses in Ophthalmology,* Series 3 (Self-Assessment Program, 1999).

Skuta GL, ed. *ProVision: Preferred Responses in Ophthalmology,* Series 2 (Self-Assessment Program, 1996).

Walsh TJ, ed. *Visual Fields: Examination and Interpretation,* Second Edition (Ophthalmology Monograph 3, 1996).

Wilson FM II, ed. *Practical Ophthalmology: A Manual for Beginning Residents* (1996).

Wirtschafter JD, Berman EL, McDonald CS. *Magnetic Resonance Imaging and Computed Tomography: Clinical Neuro-Orbital Anatomy* (Ophthalmology Monograph 6, 1992).

Multimedia

Frohman LP, Lee AG, eds. *AAO/NANOS Clinical Neuro-Ophthalmology Collection for Ophthalmic Practitioners* (CD-ROM, 1999).

ProVision Interactive: Clinical Case Studies. (Volume 1: Cornea and Neuro-Ophthalmology on CD-ROM, 1996.)

Continuing Ophthalmic Video Education

Behrens M. *Neuro-Ophthalmic Motility Disorders* (1975).

Wilson ME Jr. *Ocular Motility Evaluation of Strabismus and Myasthenia* Gravis (1993).

LEO Clinical Topic Updates

Lee AG. *Neuro-Ophthalmology* (1999).

To order any of these materials, please call the Academy's Customer Service number at (415) 561-8540.

CREDIT REPORTING FORM

BASIC AND CLINICAL SCIENCE COURSE
Section 5

1999–2000

CME Accreditation

The American Academy of Ophthalmology is accredited by the Accreditation Council for Continuing Medical Education to sponsor continuing medical education for physicians.

The American Academy of Ophthalmology designates this educational activity for a maximum of 30 hours in category 1 credit toward the AMA Physician's Recognition Award. Each physician should claim only those hours of credit that he/she has actually spent in the educational activity.

If you wish to claim continuing medical education credit for your study of this section, you must complete and return the study question answer sheet on the back of this page, along with the following signed statement, to the Academy office. This form must be received within 3 years of the date of purchase.

I hereby certify that I have spent _____ (up to 30) hours of study on the curriculum of this section, and that I have completed the study questions. (The Academy, *upon request,* will send you a transcript of the credits listed on this form.)

☐ *Please send credit verification now.*

Signature _____

Date

Name:_____

Address: _____

City and State:_____ Zip: _____

Telephone: (_____) _____ *Academy Member ID# _____
area code

* Your ID number is located following your name on any Academy mailing label, in your Membership Directory, and on your Monthly Statement of Account.

Section Evaluation

Please indicate your response to the statements listed below by placing the appropriate number to the left of each statement.

1 = agree strongly	_____ This section covers topics in enough depth and detail.
2 = agree	_____ This section's illustrations are of sufficient number and quality.
3 = no opinion	
4 = disagree	_____ The references included in the text provide an appropriate
5 = disagree	amount of additional reading.
strongly	_____ The study questions at the end of the book are useful.

In addition, please attach a separate sheet of paper to this form if you wish to elaborate on any of the statements above or to comment on other aspects of this book.

Please return completed form to: **American Academy of Ophthalmology**
P.O. Box 7424
San Francisco, CA 94120-7424
ATTN: Clinical Education Division

Question	Answer	Question	Answer
1	a b c d e	21	a b c d e
2	a b c d e	22	a b c d e
3	a b c d e	23	a b c d e
4	a b c d e	24	a b c d e
5	a b c d e	25	a b c d e
6	a b c d e	26	a b c d e
7	a b c d e	27	a b c d e
8	a b c d e	28	a b c d e
9	a b c d e	29	a b c d e
10	a b c d e	30	a b c d e
11	a b c d e	31	a b c d e
12	a b c d e	32	a b c d e
13	a b c d e	33	a b c d e
14	a b c d e	34	a b c d e
15	a b c d e	35	a b c d e
16	a b c d e	36	a b c d e
17	a b c d e	37	a b c d e
18	a b c d e	38	a b c d e
19	a b c d e	39	a b c d e
20	a b c d e	40	a b c d e

STUDY QUESTIONS

STUDY QUESTIONS

The following multiple-choice questions are designed to be used after your course of study with this book. Record your responses on the answer sheet (the back side of the Credit Reporting Form) by circling the appropriate letter. For the most effective use of this exercise, *complete the entire test* before consulting the answers.

Although a concerted effort has been made to avoid ambiguity and redundancy in these questions, the authors recognize that differences of opinion may occur regarding the "best" answer. The discussions are provided to demonstrate the rationale used to derive the answer. They may also be helpful in confirming that your approach to the problem was correct or, if necessary, in fixing the principle in your memory. Where relevant, additional textbook and journal references are given.

1. Interruption of the visual pathway in the parietal lobe is least likely to produce which of the following?

    a. Right-left confusion
    b. An asymmetric optokinetic nystagmus response
    c. Spasticity of conjugate gaze
    d. The field defect shown in A
    e. The field defect shown in B

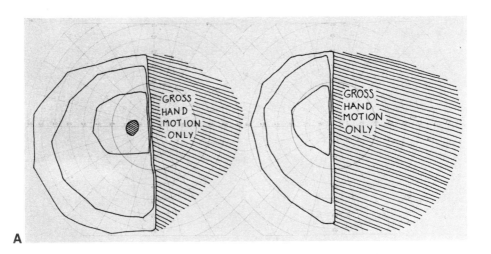

A

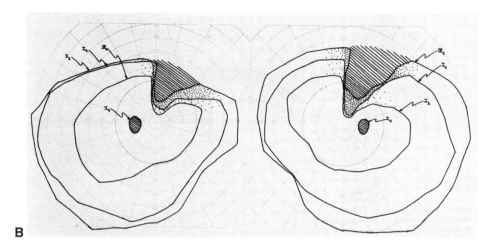

B

2. All of the following statements regarding nutritional amblyopia are true *except*

a. The peripheral visual field is usually unaffected in nutritional amblyopia.

b. There are no distinct clinical differences between nutritional amblyopia and tobacco-alcohol amblyopia.

c. Arcuate nerve fiber bundle visual field defects rarely occur in nutritional amblyopia.

d. The appearance of the fundus is usually normal initially in nutritional amblyopia despite marked central acuity depression.

e. The bilateral visual loss seen in nutritional amblyopia may mimic that seen in chiasmal syndromes.

3. A 26-year-old laboratory technician was splashed in the face with a solvent. His eyes were promptly irrigated with saline, and he was found to have a mild keratoconjunctivitis that cleared up over the next 24 hours. He has been referred to you because he complains of severe visual loss in the right eye since the incident, and a diagnosis of functional visual loss is being considered. Your initial examination finds a visual acuity of 20/200 OD and 20/20 OS. The anterior and posterior segments appear to be normal. All of the following are true *except*

a. Automated static threshold perimetry showing a dense central scotoma would rule out functional visual loss.

b. In spite of the recorded visual acuity, you expect to find no relative afferent pupillary defect in this patient with functional visual loss.

c. Before establishing a diagnosis of functional visual loss, it is important to look for possible causes of amblyopia such as marked anisometropia.

d. Testing optokinetic nystagmus monocularly with vertically moving stripes would not be helpful in establishing a diagnosis of functional visual loss.

e. It is reasonable to attempt to document better visual acuity in the right eye with a technique that deceives the patient about which eye is being tested.

4. A 30-year-old woman notices inequality of her pupils. Examination shows that the right pupil is 7 mm; it reacts minimally to light and slowly but fully to near, after which it dilates slowly to its original size. The deep tendon reflexes are generally hypoactive, especially at the ankles. The probable diagnosis is best established by instillation of which one of the following pharmacologic agents in each eye:

    a.   1% hydroxyamphetamine
    b.   0.125% (1/8%) pilocarpine
    c.   1:1000 epinephrine
    d.   1.0% pilocarpine
    e.   10% cocaine

5. A 69-year-old woman consults you regarding suddenly noticed visual loss in the left eye. Visual acuity is 20/20 OD and 20/200 OS. There is a left afferent pupillary defect and visual field testing is shown below. Biomicroscopic examination shows the patient is pseudophakic OU but is otherwise unremarkable. Fundus evaluation shows a normal disc, with a cup-to-disc ratio of 0.1 on the right and a diffusely swollen optic disc on the left. Your diagnosis is ischemic optic neuropathy. Appropriate steps include

    a.   MRI of the orbits with gadolinium enhancement
    b.   Immediate CBC and sedimentation rate and further history-taking concerning possible giant cell arteritis
    c.   Urgent treatment with a left optic nerve sheath decompression
    d.   No immediate action; ask the patient to return for a recheck in 2 weeks as nothing can be done
    e.   Lumbar puncture to rule out raised intracranial pressure

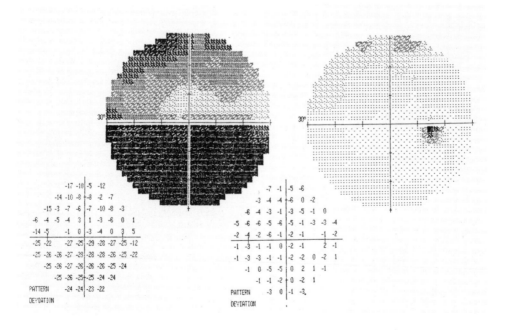

6. If the patient in question #5 also had pallor of the right optic disc and an altitudinal field defect in the right eye (not shown), which of the following is the most likely diagnosis?

    a. Diabetic papillitis
    b. Sphenoid ridge meningioma
    c. Ischemic optic neuropathy
    d. Pituitary adenoma
    e. Chronic obstructive hydrocephalus

7. A 45-year-old woman acquires the changes in her vision noted in the visual field charts below. These changes take place over a 4-year interval, with no history of any abrupt change. She denies any other symptoms of systemic disease. Of the following, the most likely diagnosis is:

    a. Tuberculum meningioma
    b. Toxic optic neuropathy
    c. Chronic perioptic neuropathy
    d. Syphilitic optic neuropathy
    e. Chiasmatic arachnoiditis

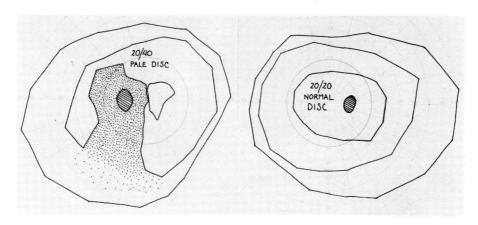

4 Years

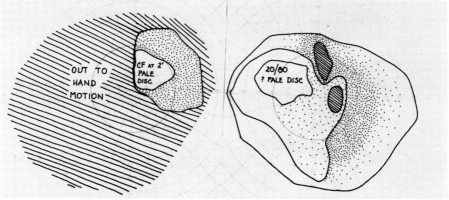

8. A 47-year-old woman presents with the visual field defect shown below. The most likely etiology is

    a. Infarction involving the monocular crescent representation in the left primary visual cortex
    b. Tilted disc syndrome
    c. Retinal detachment
    d. Tuberculum sellae meningioma
    e. Graves orbitopathy

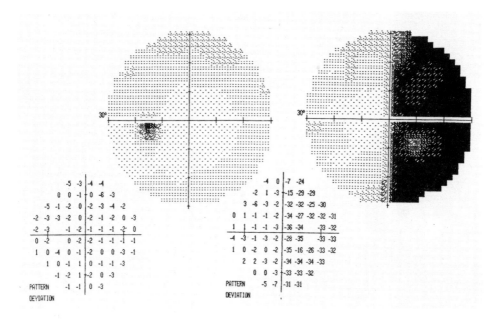

9. A 13-month-old infant is brought to your office because "his head wobbles and his eyes jiggle." You make the diagnosis as spasmus nutans. With regard to this condition, all of the following statements are true *except*:

    a. The nystagmus is fast and of low amplitude.
    b. The diagnosis can be made in the absence of head nodding.
    c. The nystagmus is often monocular or asymmetric.
    d. The nystagmus is present from birth.
    e. Neuroimaging should be obtained.

10. An 11-year-old girl is struck by a car while waiting for a school bus. You are asked to see her in the intensive care unit. One eye is higher than the other. There is no obvious cranial nerve palsy or orbital injury. You call it skew deviation. All of the following statements about skew deviation are true *except:*

    a.   Skew deviation is an acquired vertical misalignment of the eyes.

    b.   The lesion causing the skew deviation is always localized to the brain stem or cerebellum on the side of the higher eye.

    c.   Skew deviation can be a cause of transient diplopia in patients with basilar artery insufficiency.

    d.   You will see more skew deviations in the intensive care unit than in the strabismus clinic.

    e.   To make the diagnosis of skew deviation, a superior oblique palsy, blowout fracture of the orbit, or old vertical muscle imbalance must be ruled out.

11. Unilateral isolated pupillary dilation may occur with

    a.   Optic nerve lesion

    b.   Migraine or otherwise healthy cases

    c.   Middle ear disease

    d.   Optic chiasmal defect

    e.   Branch retinal artery occlusion

12. In attempting to look upward, a young man has synchronous backward jerking movements of both eyes. The nature of his difficulty will be defined best by which one of the following?

    a.   CT scan of the orbits

    b.   CT scan of the brain without contrast

    c.   Forced duction test

    d.   MRI of the brain

    e.   Cerebrospinal fluid electrophoresis

13. You are consulted on a 29-year-old, otherwise healthy, man with recent onset of horizontal diplopia worse in right gaze, a 12 D esotropia in primary gaze, and a corresponding abduction deficit in the right eye. Extraocular movements are otherwise normal. You also note that he has 1 mm of relative ptosis on the right side and that his right pupil is smaller than the left. The anisocoria is accentuated in dim light. He has no proptosis, and there is no variability of findings during the day. All of the following are true *except:*

    a.   The likely site of the pathologic lesion is the right cavernous sinus.

    b.   MRI of the brain is an appropriate diagnostic step.

    c.   He is likely to have a right facial nerve palsy.

    d.   Topical 10% cocaine solution is likely to cause greater dilation of the left pupil than the right.

    e.   Topical Paredrine (hydroxyamphetamine) is likely to cause greater dilation of the left pupil than the right.

14. All of the following statements regarding disc drusen are true *except:*

    a. They are common in darkly pigmented individuals.
    b. They are located in the prelaminar optic nerve.
    c. They are often bilateral.
    d. Field defects are often present.
    e. Central acuity loss is rare.

15. Two patients present a similar picture on motility examination (see diagram below). One is a 66-year-old man who complained of sudden dizziness and mild hemiparesis; the other is a 15-year-old girl with mild diffuse right-sided facial weakness and numbness. The locus of a single lesion involving the ocular motor system causing this deficit is

    a. Left frontal lobe
    b. Upper right midbrain involving paramedian reticular formation
    c. Right pons including the sixth nerve nucleus and the medial longitudinal fasciculus
    d. Left pons including the sixth nerve nucleus and the medial longitudinal fasciculus
    e. Right pons discretely involving medial longitudinal fasciculus

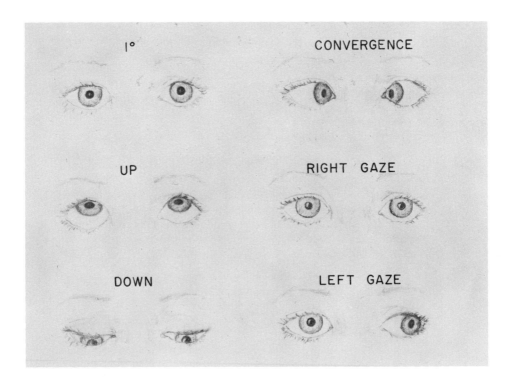

16. Concerning the two patients described in question #15, which statement is false?

    a. The motility disturbance in the 15-year-old will probably resolve.
    b. Despite the age discrepancy, the etiology is probably the same in both patients.
    c. This is a $1\frac{1}{2}$ syndrome.
    d. This is a gaze palsy combined with an internuclear ophthalmoplegia.
    e. Both patients should be immediately investigated for a mass lesion.

17. A 60-year-old retiree has severe and continuous pain on the left side of her forehead and temple of 2 days and then develops left-sided ptosis, medial rectus weakness, and immobility of the involved eye in the vertical plane. Her left pupil is equal in size to the right pupil and reacts promptly to light stimulation. Most likely, the cause of her disease is

    a. Left posterior communicating artery aneurysm
    b. Ophthalmoplegic migraine
    c. Carcinomatous meningitis
    d. Ocular myasthenia
    e. Diabetes mellitus

18. The most likely pathoetiology for the patient in question #17 is

    a. Compressive
    b. Microvascular ischemic
    c. Infiltrative neoplastic
    d. Autoimmune (neuromuscular junction)
    e. Inflammatory

19. The first diagnostic study should be

    a. Carotid angiography
    b. Tensilon test
    c. EEG
    d. Fasting blood sugar
    e. Cerebrospinal fluid cytology

20. Anatomically, the lesion described above spares the

    a. Large-caliber axons in the core of the nerve
    b. Large-caliber axons at the periphery of the nerve
    c. Large-caliber axons on the superior surface of the nerve at its exit from the brain stem
    d. Small-caliber axons in the core of the nerve
    e. Small-caliber axons at the periphery of the nerve

21. If the patient in question #17 were a known diabetic, if her left pupil were dilated and nonreactive, and if an MRI scan showed no aneurysm, a proper diagnostic work-up would include consultation with

    a. Nuclear medicine to search for a vascular-type neoplasm with radioactive scan techniques
    b. Internal medicine to evaluate for collagen vascular disease
    c. Otolaryngology to search for nasopharyngeal carcinoma
    d. Neurology to perform a Tensilon test
    e. Neuroradiology to rule out aneurysm by MRA

22. Lesions of the visual cortex may have all of the following features *except:*

    a. Homonymous field defects
    b. Formed visual hallucinations accompanied by the sensation of bad odor
    c. Perception of motion in the absence of perception of form
    d. Macular "splitting"
    e. Congruous field defects

23. The ciliary ganglion contains all of the following fibers *except:*

    a. Synapsing parasympathetic fibers to the iris sphincter
    b. Conjunctival vasoconstrictor fibers
    c. Sensory fibers from the globe
    d. Synapsing sympathetic fibers to the iris dilator
    e. Synapsing parasympathetic fibers to the ciliary muscle

24. The action of pilocarpine at the iris sphincter muscle is analogous to the action of what drug at the iris dilator muscle?

    a. Cocaine
    b. Timolol
    c. Priscoline
    d. Hydroxyamphetamine (Paredrine)
    e. Epinephrine

25. A pediatrician asks you to see a 1-day-old girl prior to hospital discharge. She was born following an unremarkable pregnancy and vaginal delivery. The infant has bilateral horizontal nystagmus. All of the following are likely to be true *except:*

    a. The nystagmus will not be visible during sleep.
    b. Given the early presentation, visual prognosis is extremely poor, and this child will be unlikely to be able to see to read.
    c. The oscillations may be relatively dampened in a particular direction of gaze.
    d. The nystagmus remains horizontal even when looking up or down.
    e. The patient may develop head oscillations.

26. Concerning arteriovenous fistulas in the cavernous sinus region, all of the following statements are true *except:*

    a. They may occur spontaneously, although they are usually a sequel to trauma.
    b. They are usually, but not always, characterized by proptosis, injection of the globe, and bruit.
    c. The third nerve is the most likely of the three ocular motor nerves to be involved.
    d. External signs are usually, but not necessarily, ipsilateral to the fistula.
    e. Hypoxic retinopathy reflects the decreased arterial and increased venous pressure consequent to the fistula and the further narrowing of the arteriovenous perfusion gradient by the IOP, which is usually elevated.

27. A 55-year-old man calls his ophthalmologist to say that he has just had three episodes of blindness in his right eye. These episodes occurred within 2 days of one another, lasted 6–7 minutes, and then cleared first in the inferior field of vision and then in the superior field. There was no associated eye pain or headache. The most likely diagnosis is

    a. Retinal migraine
    b. Transient visual obscuration from vertebrobasilar insufficiency
    c. Orthostatic hypotension
    d. Right carotid artery atheroma
    e. Impending ischemic optic neuropathy due to giant cell arteritis

28. The test that will best confirm the diagnosis in question #27 is

    a. Temporal artery biopsy
    b. Blood pressure determination
    c. Cerebral/cervical angiography
    d. Ophthalmodynamometry
    e. Therapeutic trial with propranolol

29. Pulsation of orbital contents may occur in all of the following situations *except:*

    a. Carotid cavernous fistula
    b. Orbital varix
    c. Neurofibromatosis
    d. Anterior encephalocele
    e. Blowout fracture of the orbital roof

30. A 27-year-old woman with diabetes mellitus develops fever, malaise, a left central retinal artery occlusion, and left fifth and sixth cranial nerve palsies over a 7-day period. Immediate work-up is necessary to rule out which of the following?

    a. Acute sphenoidal sinusitis
    b. Granulomatous arteritis in the cavernous sinus
    c. Diabetic neuropathy
    d. Phycomycosis (mucormycosis)
    e. Basal meningitis

31. A 77-year-old woman presents with sudden loss of visual acuity in her left eye. Vision is 20/20 in the right eye and "bare light perception" in the left eye. Ophthalmoscopy in the right eye reveals multiple cotton-wool spots surrounding a normal optic disc. Ophthalmoscopy of the left eye reveals pale swelling of the optic disc. Further history reveals that the patient has been treated for several months for "arthritis." Which of the following statements is correct?

    a. The patient probably has hypertensive retinopathy and should have a general medical examination.

    b. An ESR and temporal artery biopsy should be obtained. If either of these is abnormal, the patient should be started on corticosteroids.

    c. An ESR should be obtained immediately, and corticosteroids instituted. A temporal artery biopsy should be obtained as soon as possible.

    d. Because of the patient's age, corticosteroids should not be instituted unless temporal artery biopsy is positive.

    e. Because of the patient's age, if treatment is considered, aspirin should be used instead of corticosteroids.

32. The most likely cause of the following field defect is:

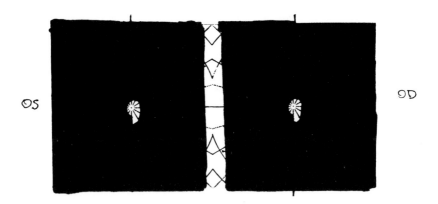

    a. Occipital infarcts
    b. Optic perineuritis
    c. Endstage glaucoma
    d. Tapetoretinal degeneration
    e. Hysteria

33. An 18-year-old woman complains of headache and blurred vision in the right eye for 2 days. The right pupil is dilated and fixed. Eye movements and eyelids are normal. Which of the following should be done first?

    a. Refer the patient to a neurologist.
    b. Patch the right eye so that medications cannot be placed in the eye; reexamine several days later.
    c. Place 0.125% pilocarpine in both eyes and observe for constriction of the right pupil.
    d. Obtain an emergency cerebral arteriogram.
    e. Place 1% pilocarpine in both eyes and observe for constriction of either pupil.

34. You are examining a 5-year-old boy who flunked his school visual screening examination. Visual acuity is 20/200 OD and 20/20 OS. There is a small right afferent pupillary defect. Fundus examination shows a smaller optic disc in the right eye, surrounded by a halo ring. The left disc and the blood vessels in both eyes are of normal size. You diagnose optic nerve hypoplasia. All of the following are true *except:*

    a. MRI of the brain may show other intracranial abnormalities.
    b. Visual field defects that don't follow either the vertical or horizontal meridians are common.
    c. A trial of full-time patching of the left eye is indicated.
    d. Optic nerve hypoplasia is associated with colobomas of the iris and retina.
    e. The halo is a result of retina and retinal pigment epithelium partially covering the lamina cribrosa.

35. Congenital ocular motor apraxia is characterized by all of the following *except:*

    a. Loss of voluntary horizontal gaze
    b. Intact vertical gaze
    c. Intact horizontal optokinetic and vestibular nystagmus
    d. Horizontal head thrusts past object of attention, with simultaneous doll's head contraversion of the eyes to achieve fixation and then return of the head to allow fixation in primary position
    e. Improvement to near normal by the end of the second decade

36. A 55-year-old woman complains of a chronically red right eye (see photo-graph). On examination the conjunctival blood vessels are markedly enlarged and tortuous. The mires of the applanation tonometer separate widely in a pulsatile fashion that corresponds to her heart rate. All of the following are likely *except:*

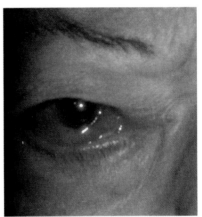

    a.   An enlarged superior ophthal-mic vein visible on a contrast CT scan of the brain

    b.   An enlarged cup-to-disc ratio in the right optic disc

    c.   A bruit heard over the right eye

    d.   Elevated T_4 and depressed TSH level

    e.   Blood visible in Schlemm's canal

37. An 80-year-old white woman sees you regarding suddenly noticed visual loss in the left eye. Visual acuity is 20/30 OD and 20/400 OS. There is a left affer-ent pupillary defect. The right eye and visual field are normal. The left eye has a swollen optic nerve head. Which of the following excludes a diagnosis of giant cell arteritis?

    a.   A sedimentation rate of 24 mm/hr and an Hgb of 14.1

    b.   Visual field loss in the left eye that crosses the horizontal meridian

    c.   Lack of any temple pain

    d.   A negative 4.5-cm left temporal artery biopsy

    e.   None of the above

38. All of the following are true about Leber hereditary optic neuropathy *except:*

    a.   There is a male predominance.

    b.   Leber optic neuropathy is inherited as a sex-linked recessive trait.

    c.   Visual loss is usually profound and permanent.

    d.   Funduscopic findings may be characteristic.

    e.   It is associated in some families with cardiac preexcitation syndromes.

39. All of the following statements are true about optic nerve gliomas *except:*

    a.   They most commonly occur in middle-aged women.

    b.   They are commonly associated with neurofibromatosis.

    c.   Visual loss is the most common presenting symptom.

    d.   The optic disc may appear either swollen or pale.

    e.   The tumor may spread to the contralateral optic nerve.

40. All of the following could be true about the patient with the lesion shown below *except:*

    a. The patient has a left homonymous hemianopia.
    b. The most likely cause of the lesion is an embolus to the middle cerebral artery.
    c. The patient may not be aware of the deficit.
    d. An EKG should be performed looking for atrial fibrillation.
    e. The macula may be spared.

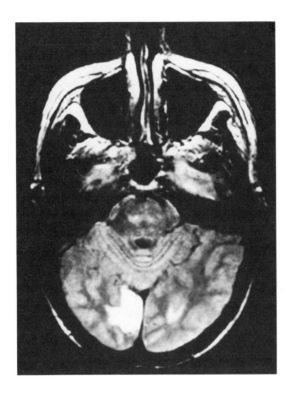

ANSWERS AND REFERENCES

1. Answer—e. The inferior retinal fiber projection is not isolated in a parietal lobe lesion (as it might be in temporal lobe lesions involving Meyer's loop, the so-called pie-in-the-sky defect depicted in drawing B). There is, of course, no localizing clue in a complete homonymous defect (d), which may occur from tract to cortex.

   See p 59.

2. Answer—d. The characteristic visual field defects seen in nutritional amblyopia, a disorder clinically indistinguishable from tobacco-alcohol amblyopia, are bilateral cecocentral scotomata. Such defects have sloping margins, may have denser nuclei of field loss between fixation and the blind spot, and may mimic the bitemporal depression seen with chiasmal compression. However, in nutritional amblyopia, the field defects do not obey the vertical meridian and assume the characteristic cecocentral form as they evolve. The fundus usually shows evidence of minimal disc edema or temporal pallor. The papillomacular bundle is often atrophic.

   See p 87.

3. Answer—a. Perimetry is frequently unreliable in patients feigning visual loss and cannot be used to exclude the diagnosis of functional visual loss. The lack of a relative afferent pupillary defect would be expected in a patient with nonorganic monocular visual loss. Functional visual loss is a diagnosis of exclusion. It is important to rule out other causes of visual loss compatible with the examination given, such as anisometropia or heterotropia. Large-target optokinetic nystagmus could be normal in a patient with this visual acuity and organic disease. Confusion and trickery in an effort to prove better than reported visual acuity is the standard method of establishing a diagnosis of monocular functional visual loss.

4. Answer—b. This patient has a tonic pupil and will exhibit denervation supersensitivity of the right pupil by responding with miosis induced by dilute pilocarpine instillation. The right pupil will also respond to 1% pilocarpine, but the left pupil would also respond to this higher concentration, and denervation supersensitivity would therefore not be as apparent. One percent pilocarpine is useful to determine if unreactive unilateral pupillary dilation is a result of mydriatic instillation; such a pupil will not respond to 1% pilocarpine. Hydroxyamphetamine, epinephrine, and cocaine are used in testing for and localization of Horner syndrome.

   Thompson HS, Kardon R. The clinical importance of pupillary inequality. In: *Focal Points: Clinical Modules for Ophthalmologists.* San Francisco: American Academy of Ophthalmology; 1992;10:10.

   Thompson HS, Pilley SFJ. Unequal pupils. A flow chart for sorting out the anisocorias. *Surv Ophthalmol.* 1976;21:45–48.

   See pp 105–111.

5. Answer—b. Ischemic optic neuropathy represents a lacunar-type infarct of the optic nerve head felt to be a result of closure of small vessels rather than embolic disease. It is important to distinguish the arteritic form, as treatment with high-dose oral corticosteroids may prevent visual loss in the opposite eye. An elevated sedimentation rate and symptoms such as scalp tenderness and jaw claudication are suggestive of giant cell arteritis. Prophylactic treatment with systemic corticosteroids and temporal artery biopsy are indicated when there are sufficient clinical symptoms of giant cell arteritis. There is no proven treatment for the nonarteritic form. The national Ischemic Optic Neuropathy Decompression Trial found that patients treated with optic nerve sheath fenestration had a worse prognosis compared to those without treatment. In a typical case of unilateral disc swelling and visual loss, there is no need for neuroimaging or lumbar puncture.

6. Answer—c. This picture of swollen nerve head on one side and a pale disc on the other must not only be interpreted as the Foster-Kennedy syndrome signifying a basofrontal tumor. In Foster-Kennedy visual acuity on the side of the swollen disc is typically normal since the etiology is papilledema. This patient has simply had a previous episode of ischemic optic neuropathy in the eye with the pale disc. This is a common cause of sudden loss of vision in the sixth and seventh decades of life.

7. Answer—a. Slowly progressive, asymmetric visual loss (with "normal" fundus examination, lens, etc.) is a subfrontal mass lesion until proven otherwise (giant parasellar aneurysm; meningioma of the optic canal, sphenoid, or tuberculum sella; pituitary tumor).

8. Answer—d. The field defect is a temporal hemianopia, confined to the right eye. Infarction of the monocular crescent representation in left primary visual cortex would produce a field defect in the right eye only, but it would be from 55° to 100° in the temporal field. Tilted disc syndrome and retinal detachment could account for a monocular temporal field cut, but it would not strictly respect the vertical meridian. Graves orbitopathy would not produce a discrete temporal field cut. Tuberculum sellae meningioma is the most likely etiology. Compression of the optic nerve just anterior to the optic chiasm can cause a temporal hemianopia. If the optic chiasm is not involved, there is no field cut in the other eye.

9. Answer—d. The nystagmus of spasmus nutans is not present at birth. It usually starts between the fourth and twelfth months of life. A picture essentially identical to the benign condition of spasmus nutans, however, may be seen with lesions of the chiasm and third ventriclar region, such as gliomas. Testing for visual loss, a relative afferent pupillary defect, and disc pallor should be performed. Neuroimaging is necessary to rule out a parachiasmal lesion.

Schulman JA, Shults WT, Jones JM. Monocular vertical nystagmus as an initial sign of chiasmal glioma. *Am J Ophthalmol.* 1979;87:87–90.

10. Answer—b. The lesion causing a skew deviation is usually not localizable to anywhere more specific than the posterior fossa, although it is more often found on the side of the lower eye. The other statements are true. Ophthalmologists seldom make the diagnosis because they do not see many comatose patients, and other specialists do not often make the diagnosis because of answer *e*.

See p 146.

11. Answer—b. No afferent defect per se causes anisocoria. An isolated unilateral dilated pupil is almost always benign.

12. Answer—d. Convergence-retraction nystagmus is part of the dorsal midbrain (Parinaud) syndrome. The usual cause of acquired dorsal midbrain syndrome in a young adult is a tumor compressing the upper midbrain. Tumors and intrinsic midbrain lesions that might result in the dorsal midbrain syndrome are best seen on MRI.

See p 138.

13. Answer—c. The patient has a right sixth nerve paresis and an ipsilateral Horner syndrome. These two nerves travel together within the cavernous sinus. MRI is the neuroimaging test of choice in this region. The seventh (facial) nerve wraps around the sixth nerve in the brain stem but is not present in the cavernous sinus. A miotic pupil caused by a third-order (postganglionic) sympathetic paresis will not dilate in response to either cocaine or Paredrine.

14. Answer—a. Drusen are very rarely seen in darkly pigmented individuals. Although peripheral field loss of variable degree is common, central field loss with consequent reduction of central vision is rare. Drusen occur in the prelaminar portion of the optic nerve.

Rosenberg MA, Savino PJ, Glaser JS. A clinical analysis of pseudopapilledema. I. Population, laterality, acuity, refractive error, ophthalmoscopic characteristics, and coincident disease. *Arch Ophthalmol.* 1979;97:65.

15. Answer—c. We show two patients, both of whom cannot look to the right with either eye and can only look to the left with the left eye. However, both medial recti, although paralyzed in gaze movements, contract normally in convergence. Therefore, the gaze palsy is of the supranuclear type. There is a total palsy of right lateral gaze, and "half" a palsy of left lateral gaze (the half contributed by the right medial rectus). C. Miller Fisher thus dubbed this the $1\frac{1}{2}$ syndrome.

Leigh RJ, Zee DS. *The Neurology of Eye Movements.* 2nd ed. Philadelphia: Davis; 1991:436–437.

Answer *a* must be incorrect since a left frontal lobe lesion would only cause a left gaze preference and no involvement of the right medial rectus (RMR). Answer *b* is wrong since a right midbrain lesion would typically involve upward gaze, convergence, or both. Answer *e* would only give the RMR weakness on left gaze and would *not* give a right gaze palsy. Answer *c* is the correct answer because involvement of the sixth nerve nucleus (also known as the horizontal gaze center) on the right side has paralyzed right gaze, and the concurrent adjacent right medial longitudinal fasciculus involvement paralyzes the RMR on left gaze. In the elderly this lesion may be caused by a single vascular accident. In the young it may be caused by a pontine glioma, AVM, or demyelinating plaque. Answer *d* gives the inverse findings of those described in the diagrams.

16. Answer—b. See explanation with #15.

17. Answer—e. Pupil-sparing third nerve palsy is most often the result of microvascular occlusion of vessels supplying the oculomotor nerve. Diabetes is a common cause of occlusive microvasculopathy. Posterior communicating artery aneurysms usually distort the subarachnoid part of the third nerve and almost always involve pupillary fibers producing pupillary dilation. Ophthalmoplegic migraine is rare and usually occurs in young patients with accompanying pupillary involvement. Carcinomatous meningitis is usually a late result of systemic malignancy, and multiple cranial nerves are often involved. While this patient's problem could be attributed to meningeal seeding of carcinoma, this is not the most likely origin of her problem. Ocular myasthenia gravis, while capable of mimicking a pupil-sparing third nerve palsy, is painless.

    See pp 152–154.

18. Answer—b. We are describing a person with a painful ophthalmoplegia involving all ocular muscles supplied by the left third nerve, but sparing the pupil. This type of pupil-sparing third nerve palsy is typical of diabetic cranial mononeuropathy and probably occurs on an acute ischemic basis.

19. Answer—d. This should be followed by a glucose tolerance test and/or hemoglobin A1c measurements. An ESR should also be obtained and the diagnosis of giant cell arteritis at least considered.

20. Answer—e. The small parasympathetic axons (for pupil sphincter and accommodation) are at the periphery of the nerve. If vaso-occlusion occurs, the fibers in the central core of the nerve get into trouble first because they are farthest from the blood supply; but if the nerve is compressed or stretched (as by an aneurysm), then the peripheral fibers will get it every time.

21. Answer—e. Once again, the importance of pupillary involvement is stressed. Angiography is indicated to settle the question of a possible posterior communicating aneurysm.

Trobe JD. Isolated pupil-sparing third nerve palsy. *Ophthalmology.* 1985; 92:58.

Trobe JD. Third nerve palsy and the pupil: footnotes to the rule. *Arch Ophthalmol.* 1988;106:601.

22. Answer—b. Formed visual hallucinations may occur after visual cortex disease, but the associated symptom of peculiar odors indicates temporal lobe disease.

23. Answer—d. The sympathetic fibers in the ciliary ganglion are postganglionic, originating in the superior cervical ganglion. They do not synapse in the ciliary ganglion, and they are not destined for the iris dilator.

24. Answer—e. Pilocarpine, like epinephrine, directly stimulates muscle receptor sites.

25. Answer—b. Visual acuity is related to the speed of the slow phase of the nystagmus (i.e., to the amount of time that a target remains on the fovea). Most patients with congenital nystagmus have moderately depressed visual acuity and are able to read. Near vision is frequently better than distance vision. The other statements are true.

26. Answer—c. The sixth nerve is more commonly involved, probably because it is typically free floating in the cavernous sinus and not within a dural fold like the other nerves. Venous pressure is increased in the affected orbit, and arterial pressure is decreased; this impairs perfusion of the eye and causes hypoxia. The hypoxic damage to the trabecular meshwork impairs aqueous outflow, raising IOP, which in turn increases resistance to perfusion even more, leading to further hypoxic damage.

27. Answer—d. Transient, painless visual loss in adults should prompt a search for carotid occlusive disease. These transient ischemic episodes may be due to microemboli from ulcerating atheromas, most commonly located at the carotid bifurcation. Screening for carotid artery disease can be performed through noninvasive testing, especially carotid duplex scanning. While the indications for surgical intervention are not universally accepted, arteriography followed by thromboendarterectomy should be considered in a relatively young person. If the patient has a known history of rheumatic fever or heart disease, a cardiac source should be considered. In either case a complete medical evaluation is indicated prior to angiography.

28. Answer—c. See explanation to #27.

29. Answer—b. It is true that an orbital varix can produce an *intermittent proptosis* with straining, Valsalva's maneuver, or bending over, but that is something quite different from the pulse-synchronous pulsation seen in answers *a, c, d,* and *e.*

30. Answer—d. In the ketotic diabetic patient, onset of orbital signs and symptoms should always raise suspicion of mucormycosis. Those cases not diagnosed early are almost universally fatal.

31. Answer—c. The most likely diagnosis by far is cranial arteritis despite the lack of severe central vision loss. Treatment should be started immediately without waiting for confirmatory laboratory data such as an elevated ESR. Temporal artery biopsy should be obtained as soon as possible.

    See pp 76–80.

32. Answer—a. The key is the *vertical* step. The fields demonstrate bilateral homonymous hemianopia with bilateral macular sparing. The vertical step does not occur in retinal or optic nerve lesions. Glaucomatous loss has a horizontal step. The congruity places the lesion in the primary visual cortex. Hysterical fields are generally round, spiraling, or tubular in character, and they lack a vertical step.

33. Answer—c. Since Adie's pupil may present this way, but denervation hypersensitivity may not develop immediately, 1% pilocarpine should be used subsequently to rule out a pharmacologic pupil if the right pupil did not constrict to dilute pilocarpine. A denervated pupil will constrict to pilocarpine, whereas a pupil dilated as a result of an atropine-like drug will not constrict.

    Thompson HS, Kardon R. The clinical importance of pupillary inequality. In: *Focal Points: Clinical Modules for Ophthalmologists.* San Francisco: American Academy of Ophthalmology; 1992;10:10.

    Thompson HS, Pilley SFJ. Unequal pupils. A flow chart for sorting out the anisocorias. *Surv Ophthalmol.* 1976;21:45–48.

34. Answer—d. Colobomas of the optic nerve are associated with colobomas of other ocular structures. Many patients with optic nerve hypoplasia have normal or near normal visual acuity potential. An evaluation for potential other causes of amblyopia and a trial of patching is warranted. If there is no response, the child should not be subjected to prolonged patching of the "good" eye. MRI shows abnormalities in the majority of patients such as absence of the septum pellucidum. Many structural abnormalities have associated systemic problems. For example, posterior pituitary ectopia is associated with hormonal deficiencies.

35. Answer—c. The fast phase of OKN and rotational nystagmus is absent in congenital ocular motor apraxia (with maintained tonic deviation) although the fast phase appears as the child "outgrows" it.

36. Answer—d. The scenario presented is that of a high-flow carotid cavernous fistula. Graves disease does not result in pulsatile IOP changes or arterialization of conjunctival vessels.

37. Answer—e. Giant cell arteritis has significant variability in presentation. The diagnosis remains a clinical one based on the physician's perception of the patient's history, physical findings, and laboratory evaluation. Presence of common symptoms, elevated Westergren sedimentation rate, and biopsy evidence of disease are helpful when present. Their absence, however, does not exclude the disease.

38. Answer—b. Leber hereditary optic neuropathy is transmitted in a pattern of maternal inheritance through defects in the mitochondrial DNA. The reason there is a male predominance of expression may relate to a modifying factor on the nuclear X chromosome. Although spontaneous recovery may occur even years after initial visual loss, the visual deficit usually remains severe and permanent. The characteristic funduscopic appearance of Leber, although not seen in all cases, includes microangiopathic telangiectasias, pseudoedema of the disc, and vascular tortuousity. In some families, especially in Finland, there are associated cardiac conduction abnormalities.

Newman NJ, Wallace DC. Mitochondria and Leber hereditary optic neuropathy. *Am J Ophthalmol.* 1990;109:726–730.

39. Answer—a. Ninety percent of optic gliomas occur in the first two decades of life. In contrast, optic nerve meningiomas occur more commonly in women and in the fifth and sixth decades of life. There is a strong association with neurofibromatosis. Presentations include visual loss, strabismus, nystagmus, and proptosis. The appearance of the disc depends on the stage of the disease. Gliomas can spread to the contralateral nerve by way of the chiasm. Surgical resection of orbital gliomas before they reach the chiasm is indicated for this reason.

40. Answer—b. This T2-weighted MRI shows a lesion in the right occipital cortex in the distribution of the right posterior cerebral artery. This will result in a left homonymous hemianopia that may be macula sparing, especially given the relative sparing of the occipital cortex seen most posteriorly (the macular representation occurs most posteriorly). Discrete occipital infarcts like this are usually the result of embolic disease. Atrial fibrillation may be a cause of embolism. Sometimes these infarcts are "silent," in that the patient remains unaware of the deficit, especially when located on the right side.

See pp 68–71.

INDEX

Abducens nerve. *See* Cranial nerve VI
Abduction
  deficit in
    sixth nerve palsy causing, 148
    in thyroid ophthalmopathy, 189–191
  extraocular muscles in, 113, 113*i*
Aberrant regeneration
  after Bell's palsy, 164
  primary, 155
  after third nerve palsy, 155, 155*i*
Absolute visual field defects, 19*t*, 22. *See
  also* Visual field defects
Accommodation, in near response, 100
Accommodative vergence (blur), 130
Accuracy, saccadic, 126–127
Acephalgic migraine (migraine equivalent),
  219
Acetazolamide, for pseudotumor
  cerebri, 75
Acetylcholine receptor antibody tests, for
  myasthenia gravis, 179–180
Acetylcholine receptor sites, in myasthenia
  gravis, 177
Acetylcholinesterases, for myasthenia
  gravis, 180
Achromatopsia, 96
Acoustic neurofibromatosis, bilateral, 183.
  See also Neurofibromatosis
Acquired immunodeficiency syndrome
  (AIDS), 222–225
Acuity, visual
  "bottom-up," in functional visual
    loss, 33
  testing, 14
  in visual rehabilitation, 233
Adduction
  deficit in, in thyroid ophthalmopathy,
    189
  extraocular muscles in, 113, 113*i*
Adenoma sebaceum, in tuberous sclerosis,
  184, 184*i*
Adie's syndrome (tonic pupil), 108–109,
  108*i*, 111*t*
Afferent limb of pupillary pathways,
  97, 98*i*
Afferent pupillary defects, 100–104
  in compressive optic neuropathy, 83

in optic neuritis, 81
  pretectal, 105
  relative (Marcus Gunn pupil), 100–104,
    101*i*, 102*i*, 103*i*
    testing for, 15, 23–24, 100, 101*i*,
      102*i*, 103*i*
Agnosia, 95
Agraphia, 95
AIDS, 222–225
AIDS dementia complex, 224
AION. *See* Anterior ischemic optic
  neuropathy
Alexia, 95
Allergic aspergillosis, 227
Alternating (swinging) light test, 23–24,
  100, 101*i*, 102*i*, 103*i*
Altitudinal visual field defects, 19*t*
  bilateral homonymous, 70
  scotoma, 65, 66*i*
Amaurosis fugax (transient monocular
  visual loss/blindness), 196, 198
  carotid disease causing, 198
Amblyopia, relative afferent pupillary
  defect and, 24
Amplitude, of visually evoked cortical
  potential, 16
Amsler grid testing, 21
  in visual rehabilitation, 233–234
Analgesic rebound headache, 220
Aneurysms, 207–211. *See also specific
  artery*
  berry (saccular), 207
  clinical presentation of, 208–209
  dissecting, 213–214, 213*t*
  laboratory investigation of, 209, 210*i*
    arteriography in, 47–49, 48*i*
    magnetic resonance angiography in,
      47, 209, 210*i*
  neuro-ophthalmic signs of, 207–211
  prognosis of, 209–210
  ruptured, 209
  treatment of, 211
Angiography
  in arteriovenous malformation
    evaluation, 211, 212*i*
  in carotid system evaluation, 202–204
  in cerebral aneurysm evaluation, 210*i*

Angioma (angiomatosis)
  cerebrofacial (encephalotrigeminal
    angiomatosis/Sturge-Weber
    syndrome), 181, 184–186, 186*i*
  racemose, in Wyburn-Mason syndrome,
    188, 188*i*
  retinal (von Hippel disease), 181,
    186–187, 187*i*
Angular gyrus, visual integration disorders
  caused by lesions of, 95
Angular magnification, 234
Anisocoria, 23, 105–109, 107*i*
Annulus of Zinn, 54
Anomia, 95
Anterior chiasmal syndrome, 66, 67*i*
Anterior communicating artery, aneurysm
  of, 208
Anterior ischemic optic neuropathy
  (AION), 76–80, 202
  arteritic, 76–79
  nonarteritic, 77*i*, 79–80
Anterograde changes, retinal disease
  causing, 51
Anticoagulation, for carotid artery
  disease, 205
Antiplatelet therapy, for carotid artery
  disease, 205
Anton syndrome, 206
Apraxia, ocular motor, 133
Arcuate scotoma, 19*t*, 65, 66*i*
Argyll Robertson pupil, 105
Arteriography, intracerebral, 47–49, 48*i*
  for cerebral aneurysm evaluation,
    209, 210*i*
  for dissecting aneurysm evaluation,
    214, 215*i*
Arteriovenous malformations, 211, 212*i*
  neuroimaging in evaluation of, 45, 46,
    211, 212*i*
  neuro-ophthalmic signs of, 211, 212*i*
  in Wyburn-Mason syndrome, 188, 189
Arteritis, giant cell (temporal), anterior
  ischemic optic neuropathy in, 76–79
"Ash-leaf spot," sebaceum, 184, 184*i*
Aspergillus (aspergillosis), 227–228
Aspirin, prophylactic, 205
Astrocytic hamartoma, in tuberous
  sclerosis, 184, 185*i*

Ataxia-telangiectasia (Louis-Bar syndrome),
  181, 187–188, 188*i*
Atherosclerosis, carotid, 202, 203*i*
Aura, migraine headache and, 218
Automated bowl perimetry, 22–23
AVMs. *See* Arteriovenous malformations
AVONEX. *See* Interferon β1a
Axoplasmic transport, obstruction of, optic
  disc edema and, 71–72

B-scan ultrasonography, orbital, 50
Bartonella henselae (*Rochalimea* sp), cat-
  scratch disease caused by, 231
Basilar artery dissection, 214
Battle's sign, seventh nerve palsy and, 165
Bell's palsy, 162–164
Bell's phenomenon, 25–26
Benedikt syndrome, 115
Benign essential blepharospasm, 165–167,
  166*t*
Benign papillophlebitis, 88
Berry aneurysm (saccular aneurysm), 207
Betaseron. *See* Interferon β1b
Bilateral acoustic neurofibromatosis, 183.
  See also Neurofibromatosis
BIMVAT. *See* Binocular Integrated
  Multicolored Vision Assessment Test
Binasal hemianopia, lateral chiasmal
  lesions causing, 67
Binding antibodies, acetylcholine receptor,
  in myasthenia gravis diagnosis, 179
Binocular diplopia, 12–13
  evaluation of, 26–27, 27*i*
Binocular eye movements, testing, 25
Binocular Integrated Multicolored Vision
  Assessment Test (BIMVAT), in
  functional visual loss evaluation,
  33–34
Binocular single vision, measuring field of,
  in diplopia evaluation, 27, 27*i*
Binocular transient visual loss, 196
Bitemporal visual field defects, 19*t*
  hemianopia, 67, 67*i*
  scotomata, 67, 67*i*
Blastomycosis (*Blastomyces dermatitidis*),
  228–229
Blepharospasm
  essential, 165–167, 166*t*
  reflex, 168

Blindness. *See also* Visual loss
  central retinal artery occlusion
    causing, 199
  cerebral/cortical, 70
    in preeclampsia, 195
    in vertebrobasilar system disease, 205
  monocular
    functional, evaluation of, 34–36
    pupillary evaluation in, 24
    transient (amaurosis fugax), 196, 198
Blindsight, 70
Blinking, seventh nerve control of, 158
Blocking antibodies, acetylcholine
  receptor, in myasthenia gravis
  diagnosis, 179–180
Blur (accommodative vergence), 130
Blurring, in vertebrobasilar system
  disease, 205
Bobbing, ocular, 138
Borrelia burgdorferi, Lyme disease caused
  by, 225
Botox. *See* Botulinum toxin type A
"Bottom-up" acuity, in functional visual
  loss, 33
Botulinum toxin type A
  for diplopia, 156–157
  for essential blepharospasm, 166
  for hemifacial spasm, 167
Bourneville syndrome (tuberous sclerosis),
  181, 184, 184*i*, 185*i*
Bowl perimetry
  automated, 22–23
  manual, 21–22
Brain stem lesions, facial movements
  affected by, 161
"Brain stones," in tuberous sclerosis,
  184, 185*i*
Branch retinal artery occlusion, 200
BRAO. *See* Branch retinal artery occlusion
Brightness comparison testing, 15
Brodmann's area 17, 60. *See also*
  Occipital cortex
Brodmann's area 18, 60
Brodmann's area 19, 60
Bruits, carotid, 202

Café-au-lait spots, in neurofibromatosis,
  182
Cajal, interstitial nucleus of, 125
Caloric testing, 25
Candida (candidiasis), 229

Cardiovascular disease, stroke and TIAs
  caused by, 202
Carotid dissection, 202
Carotid endarterectomy, 205
  for ocular ischemic syndrome, 201
Carotid occlusive disease, 200–201. *See
  also* Carotid system, disorders of
Carotid system, 203*i*
  disorders of, 198–205. *See also type*
    aneurysms, 208–209
      dissecting, 213–214, 213*t*
    clinical and laboratory evaluation of,
      202–204
    color flow Doppler imaging in
      evaluation of, 49, 50*i*
    etiologies of, 202
    neurologic symptoms and signs
      of, 202
    neuro-ophthalmic signs of, 197,
      198–205
    prognosis of, 204
    treatment of, 205
Carotidynia, 221
Cat-scratch disease, 231
Cataracts, "Christmas tree," in myotonic
  dystrophy, 180
Cavernous sinus
  fourth nerve in, 122
  neuroimaging in evaluation of, 44
  sixth nerve in, 123
  third nerve in, 117, 120*i*
Cavernous sinus thrombosis, 214–216
  septic, 214
Cecocentral scotoma, 19*t*, 65, 66*i*
Central nervous system
  candidiasis affecting, 229
  lymphoma affecting, in AIDS/HIV
    infection, 222
  mucormycosis involving, 228
Central retinal artery occlusion, 199, 200*t*
Central scotoma, 19*t*, 65, 66*i*
Central vision loss, driving and, 239
Cerebellar gain, 126
Cerebral aneurysms, 207–211
  classification of, 207, 208*t*
  clinical presentation of, 208–209, 210*i*
  dissecting, 213–214, 213*t*
  laboratory investigation of, 209
    arteriography in, 47–49, 48*i*
    magnetic resonance angiography in,
      47, 209, 210*i*

M-cells (magnocellular neurons), 57–58
Macula-sparing homonymous hemianopia, 69–70
Maddox rod testing
  in diplopia evaluation, 26–27
  double
    for cyclovertical deviation evaluation, 28
    in fourth nerve palsy, 151
  in fourth nerve palsy, 151
Magnetic resonance angiography, 47, 48*i*
  carotid, 204
  for cerebral aneurysm evaluation, 209, 210*i*
Magnetic resonance imaging, 39–41
  advantages of, 42–43
  for arteriovenous malformation evaluation, 211, 212*i*
  for cerebral aneurysm evaluation, 47, 209, 210*i*
  contraindications to, 43
  for dissecting aneurysm evaluation, 214
  functional, 49
  for intracranial tumor evaluation, 44–45
  in multiple sclerosis, 46, 175, 176*i*
  in optic neuritis, 81, 83, 173
  in orbital assessment, 43–44
  of parasellar and cavernous sinus regions, 44
  terminology associated with, 40–41
  in thyroid ophthalmopathy, 192
  for vascular lesion evaluation, 45–46
  vs. CT scanning, 41–47
Magnification
  angular, 234
  in visual rehabilitation, 234–235
Magnocellular neurons (M-cells), 57–58
Manual bowl perimetry, 21–22
Marcus Gunn jaw-winking syndrome, 161
Marcus Gunn pupil (relative afferent pupillary defect), 100–104, 101*i*, 102*i*, 103*i*
  testing for, 15, 23–24, 100, 101*i*, 102*i*, 103*i*
Mass lesions
  optic nerve hypoplasia and, 93
  optic neuropathy caused by, 83–86
Medial longitudinal fasciculus, 122, 125
Medial rectus muscle, 113
Meige syndrome, 165
Melkersson-Rosenthal syndrome, 165
Meningiomas
  chiasmal compression caused by, 94
  neuroimaging in evaluation of, 45
  optic nerve, 85–86, 86*i*
Meningitis, tuberculous, 224
Methotrexate, for multiple sclerosis, 177
Methylprednisolone, for optic neuritis, 82–83, 173
MG. *See* Myasthenia gravis
Midbrain lesions, efferent pupillary lesions caused by, 104–105
Migraine equivalent (acephalgic migraine), 75
Migraine headache, 218–220
  ophthalmoplegic, 153
Millard-Gubler syndrome, 123, 148
Minification, 235–236
Minus lenses, for minification, 235–236
Miosis, pupillary, in near response, 100
MLF. *See* Medial longitudinal fasciculus
Möbius syndrome, 149
Modulating antibodies, acetylcholine receptor, in myasthenia gravis diagnosis, 180
Molds, 227
Monocular blindness, pupillary evaluation in, 24
Monocular diplopia, 12
Monocular elevation deficiency, in thyroid ophthalmopathy, 189
Monocular eye movements, testing, 25
Monocular transient visual loss/blindness (amaurosis fugax), 196, 198
  carotid disease causing, 198
Morning glory disc, 92
de Morsier syndrome (septo-optic dysplasia), 93
Motility examination. *See* Ocular motility, evaluation of
MRA. *See* Magnetic resonance angiography
MRI. *See* Magnetic resonance imaging
MS. *See* Multiple sclerosis
Mucormycosis, 228
Multiple cranial nerve palsies, 155–156
Multiple sclerosis, 169–177
  chiasmal abnormalities in, 173
  clinical presentation of, 171
  course and prognosis of, 170
  epidemiology of, 169–170
  funduscopic abnormalities in, 174

sixth nerve, 123, 148–151
  in multiple sclerosis, 174
  work-up of, 149–151
third nerve, 152–155
  cavernous sinus disorders and,
      117–121
  clinical approach to, 153–155
  congenital, 153
  cyclical, 153
  diabetic, 117
  fascicular, 115
  ischemic, 117–121
  in multiple sclerosis, 174
  posterior communicating artery
      aneurysm causing, 117, 153
  pupillary involvement in, 106, 117,
      152, 153, 154
Pancoast syndrome, 110
Papilledema, 55, 73–74, 73*i*
  pseudodrusen and, 73, 91
  in pseudotumor cerebri, 73*i*, 74–76
Papillitis, in optic neuritis, 81
Papillophlebitis, benign, 88
Paracentral scotoma, 19*t*
Paradoxical pupillary phenomena, 104
Paralysis. *See* Palsy
Paralytic strabismus, evaluation of, 28
Parasellar regions
  neuroimaging in evaluation of, 44
  third nerve palsy caused by lesions
      of, 153
Parasympathetic pathway, pupillary, 97
  lesions of, 106–109
Parasympathomimetic agents, tonic pupil
  response to, 109
Paretic syndromes, diplopia in, 143
Parinaud dorsal midbrain syndrome, 105
  in multiple sclerosis, 174
Pars planitis, in multiple sclerosis, 174
Parvocellular neurons (P-cells), 57, 58
Paton's lines, in papilledema, 73
Pattern electroretinogram, 18. *See also*
  Electroretinogram
Pattern visually evoked cortical potentials,
  16
Pause cells, 126
  nystagmoid movements caused by
      abnormalities of, 137
PERG. *See* Pattern electroretinogram
Pericentral scotoma, 19*t*

Perimetry
  automated, 22–23
  in functional visual loss evaluation,
      35, 35*i*
  Goldmann, 21–22
  kinetic, 21, 22
  manual, 21–22
  static, 21
  terminology used in, 19*t*
Periodic alternating nystagmus, 140–141
Periodic blinking, seventh nerve control
  of, 158
Peripheral portion of facial nerve,
  158–161, 160*i*
  lesions of, 162–165
Periphlebitis, in multiple sclerosis, 174
Petrous pyramid, sixth nerve in, 123
  pathology of, 149, 150*i*
Phakomatoses, 181–189. *See also*
  specific type
Pharmacologic mydriasis, 108, 111*t*
Photisms, sound-induced, 171
Photophobia, management of, 238
Photopsias, in vertebrobasilar system
  disease, 205
Photostress recovery test, 15
Physiologic pupillary unrest, 23
Pilocarpine, for diagnosis of tonic
  pupil, 109
Pinhole visual acuity testing, 14
Pits, optic, 92
Pituitary infarction, postpartum, neuro-
  ophthalmic signs in, 196
Pituitary tumors, chiasmal compression
  caused by, 94
Platelet thrombi, retinal, 198
Plexiform neurofibroma, 182, 183*i*
PML. *See* Progressive multifocal
  leukoencephalopathy
Pneumocystis carinii infection, in
  AIDS/HIV infection, 224
POHS. *See* Presumed ocular
  histoplasmosis syndrome
Pontine lesions, facial nerve disorders
  caused by, 162
Pontine paramedian reticular formation,
  124, 125, 126
Poser criteria, for multiple sclerosis,
  174, 175*t*
Position command, 127

Posterior communicating artery aneurysm, third nerve palsy caused by, 117, 153, 208
Posterior ischemic optic neuropathy, 81
Postganglionic Horner syndrome, 110–111
  testing for, 111*t*
Postherpetic neuralgia, 221
PPRF. *See* Pontine paramedian reticular formation
Prednisone
  for giant cell arteritis, 79
  for optic neuritis, 82–83, 173
Preeclampsia, neuro-ophthalmic disorders associated with, 195
Preganglionic Horner syndrome, 111*t*
Pregnancy
  neuro-ophthalmic disorders associated with, 195–196
  toxemia of, 195
Presumed ocular histoplasmosis syndrome, 231
Pretectal afferent pupillary defects, 105
Pretectal pathway, 57
Prism cover testing, in diplopia evaluation, 26
Prisms
  for diplopia, 156–157
  full-diameter, 236
  partial, 236
  in visual rehabilitation, 236–237
Progressive multifocal leukoencephalopathy, in AIDS/HIV infection, 224–225, 226*i*
Progressive supranuclear palsy (Steele-Richardson-Olszewski syndrome), 162
  saccadic slowing in, 135
Proptosis
  evaluation of, 32
  in thyroid disease, 191–192
Prosopagnosia, 95
Prostigmin test. *See* Neostigmine methylsulfate test
Proton-density weighted images, 40
Pseudoalexia, 95
Pseudodrusen, papilledema and, 73, 91
Pseudoisochromatic color plate testing, 14–15
Pseudopapilledema, drusen and, 90–91

Pseudotumor cerebri (idiopathic intracranial hypertension), 74–76
  lateral sinus thrombosis and, 217
PSP. *See* Progressive supranuclear palsy
Ptosis
  conditions causing, differentiation of, 181*t*
  evaluation of, 32
  in myasthenia gravis, 146, 177
    edrophonium chloride (Tensilon) test and, 178, 179*i*
Pulse sequence, for MRI studies, 40
Pulvinar, 57
Pupil. *See* Pupils
Pupillary defects
  afferent, 100–104
    in compressive optic neuropathy, 83
    in optic neuritis, 81
    pretectal, 105
    relative (Marcus Gunn pupil), 100–104, 101*i*, 102*i*, 103*i*
      testing for, 15, 23–24, 100, 101*i*, 102*i*, 103*i*
  efferent (midbrain lesions), 104–105
Pupillary light reflex, 23–24
  pathways for, 97, 98*i*
Pupillary miosis, in near response, 100
Pupillary pathways, anatomy of, 97–100
Pupillary sphincter, episodic spasm of, 109
Pupillary unrest, physiologic, 23
Pupils, 97–111. *See also under* Pupillary
  abnormal, physiologic testing for, 111*t*
  Argyll Robertson, 105
  episodic phenomena affecting, 109
  examination of, 23–24
  in Horner syndrome, 109–111, 111*t*
  Marcus Gunn (relative afferent pupillary defect), 100–104, 101*i*, 102*i*, 103*i*
    testing for, 15, 23–24, 100, 101*i*, 102*i*, 103*i*
  reactivity of to light, 23–24. *See also* Pupillary light reflex
    pathways for, 97, 98*i*
  relative difference in size of (anisocoria), 105–109
  in third nerve palsy, 106, 117, 152, 153
    relative sparing of, 154
  tonic (Adie's syndrome), 108–109, 108*i*, 111*t*

Pursuit deficits, 137
Pursuit system. *See* Smooth pursuit system
Pursuit at zero velocity, 132, 137

Quadrantanopia, 19*t*

Racemose angioma, in Wyburn-Mason
    syndrome, 188, 188*i*
Radiation therapy, for thyroid
    ophthalmopathy, 194
Radiofrequency pulse, in MRI, 40
Raeder paratrigeminal syndrome, 111
Raeder syndrome, 111
Ramsay Hunt syndrome, 164, 165
RAPD. *See* Relative afferent pupillary
    defect
Reading, visual rehabilitation and, 238
Rebleeding, cerebral aneurysm rupture
    and, 210
Rebound headache (analgesic), 220
Rectus muscles, 113–114, 113*i*
    in thyroid ophthalmopathy, 189–191
Red-glass testing, in paralytic strabismus
    evaluation, 28
Red-green glasses, in functional visual loss
    evaluation, 33–34
Refixation movements, 112
Reflex blepharospasm, 168
Refraction, clinical, in visual rehabilitation,
    234
Regeneration, aberrant
    after Bell's palsy, 164
    primary, 155
    after third nerve palsy, 155, 155*i*
Rehabilitation. *See* Visual rehabilitation
Relative afferent pupillary defect (Marcus
    Gunn pupil), 100–104, 101*i*,
    102*i*, 103*i*
    testing for, 15, 23–24, 100, 101*i*,
    102*i*, 103*i*
Relative pupil sparing, in third nerve
    palsy, 154
Relative visual field defects, 19*t*, 22
Relaxation, in MRI, 40
Release hallucinations, 96
Repetition time, in MRI, 40
Repetitive nerve stimulation,
    electromyographic, in myasthenia
    gravis diagnosis, 180

Restrictive syndromes, diplopia in,
    141–142, 142*i*
Reticular formation, pontine paramedian,
    124, 125, 126
Retina, anatomy of, 51–53
Retinal angiomatosis (von Hippel disease),
    181, 186–187, 187*i*
Retinal artery
    branch, occlusion of, 200
    central, occlusion of, 199, 200*t*
Retinal nerve fibers, 51, 52*i*
Retinitis
    cytomegalovirus, in AIDS/HIV infection,
    222
    in multiple sclerosis, 174
Retinopathy
    diabetic, venous stasis retinopathy
        differentiated from, 201*t*
    venous stasis, 200–201
        diabetic retinopathy differentiated
        from, 201*t*
Retrochiasmal lesions
    in multiple sclerosis, 173
    visual field defects caused by, 68, 69*i*
Retrogeniculate lesions, visual field defects
    caused by, 68–70
Retrograde axoplasmic transport,
    obstruction of, optic disc edema and,
    71–72
Retrograde changes, retinal disease
    causing, 51–52
Reverse telescopes, for minification,
    235–236
RF pulse. *See* Radiofrequency pulse
Rhinocerebral mucormycosis, 228
Riddoch phenomenon, 70
Rostral interstitial nucleus, 125

Saccades, 126–127
    assessment of, 25, 133
        optokinetic nystagmus testing in, 26
    disorders of, in ataxia-telangiectasia,
    188
    slowing of, 135–137
        in sixth nerve palsy, 148
Saccadic dysmetria, 127
Saccadic system, 112, 126–127
    neural integrator of, 127–128, 128*i*
Saccadomania, 126
Saccular aneurysm (berry aneurysm), 207

T1 properties of tissue, in MRI, 40
T1-weighted images, 40, 41*i*
T1WI. *See* T1-weighted images
T2 properties of tissue, in MRI, 40
T2-weighted images, 40, 41*i*
T2WI. *See* T2-weighted images
Tangent screen, in visual field evaluation,
    21
  for functional visual loss evaluation, 35
Tardive dyskinesia, facial dyskinesias
    and, 168
TE. *See* Echo time
Telescopes, in visual rehabilitation, 235
  driving and, 239
Temporal arteritis. *See* Giant cell arteritis
Temporal crescent, 60
Temporomandibular joint syndrome, 221
Tensilon test. *See* Edrophonium chloride
    test
Tension-type headache, 218–220
  treatment of, 219–220
Tensor tympani dysfunction, 31
Third cranial nerve. *See* Cranial nerve III
Third nerve palsy, 152–155
  cavernous sinus disorders and, 117–121
  clinical approach to, 153–155
  congenital, 153
  cyclical, 153
  diabetic, 117
  fascicular, 115
  ischemic, 117–121
  in multiple sclerosis, 174
  posterior communicating artery
    aneurysm causing, 117, 153
  pupillary involvement in, 106, 117, 152,
    153, 154
Third-order neuron lesions, Horner
    syndrome caused by, 110
Three-part reflex, testing, 133
Three-step test, in cyclovertical deviation
    evaluation, 28, 29*i*
Threshold of vision, 22
Thrombosis
  cavernous sinus, 214–216
  lateral (transverse) sinus, 216–217
Thymectomy, for myasthenia gravis, 180
Thyroid ophthalmopathy (Graves disease),
    181*t*, 189–195
  clinical presentation and diagnosis of,
    189–192

  eyelid signs of, 189, 190*i*, 191*i*
  treatment of, 192–195
TIAs. *See* Transient ischemic attacks
Tic douloureux (trigeminal neuralgia), 221
Tilted optic disc, 91, 91*i*
Time of flight magnetic resonance
    angiography, 47, 48*i*
Todd's paralysis, 168
Tolosa-Hunt syndrome, 156
Tonic pupil (Adie's syndrome), 108–109,
    108*i*, 111*t*
Toxemia of pregnancy, neuro-ophthalmic
    disorders associated with, 195
Toxic optic neuropathy, 87
Toxoplasmosis, in AIDS/HIV infection,
    225, 226*i*
TR. *See* Repetition time
Transient ischemic attacks, 197, 202, 206
Transient visual loss, 196–197
  binocular, 196
  monocular (amaurosis fugax), 196, 198
    carotid disease causing, 198
Transient visual obscurations, in
    papilledema, 74
Transient visually evoked cortical
    potentials, 16
Transverse sinus thrombosis (lateral sinus
    thrombosis), 216–217
Traumatic dissection, carotid, 213, 213*t*
Traumatic mydriasis, 106–108
Trigeminal nerve. *See* Cranial nerve V
Trigeminal neuralgia (tic douloureux), 221
Trochlear nerve. *See* Cranial nerve IV
Tuberculous meningitis, 224
Tuberous sclerosis (Bourneville syndrome),
    181, 184, 184*i*, 185*i*

Uhthoff's phenomenon/symptom, 81, 171
Ultrasonography (ultrasound)
  B-scan, of orbit, 50
  carotid, 204
  in thyroid ophthalmopathy, 192
Uncal herniation, third nerve damage
    in, 117
Upbeat nystagmus, 139–140
Uveitis
  ischemic, 201
  in multiple sclerosis, 174

V1 (striate cortex), 60, 61*i*, 62*i*
V2 through 5 (extrastriate visual area), 60, 61*i*, 62*i*
Vascular lesions, neuroimaging in evaluation of, 45–46
Vasospasm, cerebral aneurysm rupture and, 210
VECP. *See* Visually evoked cortical potentials
Velocity
  pursuit, 128
  saccadic, 126
Velocity command, 127
Venous stasis retinopathy, 200–201
  diabetic retinopathy differentiated from, 201*t*
VEP. *See* Visually evoked cortical potentials
VER (visually evoked response). *See* Visually evoked cortical potentials
Vergence system, 112, 130
  assessment of, 133
Versions, testing, 25
Vertebral artery dissection, 214
Vertebrobasilar circulation, 203*i*
  disorders of, 205–207
    clinical features of, 206
    clinical and laboratory evaluation of, 207
    dissecting aneurysms, 213–214
    etiologies of, 206–207
    neuro-ophthalmic signs of, 197, 205–207
Vertical diplopia, fourth nerve palsy causing, 151, 152*i*
Vertical gaze centers, 125
Vertical gaze palsies, 135, 136*i*
Vertical rectus muscles, 113
Vertigo, in vertebrobasilar system disease, 205
Vestibular nystagmus, 126, 139, 140*t*
  horizontal, 140
  periodic alternating, 140–141
  vertical, 140
Vestibular subnuclei, in ocular motility, 125–126
Vestibulo-ocular reflex, 129–130
  assessment of, 25, 132
  in gaze palsy and preference, 134
Vestibulo-ocular system, 112, 129–130

Vision, threshold of, 22
Visual acuity
  "bottom-up," in functional visual loss, 33
  testing, 14
  in visual rehabilitation, 233
Visual cortex, anatomy of, 60, 61*i*, 62*i*
Visual extinction, 95
Visual field defects, 65–71
  absolute, 19*t*, 22
  in anterior ischemic optic neuropathy, 76, 77*i*
  arteriovenous malformations causing, 211, 212*i*
  constriction, prisms for, 237
  drusen causing, 90, 90*i*
  evaluation of, 18–23. *See also* Visual field testing
  in multiple sclerosis, 173
  optic chiasm lesions causing, 66–68, 67*i*
  optic disc/optic nerve lesions causing, 65, 66*i*
  optic tract lesions causing, 68, 69*i*
  relative, 19*t*, 22
  retrogeniculate lesions causing, 68–70
  terms describing, 19*t*
  in tilted optic disc, 91, 91*i*
  in vertebrobasilar system disease, 205
Visual field testing, 18–23. *See also* Perimetry
  Amsler grid, 21
  automated bowl perimetry, 22–23
  confrontation, 20–21
  in functional visual loss evaluation, 35, 35*i*
  historical events in, 3–9
  manual bowl perimetry, 21–22
  tangent screen, 21
  terminology used in, 19*t*
Visual hallucinations
  formed and unformed, 70
  ictal, 96
  release, 96
Visual integration, disorders of, 95–96
Visual loss. *See also* Blindness
  carotid dissection causing, 213
  central, driving and, 239
  functional
    history-taking in, 13
    verification of, 32–36

ILLUSTRATIONS

The authors submitted the following figures for this revision. (Illustrations that were reproduced from other sources or submitted by contributors not on the committee are credited in the captions.)

Deborah I. Friedman, MD: Fig VIII-20, Fig VIII-23, Fig VIII-24

Thomas R. Hedges III, MD: Fig II-7, Fig VIII-2

Jonathan C. Horton, MD, PhD: Fig III-12B, Fig III-22, Fig III-23, Fig III-24

Steven A. Newman, MD: Fig I-4, Fig VI-1, Fig VI-2, Fig VI-3, Fig VI-4, Fig VI-5, Fig VI-6, Fig VI-7, Fig VI-8, Fig VI-9, Fig VI-10, Fig VI-11, Fig VI-12

Gerald G. Striph, MD: Fig II-1, Fig II-2, Fig II-3, Fig II-4, Fig II-5, Fig II-6

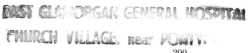